Microbial Perturbation of Host Defences

The third of a series of occasional colloquia on aspects of infection which are of current concern to clinicians and scientists.

Medical Society of London
17th–19th September 1980

To the memory of
Don Goodchild, 1917–1980
who conceived and propelled the Beecham Colloquia

Microbial Perturbation of Host Defences

Editors

FRANCIS O'GRADY

Professor of Microbiology
University of Nottingham

HARRY SMITH

Professor of Microbiology
University of Birmingham

1981

ACADEMIC PRESS
A Subsidiary of Harcourt Brace Jovanovich, Publishers

London New York Toronto Sydney San Francisco

ACADEMIC PRESS INC. (LONDON) LTD.
24/28 Oval Road,
London NW1

United States Edition published by
ACADEMIC PRESS INC.
111 Fifth Avenue
New York, New York 10003

British Library Cataloguing in Publication Data

Microbial perturbation of host defences.
1. Immune response—Congresses
2. Micro-organisms, Pathogenic—Congresses
I. O'Grady, F. II. Smith, H.
616'.01 QR175

ISBN 0–12–524750–8

Typeset in Great Britain by Phoenix Photosetting, Chatham
Printed in Great Britain by Mackays of Chatham Ltd

Preface

The great effort devoted over the years to mechanistic analyses of microbial pathogenicity and host defences has moved progressively closer to the molecular level. At the Third Beecham Colloquium we wanted to deal with some aspect of the large area of host–parasite interaction and, being anxious to focus our attentions, chose to look not at what the parasite does to the host or what the host does to the parasite, but what the parasite does to the host to stop the host doing much to the parasite.

The meeting followed the pattern of its predecessors in being held at the Medical Society of London, where a small international group talked through and around the subject almost continuously over three days. Each topic was briefly introduced by the main speaker who also provided a full paper which is published here. Most of the time was taken up by discussion which was converted into typescript with such commendable speed that at the end of each session the speakers were able to adjust the elegance of their remarks—but not allowed to write what they wished they had said. This they did so well that the editors have had to do little more than put the contributions together.

The planning of what proved to be a most enjoyable and successful meeting was marred by the death of Don Goodchild who over the years brought meetings sponsored by Beecham to a standard of excellence which was widely acclaimed. He regarded the Colloquia as the ultimate expression of his organizational skill and it was particularly sad that he did not live to enjoy the success of the third meeting. To have the main organizer die with preparations for an international meeting incomplete is a major disaster and tribute must be paid to Mrs Eileen Beirne, for many years Mr Goodchild's business associate and to his successor, Mr Ken Fergusson, who, guided by Mr Bill Burns, kept all the arrangements on course and on time to the point where only those at the centre had any inkling that anything untoward had happened A particular debt is due to Beecham Research Laboratories who continue to sponsor the Colloquia despite the escalating cost.

We are much indebted to Miss Diana Nisbet, who constructed virtually faultless text from manuscripts of the discussion, corrected and recorrected in places to the point of near obliteration and to Academic Press for the expeditious processing and prompt appearance of the proceedings which are so essential to publications in a rapidly moving field.

Sir Charles Stuart-Harris
Professor H. P. Lambert
Professor C. A. Mims
Professor F. W. O'Grady
Professor H. Smith
Professor J. D. Williams
Professor C. B. S. Wood
The late Mr D. Goodchild

List of Participants

M. J. Anderson, King's College Hospital Medical School, Denmark Hill, London SE5 8RX, UK

J. P. Arbuthnott, Department of Microbiology, Moyne Institute, Trinity College, Dublin 2, UK

A. J. Beale, The Wellcome Research Laboratories, Langley Court, Beckenham, Kent BR3 3BS, UK

Abraham I. Braude University Hospital, 225 West Dickinson Street, San Diego, California 92103, USA

M. Campa, Institute of Microbiology, University of Pisa, 56100 Pisa, Italy

P. Draper, National Institute for Medical Research, Mill Hill, London NW7, UK

C. Easmon, Wright-Fleming Institute, St Mary's Hospital Medical School, London W2 1PG, UK

G. Falcone, Institute of Microbiology, University of Pisa, 56100 Pisa, Italy

R. van Furth, Department of Infectious Diseases, Academisch Ziekenhuis Leiden, Rijnsburgerweg 10, 2333 AA Leiden, Holland

J. Jeljaszewicz, National Institute of Hygiene, 24 Chocimska Street, 00-791 Warsaw 36, Poland

H. P. Lambert, St George's Hospital, Blackshaw Road, Tooting, London SW17 0QT, UK

C. A. Mims, Department of Microbiology, Guy's Hospital, London SE1 9RT, UK

S. Mogensen, Institute of Medical Microbiology, Bartholin Building, University of Aarhus, Denmark

F. W. O'Grady, Department of Microbiology, University Hospital, Queen's Medical Centre, Nottingham NG7 2UH, UK

D. K. Peters, Royal Postgraduate Medical School, Hammersmith Hospital, Ducane Road, London W12, UK

C. Potter, Department of Virology, University of Sheffield Medical School, Beech Hill Road, Sheffield S10 2RX, UK

Paul G. Quie, Department of Pediatrics, University of Minnesota Medical School, Box

483, Mayo Memorial Building, 420 Delaware Street, S.E., Minneapolis, Minnesota 55455, USA

H. Smith, Department of Microbiology, SW Campus, The University of Birmingham, PO Box 363, Birmingham B15 2TT, UK

Sir Charles Stuart-Harris, Department of Medical Microbiology, University of Sheffield Medical School, Beech Hill Road, Sheffield S10 2RX, UK

C. Sweet, Department of Microbiology, SW Campus, The University of Birmingham, PO Box 363, Birmingham B15 2TT, UK

H. Valdimarsson, Department of Immunology, St Mary's Hospital Medical School, London W2 1PG, UK

J. D. Williams, Department of Medical Microbiology, The London Hospital Medical College, Turner Street, London E1, UK

J. M. A. Wilton, Department of Oral Immunology and Microbiology, Guy's Hospital, London SE1 9RT, UK

C. B. S. Wood, Department of Child Health, Queen Elizabeth's Hospital for Children, Hackney Road, London E2 8PS, UK

ORGANIZING COMMITTEE

Chairman—Sir Charles Stuart-Harris, CBE

Professor H. P. Lambert

Professor C. A. Mims

Professor F. W. O'Grady

Professor H. Smith

Professor J. D. Williams

Professor C. B. S. Wood

The late Mr D. Goodchild

Contents

Introduction by Sir Charles Stuart-Harris

The programme of this meeting was drawn up by the members of the Organizing Committee. In January of this year, we reached the stage of deciding that we would like to have our third colloquium on the general subject of microbial pathogenicity. But our problem was that we knew that within two days we could not possibly discuss the whole subject. We had not then narrowed the choice to one aspect, knowing that there were about four symposia planned on microbial pathogenicity and we did not then know their subject matter. Therefore I had to leave it to my colleagues to make the ultimate choice.

Infection is surely nowadays regarded as an interaction between two or more species. The outward and visible manifestations of infection are seen in the form of the pathological changes occuring in the host. Microbial species occupy the air, the sea and the soil throughout the earth in incredible numbers and varieties and some live along with the higher organisms in the form of mutual benefit.

Thus pathogenicity of microoganisms is a subject of intense medical importance and yet one which seems at times to have been relatively neglected; it would have required at least a week of meetings to discuss its various aspects. We might have chosen to discuss morphology, or genetics of pathogenic microoganisms, or the range of pathological changes in the host which they induce. Instead the Committee requested participants to discuss the subject which is at the very heart of the interaction between parasite and host, and the manner in which the parasite manipulates the defences possessed by the host against attack.

In spite of its large vocabulary, English has limitations inherent in its origins. I suggest that "attack" and "counter attack" are words which conjure up visual images. In this violent age in which we live, an attack has all the emotional connotations of battle or at least conflict. The consequences of any conflict may be trivial or fatal. There may be destruction in various degrees, either of the host or of the organismal parasite, during the attacks of infectious disease. I find myself somewhat distressed, therefore, by the word "perturbation" in our title for it conveys no imagery to me other than a gentle disturbance. The dictionary definition of the verb "to perturb" is to throw into confusion, to disturb mentally, to agitate, to induce bewilderment. If pathogenic microorganisms do no more than disturb the peaceful existence of the host, then I suggested that we need not discuss them further.

The Committee felt that "destruction" was too violent a noun to use: it might imply that we would only be discussing matters bound to lead to fatal consequences. I am tempted to suggest that their use of the word "perturbation" in part arose from the fact that they realized that there was a terrible amount of ignorance in the subject which they devised!

From the initial abstracts that I received it was clear that some of our invited speakers had interpreted their role by discussing first and foremost the host defences and the manner in which the various forms of defence may be attacked. This struck me as an excellent way to proceed, particularly as the programme was devised on a sessional basis, roughly sub-divided according to the mechanisms of defence. Whatever our individual contributions, though, great attention was paid to the clinical relevance of our subject whenever possible.

Some Reasons for Clinical Concern

C. B. S. WOOD

Department of Child Health,
Medical Colleges of St Bartholomew's
and the London Hospitals, London, UK.

The microbial perturbation or disruption of host defences finds a context and a relevance against a background of some current clinical, epidemiological, immunological and genetic aspects of infectious disease. The consequences of interaction between our species and microbial pathogens are influenced by the biological characteristics of the protagonists, and by broader environmental factors. Biological factors at the site of infection are outside the scope of this chapter, but will be the content of others. This introduction deals with general factors, environmental and genetic matters and relevant changes in function and behaviour which are used to combat virulence. Apart from the innate and self-protective properties of the host, certain deliberate behavioural modifications in preventive medicine affect this interaction and may therefore be given biological and selective weight. These, together with the currently successful use of antimicrobial medication, have allowed the clinical mind to largely ignore the study of factors contributing to virulence and to perturbation as considered by this conference. Epidemiological matters, however, continue to assist our species in keeping the balance of the contest in our favour and it must be our concern to understand them.

Historically, the situation had been much less favourable to us and early records in Great Britain reveal a very high mortality in childhood, extending beyond infancy, which was apparently even more destructive in major cities. The late Professor A. V. Neale (1964) summarized and restated much earlier information, quoting both Dr W. Farr (1805–1887, British statistician), and official records, which related to a society not yet very much affected by industrialization or by therapeutic and preventive options.

By the 1840s there was already public concern at what might be described as uncontrolled perturbation of host defences by disease. It appeared that much of the toll (Table I) was due to what is now regarded as infectious disease. To Dr Farr it seemed that infectious diseases may simply follow one another where conditions for healthy life are lacking.

TABLE I.
Births and deaths under 5 years of age.

	England and Wales	London	
	Early 20th century (1915–1924)	Mid 17th century (1730–1749)	End of 17th century (1790–1809)
Total births	927 473	315 456	386 393
Percentage dying under 5 years of age	13·8	74·5	41·3

After Neale (1964).

Neale (1964) had found that the development of concepts aimed at the control of threats to public health had begun earlier, and quotes that J. H. Rahn had proposed in 1799 that in Zurich professors should be appointed to be responsible for the following areas where a preventive influence might be brought to bear:

Medical institutions
Nutrition
Housing
Clothing
Procreation
Protection of mothers and infants
Prevention and control of epidemics

Measures against animal disease
Health education
Supervision of workhouses and orphanages

These radically modern proposals were made before microbiological science had developed, although Fracastoro of Verona (1484–1553) had already proposed a microbiological theory of disease.

INFLUENCE OF ENVIRONMENTAL FACTORS

Reducing the number and extent of opportunities for host–parasite interaction has had obvious potential in preventing and ameliorating infection. The importance of water as a vehicle of infection had been recognized by Snow in 1855 and by Budd in 1956, in cholera and typhoid fever respectively. The separation of water supply from sewerage and the securing of clean water supply were necessary for the control of hitherto prevalent infection. Currently it is recognized that in parts of the underdeveloped world, gross water pollution is still common. In the rainy season, Barrell and Rowland (1980) report that in a typical Gambian village, faecal coliforms and streptococci may reach counts of 10^5 per 100 ml in drinking water. Contamination of both traditional milk substitutes, and imported dried milk feeds which require to be reconstituted with waters, is then inevitable. In contrast, in modern England and Wales, good quality water is required to yield not more than 1 microorganism per 100 ml from 50% of samples per year. Gross contamination of infant feeding preparations was frequent in Great Britain until the twentieth century, and even after water supplies were secured, contamination still occurred because of poor hygiene in food handling. In the undefended environment, the intrinsic microbial factors which enhance virulence then decimated the child population. In the early twentieth century overcrowding, which was directly related to family size, was also related to pertussis and measles mortality.

PHYSIOLOGICAL, NUTRITIONAL, AND IMMUNOLOGICAL FACTORS

The physiological reactions to infection have now been extensively studied in the context of immune response. Other physiological phenomena associated with infection include fever; while it has become common to suppress fever to achieve comfort, it is still not plain what may be the benefit to the host of febrile reaction.

The very old, very young, preterm and very ill are characteristically less able than others to mount a febrile response. Mortality in experimental infections is increased in hypothermia. Leukocyte mobility may be reduced, and penicillin and methicillin may be more active against faecal streptococci at higher temperatures (Roberts, 1979).

Complex relationships exist between nutrition and vulnerability to infection. While iron deficiency has traditionally been considered to be associated with increased risks of bacterial infection, saturation of iron bearing proteins in serum and breast milk may permit more iron to be available for microbial metabolic needs, thus encouraging microbial growth (Weinberg, 1978). Nevertheless, iron deficiency may diminish phagocyte functions (Chandra and Newberne, 1977). Nor can it be asserted that protein and calorie shortage inevitably lead to increased rates of infection in children suffering from nutritional deficits. Gross undernutrition, however, diminishes thymus dependent lymphocyte function and phagocytic killing of *Candida*, although antibody formation may continue.

The successful application of principles of antigen-specific immunity in the prevention of disease has continued to yield successful vaccines for the prevention of epidemic disease. Recently, more emphasis has been placed on determining and using the relevant microbiological antigens, rather than directing immunity against virulence or toxic factors, so that antitoxic immunity is rarely employed in the traditional sense of diphtheria or tetanus antitoxin. The delivery and acceptance of vaccine programmes involves successful administra-

TABLE II.
Newly diagnosed episodes of respiratory disease (1979). Notifications from General Practice, England and Wales
(Average weekly rate per 100 000 population).

Period	1st Quarter	2nd Quarter	3rd Quarter	4th Quarter
Common cold	170	104·6	65·3	125·3
Influenza-like illness	148·2	64·8	41·9	70·6
Acute sinusitis	40	34·6	24·4	33·7
Sore throat/tonsillitis	153	137·1	115·9	139·9
Laryngitis and tracheitis	38·6	28·6	18·6	24·9
Acute bronchitis	110·7	76·2	54·7	81·6
Epidemic influenza	50·1	15·4	2·1	7·3
Pneumonia/pneumonitis	7·9	4·8	3·3	3·6

Reproduced from OPCS. Crown copyright.

tion, and husbanding of sometimes scarce resources and persuasion, through health education, if the best results are to be obtained. The management skills of prevention need to be married to the skills of immunology. It is now likely that fall in acceptance rates associated with negative publicity in relation to pertussis vaccine has now been corrected. Morley (1974) has pointed out that in certain underdeveloped societies, omitting the commitment of resources to Mantoux testing, and delivering BCG vaccine to the home, may result in a more widespread and therefore effective distribution of vaccine without causing costs to increase.

How effectively does a developed society resist infection? Considerable vulnerability remains to common place and predominantly virus infectious (Table II). The figures quoted are derived from primary health care records, and are therefore probably an underestimate, since minor cases, self treated, are not easily recorded.

It is customary in the UK to highlight the considerable influenza morbidity, for which the Department of Health and Social Security publish records of working days lost and hence periods for which sickness benefit is claimable (Table III, Fig 1). Virulence factors for influenza viruses, which are particularly hazardous for the old and very young and perhaps the fetus, are reviewed by Sweet and Smith (1980).

TABLE III.
Sickness and invalidity benefits (millions): England and Wales.

	New Periods		Days	
	All cases	Influenza	All cases	Influenza
1972–1973				
Male	7·0	1·0	250	11
Female	2·4	0·3	70	3
1974–1975				
Male	6·6	0·7	244	7
Female	2·3	0·2	66	2
1976–1977				
Male	6·7	0·8	256	5
Female	2·5	0·2	65	2

Reproduced with permission from the Chief Medical Officer's Report to the Secretary of State for Health and Social Security on the State of the Public Health for the year 1978.

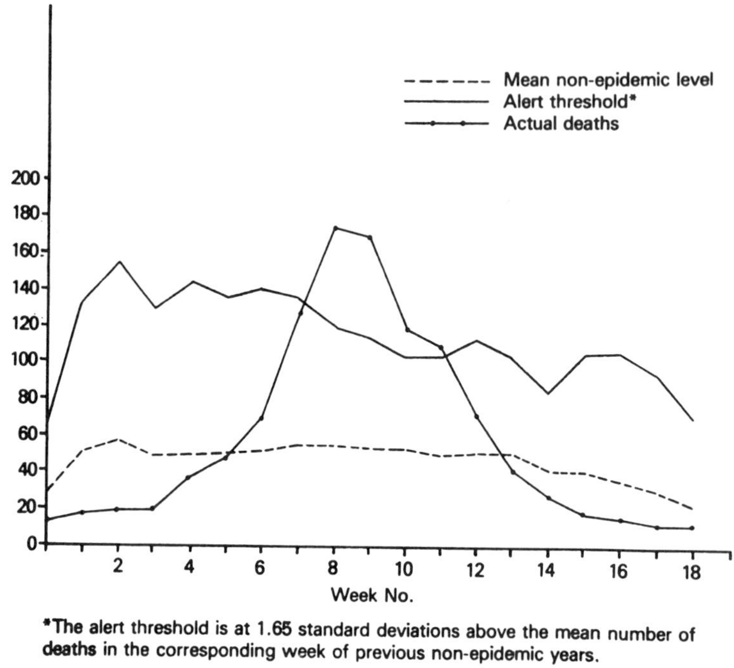

Fig. 1 Mortality from influenza: England and Wales, 1978. Reproduced with permission from the Chief Medical Officer's Report to the Secretary of State for Health and Social Security. On the State of Public Health for the year 1978, Crown Copyright.

Epidemiological aspects of bacterial infections traditionally considered to threaten developed societies have attracted less interest than formerly, and less than more recently recognized infections, such as that due to *Legionella*.

This must be seen as a consequence of the success of modern antibacterial treatment. The observed fall of case fatality for pertussis in infancy from 0·8% (1967–1968) to 0·22% (1977–1978) (CMO Report, 1978) is welcome, if little known, and may ease one aspect of the vaccine controversy.

The continuing development of various applications of intensive therapy prompts careful recording of infection occurrence and this is successfully achieved in the Public Health Laboratory Service Communicable Disease reports. In Table IV material from this source illustrates the continuing scale and severity of bloodstream infections. Particularly threatened are those in the extremes of life, including the low birth-weight infant, and those affected by trauma, surgical intervention, immunosuppression and malignancy.

Organs with special kinds of local vulnerability, e.g. the brain, or affording

TABLE IV.
Significant positive blood cultures: England, Wales and Ireland, January–March 1979.

	Total	Deaths	
Haemophilus influenzae, type b and untyped	57	6	
Bacteroides corrodens	2	1	
fragilis	50	14	
melaninogenicus	1	1	
others	1	1	
Bacteroides spp.	26	4	
Staphylococcus aureus	392	70	
Streptococcus			
group A	51	14	
group B	39	5	
group C	12	1	
group D	62	8	
group G	22	6	
Streptococcus faecalis	25	53	
Streptococcus pneumoniae	250	56	
Klebsiella aerogenes	59	17	
pneumoniae	38	12	
species	41	8	
Escherichia coli	493	83	
Proteus mirabilis	77	12	
Pseudomonas aeruginosa	47	20	
Total	1745	342	(19·6%)

Reproduced with permission—Communicable Disease Surveillance Centre from PHLS unpublished quarterly tabulations. 1st quarter 1979.

particular opportunities for invasion, e.g. the lung or gut, are of concern. The clinician has hitherto, however, concentrated more on the characteristics of the host than on the virulence factors of organisms, of which he will usually have no specialized knowledge.

MECHANISMS FOR CHANGE

The consequences of the enormous difference in generation times of our species and those of bacteria put us at a disadvantage in basic aspects of adaptive evolution. Nevertheless, the discontinous variations of phenotype which are genetic polymorphisms (which may be defined as the existence of two or more alleles at a given locus such that the gene frequency of the least numerous cannot be maintained by random mutation alone) offer opportunities for selective pressures which may enhance biological fitness.

Polymorphisms exist among immunoglobulin heavy chains (Natvig and Kunkel, 1968) and many complement components, the HLA systems of tissue antigens, and perhaps related to HLA, the immune response genes. Many others exist in structural and plasma proteins.

Not all polymorphic systems may be significant in a selective sense, and some may represent a phylogenetic pattern of gene replication and diversification (Lefranc *et al.*, 1979; Bodmer, 1973; Ohno, 1970; Britten and Kohne, 1968).

The Gm polymorphism of heavy chain (γ) of IgG molecules has recently been associated with differences in specific humoral antibody responses (Pandey *et al.*, 1979). A *Haemophilus influenzae* type B vaccine (polyribose phosphate) and meningococcal polysaccharide types A and C vaccines were given with triple vaccine (diphtheria, tetanus and pertussis). Differing strengths of antibody response were apparently associated with both heavy and light chain polymorphisms. Significantly stronger responses to the haemophilus antigen were found in the phenotype Gm 1,2,3,17, : 5,13,14,21 than others.

Similar differences were associated with the kappa light chain polymorphism: the Km 1− phenotype was associated with an antibody response, but the Km 1+ phenotype was not: reverse findings were associated with the meningococcal polysaccharide type C.

A similar differential response was reported by Mackay *et al.* (1975) who found high levels of H antigen of *Salmonella* in those whose phenotype contained Gm 1,21.

That polymorphic variation of this and other kinds may affect biological fitness was suggested by assessment of certain gene frequencies in an isolated Dutch population founded in Surinam in 1840 (de Vries *et al.*, 1979). Selective pressure may have been enforced by epidemics of enteric fever in 1840, which killed 49% of the group, and yellow fever which killed a further 20%, 2 years later. The isolation of the population make it unlikely that the observed changes in gene frequency could be due to genetic drift or intermarriage. In the study group the Gm haplotype 4,23,3,5, has apparently increased when compared with a contemporary Dutch population not exposed to such stresses, and Gm 4,35,1,17,10, and 21 has declined. Similarly, the gene frequencies of HLA AW30 and CW3 have increased significantly as has the C3 complement allotype F.

This relatively complex area of investigation, with arguments based on hypothesis and inference, has its origins in genetic and evolutionary theory, and in elementary aspects of modern immunogenetics. Our prolonged generation time, our ethical and social sensibilities, and the personal scruples which guide our pattern of assortive mating, make our biological adaption to microbiological threat very slow. In a developed society, selection pressure is fortunately reduced, although no such relaxation can be assumed to influence our microbiological adversaries, unless it be true that the more successful parasite will trouble the resilient less grieviously. Our supreme adaption has been a behavioural one, in which a succession of public health and preventive schemes based in applied microbiology can be seen to grossly override the braking effect of generation time, and through education and patterning to have a Lamarckian-like effect. The perturbative weapons and virulence factors of the organism are outflanked and public health legislation, Act by Act, can be compared to point mutation, continually to be reviewed and renewed.

In the words of Sir John Simon, first medical officer of health of the City of London, "the grammar of common sanitary legislation acquired the word virtue of an imperative mood".

REFERENCES

Barrell, R. A. E. and Rowland, M. G. M. (1979). The relationship between rainfall and well water pollution in a West African Village (Gambian). *Journal of Hygiene (Cambridge)* **83**, 143–150.

Bodmer, W. F. (1963). A new genetic model for allelism at histocompatibility and other complex loci: polymorphism for control of gene expression. *Transplantation Proceedings* **5**, 1471–1475.

Britten, R. J. and Kohne, D. E. (1968). Repeated sequences in DNA. *Science* **161**, 529–540.

Chandra, R. K. and Newberne, P. M. (1977). "Nutrition, Immunity and Infection: Mechanisms of Interaction", pp. 67–127. Plenum Press, New York and London.

HMSO (1978) Chief Medical Officer's Report on the State of the Public Health for the year 1978, pp. 29, 31, 48, 51. HMSO, London.

Lefranc, G., Dumitresco, S. M., Salier, J. P., Rivat, L., De Lange, G., Van Loghem, E., Loiselet, J. (1979). Familial lack of IgG 3 subclass. Gene elimination or turning off expression and neutral evolution in the immune system. *Journal of Immunogenetics* **6**, 215–221.

Mackay, I. R., Well, J. V. and Fudenberg, H. H. (1975). *Clinical Immunology and Immunopathology* **3**, 408.

Morley, D. (1974). "Paediatric priorities in the developing world", pp. 271–275. Butterworth, London.

Natvig, J. B. and Kunkel, H. G. (1968). Genetic markers of human immunoglobulus. The Gm and Inv systems. *Series Haematologica* **1**, 66–96.

Neale, A. V. (1964). "The advancement of child health", pp. 1–36. The Athlone Press, London.

Ohno, S. (1972). An argument for the genetic simplicity of man and other mammals. *Journal of Human Evolution* 1, 651–662.

Pandey, J. P., Fudenberg, H. H., Virella, G., Kyong, C. V., Loadholt, C. B., Galbraith, R. M., Gotschlick, E. C., Parkee, J. C. (1979). Association between Ig allotypes and immune responses to haemophilus influenza and meningoccal poly saccharides. *Lancet* 190–192.

Roberts, N. J., Jr (1979). Temperature and host defence. *Microbiological Reviews* 43, 241–259.

Sweet, C. and Smith, H. (1980). Pathogenicity of influenza virus. *Microbiological Reviews* 44, 303–330.

De Vries, R. R. P., Meera Khan, P., Bernini, L. F., Van Loghem, E., Van Rood, J. J. (1979). Genetic control of survival in epidemics. *Journal of Immunogenetics* 6, 271–287.

Weinburg, E. D. (1978). Iron and infection. *Microbiological Reviews* 42, 45–66.

DISCUSSION

Quie It is interesting that newborn infants are compromised in almost all aspects of host defence in a minor sort of way. There is a general delayed development in terms of our concept of a fully mature immune system, yet they cope with a host of microbes in those first days of life. One strain of *Escherichia coli*, the K-1 serotype, accounts for a high percentage of meningitis and septicaemia—that fact should provide a guideline for investigation of microbial factors involved in serious disease. A myriad of microorganisms colonize young individuals yet K-1 strains of *E. coli* and Group B streptococci are associated most frequently with serious disease. Knowledge about their microbial surfaces might suggest mechanisms of defence.

Wood One would like to know whether that particular pathogen had any recognizable effect on neutrophil mobility and whether this has been looked at *in vitro*.

It is now nearly a decade since Miller reported that the neutrophils of the newborn were relatively ineffective in responding to the chemotatic stimuli of bacterial endotoxin, including that of coliform organisms. I do not think that that work has been widely re-examined, but it seems to me important and may not be restricted to coliform bacteria.

There are a number of observations being made now about the changes in polymorph mobility and their appearance in dark ground microscopy when in the presence of microorganisms such as Capnocytophaga. I do not know whether anyone would like to take that on but certainly that is an area which the clinician feels is of some interest.

Quie Dr Miller's observations on depressed locomotion of neonate neutrophils has been confirmed in several laboratories and this observation seems to be a consistent finding in a field that is filled with inconsistency. The role of neutrophils in neonate susceptibility, however, continues to be a subject of some controversy.

The influence of components of K-1 *E. coli* products on neutrophil function is unknown. I think the surface of these organisms prevent activation of complement so they are poorly opsonized.

Wood In Group B streptococcal infections in the newborn it is quite characteristic to find low neutrophil counts. This may be loosely interpreted as a specific consequence of infection with that particular organism.

Quie Neutropenia may be considered a consequence of infection with that particular organism, but not a basis for susceptibility. Infants with Group B sepsis have neutrophils with compromised intracellular killing capacity. Stress of any kind seems to compromise neonatal neutrophils much more easily than at other times in life. Neutrophil function may be slightly decreased in well neonates but markedly decreased during infection or other stress.

Van Furth I just want to ask Professor Wood whether anything is known about the association of *E. coli* and Group B streptococci and HLA or G_m groups. Apparently most of the neonates can cope well with these microorganisms. The results of such a study may have some implications for their prevention.

Wood The G_m situation would be difficult in the newborn because most of the allotypic variants detectable in cord blood would be maternal, but this would not apply of course to HLA antigen and the complement allotypes will be the fetus's own. I do not know whether it is because we have not managed to gird up our loins enough to do the relevant studies, but there is a certain amount of scepticism about the relationship between immune response genes and the polymorphisms which we have talked about. Indeed, the things that I have mentioned are among the relatively few positive observations. The links between immune response and G_m genes look to me to be scanty at the moment.

Wilton Could I ask Paul Quie a couple of things? The neutropenia that you have alluded to in the Group B streptococcal infections—is there any knowledge of the mechanism of this? Is it perhaps due to increased margination or is it in some way the failure of the marrow to deliver the mature granulocyte pool?

Secondly, is there any work that has been done with capsular material and the influence of the material on neutrophil or phagocyte mobility in general? You suggested, I think, that with *E. coli* it is something to do with complement opsonization and that is, of course, something we shall presumably be talking about a lot later; but do you have any ideas about the neutropenia?

Quie I think neonates have neutropenia as a consequence of most infectious agents. There may not be anything specific about Group B streptococci or K-1

E. coli in terms of the neutropenia. The storage pool of neutrophils in normal neonates is much smaller than in older individuals. During septicaemia there may be activation of complement and margination of neutrophils; also the limited number of neutrophils may be in tissues where they are functioning. I believe neutropenia is a rather nonspecific response.

Wilton So what you are almost suggesting is that it is a general host phenomenon at that age and there is perhaps something less specific than Professor Wood has said about K-1 *E. coli* and Group B streptococci.

Quie In terms of the neutropenia, right.

Wilton Therefore, why is there this presumably strong clinical and epidemiological evidence regarding the K-1 *E. coli* and Group B streptococci? It suggests that there are two processes going on, one involving the host and the other the microbe. I think that is going to be one of the things which will come out of our discussion. We know a lot about one aspect but not the other.

Wood May I make a comment which in a sense disagrees with some of this? We look at the neutrophil count in the dyspnoeic newborn, perhaps 36 hours old, as a way of making up our minds clinically, before there is any positive culture available, between the likelihood of the dyspnoea being due to hyaline membrane or to Group B streptococcal septicaemia. Now it seems to me that hyaline membrane disease is quite stressful, admittedly in a different way, in that within a few hours there will be a kind of inflammatory response in the lung. Therefore, I am not sure that a general concept of stress as a cause of neutropenia is applicable and I would certainly like to examine further the causal relationship with this pathogen specifically.

Easmon To come back to the organism, and particularly the surface of the organism, we have been talking about K-1 *E. coli* and Group B streptococci of which there are several types. These typing systems have been designed to identify bacteria and are not necessarily a complete reflection of their surface structure. Organisms growing *in vivo* may be rather different from those that we culture by convenience *in vitro*. I think that some of the recent work on Group B streptococci, for instance, has suggested that even if one takes various strains of a single "type" of organism there is a considerable difference in the ability of these individual strains to resist phagocytosis using a common source of serum and cells. This suggests, I think, that the surface factors on the organism, which may be antiphagocytic factors, may be much more complicated than we fully realize at the moment. There may be some point in looking very much more closely at the surface of organisms that cause infection as compared, perhaps, with the colonizing strains to see if there are specific surface virulence factors that we simply have not yet recognized, and if this can aid us in looking to see why only certain babies get infected.

Braude To change the subject a little bit, do I understand, Professor

Wood, that the child whose ulcers you showed had a *Pseudomonas* infection in the wound?

Wood That is right.

Braude I am very intrigued with this because it brings to my mind a means by which microorganisms may elude or perturb host defences that had not occurred to me in preparing my talk. We have been very interested in the fact that *Pseudomonas* causes a lot of tissue injury by invading blood vessel walls and producing vasculitis manifest by ecthyma gangrenosum. This is often seen in patients who are neutropenic and who are not able to mount an inflammatory response in the vessel. I do not know whether you did a biopsy here to see if there was vasculitis. The thing that intrigues me—and I speak mainly from our experimental observations in rabbits—is that the *Pseudomonas*, unlike almost every other organism, makes a beeline for the vessel wall. It is chemotactically attracted in some way, invades the vessel wall, and then uses this as a sanctuary to protect itself from the defence reactions of the individual. Hiding in the vessel wall is an interesting way in which organisms may be able to elude host defences.

Wood We did not have a biopsy but in the last few days of that child's illness there was a clinical appearance which very much supports your suggestion in that, almost by the hour, it was possible to recognize areas of superficial skin necrosis with purpura which were not unlike the lesions of Henloch Schoenlein purpura, which is a vasculitis. This advanced very rapidly, so that the density of these lesions ultimately might be four or five in an area of 4 cm^2. This was at a time when antibiotic treatment was being given very intensively, as it was throughout. The curious thing in both the affected children in the family was that *Pseudomonas* appeared to be untreatable. They probably did not get it from the same source and they were about two or three years apart in age. The second child, however, responded to treatment for both pneumococcal meningitis and staphylococcal abscesses.

Jeljaszewicz We have recently investigated some extracellular products of *Pseudomonas* and besides confirming that *Pseudomonas* excretes at least five proteolytic enzymes, described mainly by Japanese workers, we have isolated some hitherto undescribed proteolytic enzymes. They have the ability of nonspecific prothrombin activation and may explain the affinity for the vessel wall through the generation of thrombin.

Mims As we are talking in a rather general way, may I bring up another point about infant susceptibility to infection: that is infant *in*susceptibility to infection? This bring me to a fluid, milk, that is greatly neglected by microbiologists. There is no doubt at all that there are a lot of factors present in human milk which protect against virus infection which are not immunoglobulins. This is true of the rotaviruses and for some arthropod-borne viruses and the virus inhibitors are sometimes identified as lipoproteins. Microbiologists should go into this more, because the susceptibility of a given infant to some bacterial and other infections may merely reflect the composition of its mother's milk, which perhaps lacks one of these as yet unidentified antimicrobial nonantibody types of protective factors.

Wood I agree that the newborn is surprisingly resistant to infection, considering the way that he is suddenly faced with it. Surprisingly, he escapes, in an ordinary working environment from much infection.

With regard to milk, I do not know, and perhaps Professor Mims will tell us whether the substances to which he is referring are well characterized. I recall Matthews' observations at Northwick Park which I think had not advanced to the stage of characterization of the antiviral factors, which were heat-labile and present in breast milk and not in cows' milk. There are other relevant things concerned with lipid composition of breast milk which appeared to offer advantages compared with cows' milk; yet cows' milk is better supplied with peroxidases than is breast milk and these variations, I suppose, may reflect the evolutionary experience of the different species.

I do not know whether it is realized that human milk is now a mini-industry and that many hospitals have elaborate ways of collecting the milk. Much argument exists about how it should be processed. The real milk men think that we are crazy because we do not take enough trouble to make sure that breast milk is bacteriologically "pure". We just screen some of it, freeze most of it and feed nearly all of it, whereas the real dairy men, who deal, after all, with a somewhat different range of contaminants and a rather different animal, have to satisfy much more restrictive legislation and they heat it all. If we did that to breast milk we might as well not bother with it.

Mims I am sure you are right and that most of these antimicrobial factors are not identified. There are many interesting possibilities, such as the fact that the fat globules in milk are covered with cell-derived membranes, bearing in some cases histocompatibility antigens on the surface. Perhaps these are capable of absorbing out certain viruses and preventing infection. I hope that the antimicrobial factors are going to be well studied in the next few years.

The problems with milk banks, as implied by Professor Wood, are that all the more vigorous types of treatment of milk are likely to destroy these antimicrobial factors. Another possibility is that in pooling milk from a dozen or two mothers one pools anything nasty that may be present in milk. We know that human cytomegalovirus and at times rubella virus can be present in human milk. There are important things to think about microbiologically in regard to milk banks.

Peters It seems to me, without having any special experience of the value of breast or bottle feeding, that the adaptive value of this can only be quite small in relation to other much more important events affecting the newborn.

Mims On the contrary, if we are thinking of the transfer of secretory immunoglobulin, the standard doctrine is that this is of immense importance in protecting the newborn infant against a whole variety of infectious diseases in those species, such as pigs, where colostrum is a very important method of transfer of the antibody.

Peters I am referring to the human, of course.

Wood What Professor Peters says is quite right, and here I return to the public health theme. It is since we have had clean water, trained health visitors and health education that cow milk-based feeding preparations are safe. It is only 70 years since that has been so and the mortality of the bottle-fed baby in the first decade of this century in this country was 50%. In Paris in the 1870s the "milky way" was the way to the cemetery. Now that is no longer so, but the traces of the evolutionary mechanism of the benefit of breast feeding can be detected. This is what is now being referred to as the enterothelic axis, where it appears that certainly with some species of microorganism—*Salmonella* and some coliforms—one may detect in the breast milk of the mother the specific IgA antibodies to those organisms which she has ingested. Such antibodies offer her baby protection against the faecal contamination inevitable during a normal process of delivery.

Stuart-Harris You mentioned nutrition and the sort of way in which one always looks on the well-nourished person as being resistant. If we think of tuberculosis there is no question but that you are right. In general, I suppose, it is quite true that the well-nourished person resists other infections. However, there are some very notable exceptions. It is a very old observation that foot and mouth disease always goes for the cattle that are well nourished and rather tends to ignore the emaciated ones. Poliomyelitis is well known as attacking the well-grown and well-nourished infant or child. I do not know whether you would like to take this up and say that it is simply because of X, Y and Z. I do not personally think that we know the answers.

Wood I also do not think we know the answers, but I have recently begun to consider that the relatively low haemoglobins detected in the normal infant during the period from, say, three months until three or four years old are not the result of the incompetence of nature but show the skill of nature in sharing iron rather more meanly with the microorganisms which may infect the young.

Microbial Interference with Mucosal Defences

R. VAN FURTH

Department of Infectious Diseases,
University Hospital,
Leiden,
The Netherlands.

INTRODUCTION

Under normal circumstances there is an equilibrium in the interaction between the host and the microorganisms on the skin, mucosal membranes and ambient air (Fig. 1). When this equilibrium becomes disturbed infection may occur. An infection is defined as the composite of reactions of the host to microorganisms or multicellular parasites that have invaded and multiplied in the host. An infection may occur when the host comes into contact with microorganisms that are new to it and to which it has no specific immunity as yet; or when the number of microorganisms on the skin, mucosal membrane or in the ambient air is markedly increased; or when the host defence mechanisms are greatly impaired.

Approximately 10^8 bacteria are present on the total skin area of adult humans. These are mainly staphylococci, micrococci and corynebacteria that occur in microcolonies between the toes, in the axillae and on the perineum. In

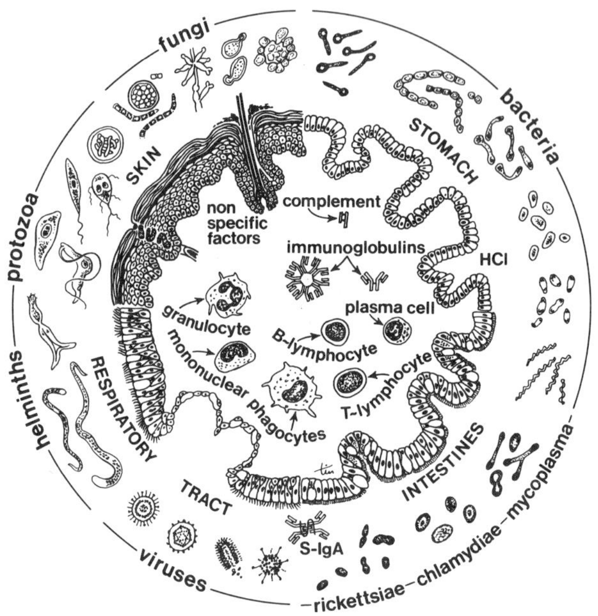

Fig. 1 The inner ring represents the integument; the (micro-)organisms that may invade the body have been indicated in the outer ring; the host defence mechanisms are depicted inside the inner ring.

the mouth streptococci predominate; one millilitre of saliva contains 10^8 bacteria. In the digestive tract bacteria occur in largest numbers in the colon (in total, 10^{14})—mainly anaerobic bacteria, Enterobacteriaceae and streptococci. The ambient air contains only 100 bacteria per cubic metre under normal conditions.

HOST DEFENCE MECHANISMS AT THE MUCOSAL MEMBRANES

The first line of defence against microorganisms is formed by an intact surface, i.e. the skin and mucous membranes (Table I). The skin is not simply a mechanical barrier; the fatty acids secreted by the sebaceous glands and the lactic acid in sweat restrict microbial colonization of the skin. The defences of the mucosal membranes are different for the various tracts: (a) in the respiratory tract mucus formed and secreted by epithelial cells, ciliary movement, respiration and coughing keeps the air passages below the glottis sterile under normal conditions; (b) Gastric acid, produced by parietal cells, and intestinal motility limit bacterial growth in the digestive tract; (c) in the urinary tract mechanical elimination is the most important factor. The surfaces of the various mucous membranes also carry substances which inhibit microbial growth; e.g. the enzyme, lysozyme, is secreted by macrophages, granulocytes, and Paneth cells (McClelland and van Furth, 1975) and splits glycopeptides in the cell wall of Gram positive bacteria, after which they are lysed osmotically. Also lactoferrin and transferrin, which are proteins that inhibit bacterial growth by binding of the iron necessary for the multiplication of bacteria, are present on the mucosal surface.

TABLE I.
Factors involved in the host defence mechanisms at the mucosal membranes.

1	Surface	Mechanical barrier Factors in secretion (mucus, lysozyme, lactoferrin) Gastric acidity
2	Mechanical elimination	Ciliary movement Coughing Peristaltic movement Micturition
3	Immunological humoral defence system	Immunoglobulins local: secretory IgA; IgM; IgG; IgE plasma: IgG; IgM; IgE Complement factors
4	Phagocytic cells	Granulocytes Monocytes and macrophages
5	Cell-mediated immunity	Macrophages plus T lymphocytes
6	Vascularization	

IgA is the most important immunoglobulin on the mucosal membranes, although IgG and IgM are also present; all three immunoglobulins are produced locally by plasma cells in the mucosa (Lai A Fat *et al.*, 1976). IgA is special because it is present in secretions of the nasal mucosa and gastrointestinal and respiratory tracts, as well as in tears and saliva, in relatively higher concentrations than in serum: it is present in a special molecular form called secretory IgA. Secretory IgA is synthesized locally, the IgA by the plasma cells in the mucosa and secretory component by epithelial cells (Lai A Fat *et al.*,

1976; Brandtzaeg and Baklien, 1977). Once produced, these proteins are secreted and combine to form a single molecule. The secretory IgA, a dimer of two IgA molecules coupled in one molecule to secretory component and the J chain, is more resistant to proteolytic enzymes such as those present in the gastrointestinal tracts, than serum proteins are. Only a very minute amount of secretory IgA synthesized in the mucosal membranes is present in the serum, whereas serum IgA is synthesized in the bone marrow, spleen, and lymph nodes (van Furth *et al.*, 1966).

Secretory IgA antibodies can contribute very effectively to the defence against penetrating microorganisms because of their special functions, which are summarized in Table II. In the tissues specific antibodies (i.e. immunoglobulins) have the capacity, often in combination with complement components, to opsonize microorganisms for phagocytosis, to neutralize or to kill noningested microorganisms, and also to neutralize endo- and exotoxins of microorganisms. Secretory IgA lacks most of these functions.

TABLE II.
Functions of secretory IgA.

No bactericidal activity except when complement and lysozyme are present
No opsonization of microorganisms
Complement activation by alternative pathway; not by classical pathway
Prevention of adhesion of bacteria to mucosal surface
Inhibition of motility of bacteria
Agglutination of bacteria
Inhibition of antigen uptake by mucosa
Neutralization of enterotoxins
Virus neutralization

The cellular defence mechanism is exerted by phagocytic cells, i.e. granulocytes and macrophages, because the body can only dispose of deleterious material by phagocytosis. Both kinds of phagocytic cells occur in the mucosa; the granulocytes also at the mucosal surfaces. The accumulation of granulocytes and macrophages at sites of infection is governed by chemotactic factors.

Phagocytosis can be divided into several phases: opsonization, recognition and attachment, ingestion, fusion of lysosomes with the phagosome, degranulation, intracellular killing of microorganisms, and enzymatic digestion and disposal of degraded material. Phagocytosis mediated by immunoglobulins with or without complement is called immune phagocytosis. The monocytes, macrophages, and granulocytes, carrying immunoglobulin (Fc) and complement (C3) receptors on the cell surface, are called professional phagocytes (Rabinovitch, 1975).

Cell-mediated immunity is a condition of changed microbicidal action of macrophages. When sensitized T lymphocytes re-encounter the antigen they produce lymphokines, which activate macrophages. Activated macrophages show both enhanced phagocytosis and intracellular killing of phagocytosed microorganisms. This type of reaction is important for defence against infections caused by facultative and obligate intracellular microorganisms, e.g. mycobacteria, *Salmonella* spp., *Listeria, Yersinia, Brucella* spp., *Candida* spp. and other fungi, *Chlamydia*, rickettsiae, several viruses, and protozoa (Sharma and Remington, 1980).

EVIDENCE FOR THE IMPORTANCE OF DEFENCE FACTORS AT THE MUCOSAL MEMBRANES

In man, evidence of the importance of host factors in the defence against microorganisms at the level of mucosal membranes has come from congenital or acquired disorders. For example, patients with granulocytopenia often develop enterobacterial septicaemia, and such infections very frequently originate from the gastrointestinal tract. It is not known whether the main site of granulocyte function is the mucosa or the lumen of the gastrointestinal tract. There is evidence that granulocytes in the mouth are functionally adequate, but it has not been demonstrated that granulocytes in the gastrointestinal tract, below the stomach, are functionally active. Most of the bacteria reaching the stomach cannot survive the low pH conditions there, but in cases of hypo- or achlorhydria this kind of host defence is impaired, and gastrointestinal infections, e.g. with *Salmonella* spp., occur more frequently (McClelland, 1979). The role of immunoglobulins is easily shown in agammaglobulinaemia since these patients repeatedly develop respiratory infections caused by *Streptococcus pneumoniae, Haemophilus influenzae,* β-haemolytic streptococci, and intestinal infections with *Giardia lamblia* (Hermans *et al.*, 1966; Root and Hierholzer, 1978, Stevens and Mahmoud, 1980).

INTERFERENCE BY MICROORGANISMS WITH DEFENCES AT THE MUCOSAL MEMBRANES

The mucosal membranes usually attacked by microorganisms are those in the oral–pharyngeal area, the upper respiratory tract, the digestive tract, and the genital tract: the lower respiratory tract and the urinary tract are normally sterile. The interactions between microorganisms and host defence factors involve the attachment, penetration, multiplication, and spreading of microorganisms as well as tissue destruction by enzymes produced by microorganisms.

Surface components of bacteria contributing to their adherence to mucous membranes include carbohydrates, glycoproteins, glycolipids, K antigens, M proteins, and pili (Smith, 1977; Arbuthnot and Smyth, 1979). All of these factors promote the entry of microorganisms into the mucosal membranes.

Little is known about the interaction between microorganisms and the humoral defence mechanisms. Recently, it has been shown that some bacteria (*Neisseria gonorrhoeae, N. meningitides*, and *Streptococcus sanguis*) produce an enzyme that cleaves IgA and secretory IgA. However, this enzyme does not split IgA_2 (Plaut *et al.*, 1977; Plaut, 1978; Mulks and Plaut, 1978; Blake *et al.*, 1979). The extent to which this mechanism interferes with the humoral immunity to infection on secretory surfaces is not yet known. It has also been reported that *Trypanosoma cruzi* contains an enzyme that splits IgG (Eisen, pers. comm., 1981), which means that opsonization, and thus phagocytosis, would be evaded.

Bacterial surface components can interfere with ingestion of invading microorganisms by phagocytic cells (Glynn, 1972; Smith, 1977; Arbuthnott and Smyth, 1979; Horwitz, 1981). These antiphagocytic factors include the polysaccharides of meningococci and pneumococci, the M protein and hyaluronic acid of streptococci, and protein A of staphylococci. Also of importance in this respect are the K antigens of *Escherichia coli*, Vi antigens of *Salmonella typhi*, and O antigens of other Enterobacteriaceae. Mucoid strains of *Pseudomonas aeruginosa* resist phagocytosis even in the presence of opsonizing antisera (Baltimore and Mitchell, 1980). Recently, it was reported that capnocytophaga can reduce the locomotion of granulocytes Shurin *et el.*, 1979; Ward, 1979).

Many microorganisms and their toxins can kill host cells and thus weaken effective defences (Graig, 1972; Mims, 1977; Horwitz, 1981). For example, both leukocidin of *Staphylococcus aureus* and certain strains of *Pseudomonas aeruginosa*, and streptolysins of *Streptococcus pyogenes* kill phagocytes; toxins of *Bordetella pertussis* cause ciliary damage; α toxins of *Clostridium welchii* cause cell necrosis and haemolysis; and enterotoxins produced by *Vibrio cholerae* and by certain strains of *E. coli* affect the intestinal epithelial cells in a way which leads to loss of water and electrolytes. *Shigella dysenteriae* penetrates the colonic epithelium and produces locally an enterotoxin that kills such cells and leads to mucosal ulcers. One part of the components of the outer layer of all Gram negative microorganisms is endotoxin, the toxic actions of which, on release after bacterial death and disentegration, are manifold.

Viral infections of the mucosal lining can cause local cell death and thus destroy the integrity of the integement. A good example of this kind of viral–host defence interaction is infection with influenza virus. Such infections lead to epithelial lesions of trachea and bronchial tree, which facilitate the penetration of *Staphylococcus aureus* and *Streptococcus pneumoniae*, together with *Haemophilus influenzae*. Secondary infections with these bacteria are frequent and are often fatal (Mulder and Hers, 1972). It is also possible that other viral infections, not only in the respiratory tract but also in the gastrointestinal and urogenital tracts, prepare the way for (secondary) bacterial infections. Little is known about these situations, because of the difficulties associated with rapid diagnosis of viral infections.

REFERENCES

Arbuthnott, J. P. and Smyth, C. J. (1979). Bacterial adhesion in host/pathogen interactions in animals. *In* "Adhesion of Microorganisms to Surfaces" (Eds D. C. Ellwood, J. Melling and P. Rutter), p. 165. Academic Press, London and New York.

Baltimore, R. S. and Mitchell, M. (1980). Immunological investigation of mucoid strains of Pseudomonas aeruginosa: comparison of susceptibility of opsonic antibody in mucoid and nonmucoid strains. *Journal of Infectious Diseases* **141**, 238.

Blake, M., Holmes, K. K. and Swanson, J. (1979). Studies on *Gonococcus* infection. XVII. IgA_1-cleaving protease in vaginal washings from women with gonorrhea. *Journal of Infectious Diseases* **139**, 89.

Brandtzaeg, P. and Baklien, K. (1977). Intestinal secretion of IgA and IgM: a hypothetical model. *In* "Immunology of the Gut" p. 77. Elsevier Excerpta Medica North-Holland, Amsterdam, Oxford, New York.

van Furth, R., Schuit, H. R. E. and Hijmans, W. (1966). The formation of immunoglobulins by human tissues *in vitro*. III. Spleen, bone marrow, lymph nodes and thymus. *Immunology* **11**, 19.

Glynn, A. A. (1972). Bacterial factors inhibiting host defence mechanisms. *In* "Microbial Pathogenicity in Man and Animals" (Eds H. Smith and J. H. Pearce), p. 75. Cambridge University Press.

Graig, J. P. (1972). The enterotoxic enteropathies. *In* "Microbial Pathogenicity in Man and Animals" (Eds H. Smith and J. H. Pearce), p. 78. Cambridge University Press.

Hermans, P. E., Huizinga, K. A., Hoffman, H. N., Brown, A. L. and Markowitz, H. (1966). Dysgammaglobulinemia associated with nodular hyperplasia of the small intestine. *American Journal of Medicine* **20**, 329.

Horwitz, M. A. (1981). Phagocytosis of microorganisms. *Reviews of Infectious Diseases*, in press.

Lai A Fat, R. F. M., McClelland, D. B. L. and van Furth, R. (1976). *In vitro* synthesis of immunoglobulins, secretory component, complement and lysozyme by human gastro-intestinal tissues I. Normal tissues. *Journal of Clinical and Experimental Immunology* **23**, 9.

McClelland, D. B. L. (1979). Bacterial and viral infections of the gastro-intestinal tract. *In* "Immunology of the Gastrointestinal Tract" (Ed. P. Asquith), p. 214. Churchill Livingstone, Edinburgh, London, New York.

McClelland, D. B. L. and van Furth, R. (1975). *In vitro* synthesis of lysozyme by human and mouse tissues and leucocytes. *Immunology* **28,** 1099.

Mims, C. A. (1977). "The Pathogenesis of Infectious Diseases." Academic Press. London and New York.

Mulder, J. and Hers, J. F. Ph. (1972). "Influenza." Wolters-Noordhoff, Groningen.

Mulks, M. H. and Plaut, A. G. (1978). IgA protease production as a characteristic distinguishing pathogenic from harmless neisseriaceae. *New England Journal of Medicine* **299,** 973.

Plaut, A. G. (1978). Microbial IgA proteases. *New England Journal of Medicine.* **298,** 1459.

Plaut, A. G., Gilbert, J. V. and Wistar Jr, R. (1977). Loss of antibody activity in human immunoglobulin A exposed to extracellular immunoglobulin A proteases of Neisseria gonorrhoeae and Streptococcus sanguis. *Infection and Immunity* **17,** 130.

Rabinovitch, M. (1975). Macrophage spreading *in vitro. In* "Mononuclear Phagocytes in Immunity, Infection and Pathology" (Ed. R. van Furth), p. 369. Blackwell Scientific, Oxford.

Root, R. K. and Hierholzer Jr, W. J. (1978). Infectious Diseases. *In* "Clinical Pharmacology. Basic Principles in Therapeutics" (Eds K. L. Melmon, and H. F. Morrelli), p. 709. Macmillan Publishing, New York Collier Macmillan Canada, Toronto Baillière-Tindall, London.

Sharma, S. D. and Remington, J. S. (1980). The role of cell-mediated immunity in resistance to infection in the immunocompromised host. *In* "Infections in the Immunocompromised Host. Pathogenesis, Prevention and Therapy" (Eds J. Verhoef, P. K. Peterson and P. G. Quie), p. 59. Elsevier/North-Holland Biomedical Press, Amsterdam, New York, Oxford.

Shurin, S. B., Socransky, S. S., Sweeney, E. and Stossel, T. P. (1979). A neutrophil disorder induced by capnocytophaga, a dental micro-organism. *New England Journal of Medicine* **301,** 849.

Smith, H. (1977). Microbial surfaces in relation to pathogenicity. *Bacterial Reviews* **41,** 475.

Stevens, D. P. and Mahmoud, A. A. F. (1980). Giardiasis: the rediscovery of an ancient pathogen. *In* "Current Clinical Topics in Infectious Diseases" (Eds J. S. Remington and M. N. Swartz), p. 195. McGraw-Hill, New York.

Ward, P. A. (1979). Those venerable notions. *New England Journal of Medicine* **301,** 888.

Weir, D. M. and Ögmundsdóttir, H. M. (1980). Cellular recognition by phagocytes: role of lectin-like receptor(s). *In* "Mononuclear Phagocytes. Functional Aspects" (Ed. R. van Furth), p. 865. Martinus Nijhoff, The Hague.

DISCUSSION

Stuart-Harris It seems to me that the relationship between influenza infection and subsequent bacterial infection is not as simple as might at first sight appear. If it is just a matter of unlocking the mechanical defence of the ciliated epithelium, why does the infection more commonly occur after the peak of cellular destruction? Thus, in the case of influenza virus infection followed by *Pneumococcus* infection, why does it not occur at the height of the virus lesion, as in the case of *Staphylococcus*? It is a fact, I think, that postinfluenzal pneumococcal pneumonia does not begin until at least a week, and maybe even up to three weeks or a month, following the initial influenza. That has been a well documented and well-accepted fact. Why this delay? And why not a similar delay in the case of staphylococcal infection of the lung? Instead, this latter is almost synchronous with the virus infection. So I cannot see that we have any right to think this is a simple mechanical process and, if it is not a mechanical process, what is it?

Mims One interesting thing is that Dr Shelakov and his colleagues from San Antonio have shown that certain bacteria will adhere specifically to influenza virus-infected cells but not to the same extent to uninfected cells. So there, in principle, is a mechanism by which, say, a staphylococcus, might have an edge on some other microorganisms.

Sweet I believe I am correct in saying that they studied strains of streptococci. However, unfortunately they were strains that were not associated with bacterial superinfection in clinical cases of influenza so, although the mechanism is quite attractive, it may not be terribly relevant. Just to add a bit more to what Sir Charles said, I think there is good evidence—although it is rather old—that mucociliary clearance mechanisms appear unimpaired even in areas of the lung where damage to the ciliated epithelium is quite severe. It seems that mechanical impairment is not the explanation for bacterial superinfection. The weight of evidence suggests that the phagocytes are defective.

van Furth In post mortem cases you will see that the epithelia are completely denuded; also in experimental infections in animals there is no longer any epithelium present. With regard to the influenza virus and the phagocytes, I would comment that a number of these studies are done *in vitro* and I do not know how relevant that is. Adding the virus to the phagocytes *in vitro* does not represent the situation *in vivo*, since there is no viraemia during influenza, thus there cannot be an interaction of the virus and the polymorphs in the circulation, except at the site of infection. I think most of these studies do not have a real relevance because usually normal peripheral blood of donors is used. Furthermore, I find it difficult to understand how the virus only present in the respiratory tract can interact with circulating neutrophils; perhaps other factors released from the site of infection interact with them.

Anderson I think some of these studies have been done with alveolar macrophages taken from animals infected with respiratory tract viruses. This work shows impairment of phagocytic activity.

Stuart-Harris I think there have also been some with human cells.

Lambert I may have misheard, but I seemed to hear the cilia being rather demoted. There is certainly one experiment of nature in which they show themselves to be very important and that is Kartagener's syndrome, in which I recall the dynein arms of the ciliary microtubules are deficient and this deficiency is closely linked with impairment of ciliary function. I do not know whether these patients have any specificity in their susceptibility to microbial infection, but susceptible they certainly are.

Mims Is it not that they are susceptible to chronic sinusitis and so on in a nonspecific way—just as they are infertile?

Lambert Yes, indeed. The problem is that we do not know what are the initiating factors of that vicious circle.

Quie We have an animal model for studying the interaction of influenza virus and *Streptococcus pneumoniae* in otitis media. Chinchillas are good experimental animals since they are not normally colonized with pneumococci. When animals are colonized with pneumococci and challenged with influenza virus most of them develop otitis media after several days. Interestingly enough, neutrophils from these animals are virtually incapable of chemotactic responsiveness to several stimuli and the metabolic response of these neutrophils is markedly diminished.

Potter We have been working with a model originally acquired from a Dr Michaels who worked in our laboratory. He was interested in the mechanism of pathogenicity of *Haemophilus influenza* and had titrated a pathogenic strain in rats aged 48 h to determine the infecting dose. In our laboratory we were particularly interested to see if prior infection with influenza viruses would promote subsequent bacterial infection by *Haemophilus influenzae.* We found that it did. We have used this model in two different ways. Firstly, we have studied some 40 different influenza A virus strains to determine what effect they have on subsequent bacteraemia and meningitis caused by *Haemophilus influenza.* We have obtained a very good correlation between the virulence of the viruses for man and the ability of these viruses to promote subsequent bacteraemia. We are rather excited to have a good laboratory model to measure human virulence. A second use for this model is to study antiviral agents and the ability of these agents to prevent the cytopathic effects of virus infection. We have shown that amantadine, given by a number of routes, is capable of limiting the influenza-induced effects in rats that subsequently lead to enhanced bacterial infection. The best effect is when the compound is given intranasally but it is also active when given by other routes. The model is an interesting one, since it can be exploited in a direction more relevant to this symposium. We could study what the virus does to the respiratory surfaces to facilitate the subsequent bacterial infection.

Stuart-Harris Could you tell us exactly where and when you put the bacteria and viruses in terms of time relationships and anatomy?

Potter The rats are used at age 48 h. We inoculate intranasally with virus at this age with a Hamilton syringe, which is quite easily controlled. The virus replicates and peak titres occur at about 48 h when the animal is 4 days old. At this time, we inoculate the rats in exactly the same way with *Haemophilus influenzae.* The strain used is passed intraperitoneally five times in order to give a strain of high pathogenicity. We assess the bacteraemia 48 h after bacterial inoculation, when the animals are killed, blood is taken for viable counts and brains are examined for histological evidence of meningitis.

Braude I do not know whether the others here who take care of adults will agree with my experience that, in contrast to children who get all kinds of bacterial infections along with influenza, the thing that is striking about adults is that staphylococcal infection of the lung has a special association with influenza. I would say that in the otherwise healthy adult the only time that he gets staphylococcal pneumonia is after influenza. I do not question the increased susceptibility to other organisms, but the unique thing about adults is that they do not develop staphylococcal pneumonia unless there is an underlying influenza infection. So I think that any theory about how influenza virus promotes superinfection by bacteria has to explain this unique susceptibility to the staphylococcus. I have been groping with this for many years and I was happy to see protein A come along because it gives us a theory, even though we do not have too much data to go on. Our theory in San Diego is that IgG specific for influenza virus attaches to the respiratory mucosa through the Fab portion and provides a trap, if you will, for staphylococci which may be present in the nasopharynx. They become anchored through the Fc portion to the respiratory epithelium. I do not know if there is anything to this, but it is a speculative approach to the specific association with the staphylococcus. I would be interested in whether anybody here has any data that might support or demolish this.

Potter I feel that the infant rat model that I described could be used to investigate this particular point. We have only used *Haemophilus influenzae* as a bacterial infection, but there is no reason why we should be limited to this organism and staphylococci could be tested in the system.

Anderson As well as staphylococci having receptors for the majority of the IgG classes, there are also certain streptococci which have receptors for immunoglobulins, including IgA.

Jeljaszewicz Our working hypothesis is that the clumping factor of *Staphylococcus* is worthy of more attention than protein A. We think the clumping factor, which we have isolated and characterized as a pure substance, may be involved in the initial stage of establishment of a staphylococcus, especially in tissue damaged in various ways.

van Furth I want to question whether Dr Braude's hypothesis is really true. I think it is an attractive idea. We know that the amount of protein A in the different strains of staphylococci is very different and that should be tested.

Until very recently we still had all the staphylococci from the outbreak in 1957. Six months ago because we did not have any idea what to do with them we threw them away. If I had succeeded in saving them we could have tested this hypothesis retrospectively. If a laboratory is willing to determine protein A in a similar series of strains you could get clinical evidence in support of your idea.

Wilton One of the things that has been known, I think for a long time, is that herpes simplex virus-infected cells express an Fc receptor and—thinking about the problem of superinfection of facial herpes simplex infections in rather the same way that Dr Braude talked about pneumonia—we reasoned that if staphylococci have protein A and therefore are able to bind Fc IgG, they would possibly bind and attach to herpesvirus infected cells and this might be one of the mechanisms of superinfection. The difficulty, of course, is that if you have antibodies in an inflammatory exudate to staphylococci they are going to attach the wrong way round as much as they are going to attach the right way round. George Cimosani in Geneva prepared for us human IgG cleaved by neutrophil elastase which binds very well to protein A and permits staphylococci to adhere very tenaciously to herpes simplex virus infected cells. That is the first thing.

That then led me to think in terms of other mechanisms whereby these immunological fragments, particularly immunoglobulin fragments, might work. They are often dismissed as being ineffective. I think that is perhaps a bit premature because using the same elastase-digested IgG (which does not, of course, give the same sort of Fc/ $(Fab^1)_2$ split as pepsin or papain) we have some initial experiments showing quite clearly that Fc receptor-positive streptococci are phagocytosed very easily in the absence of $(Fab^1)_2$ and Fc receptor-negative streptococci are not. I think that phagocytosis, at least by neutrophils, can be mediated by fragments of IgG provided that the Fc receptor binding moiety of the fragment is preserved. It may be, since the early events of any mucosal infection are hyperaemia and increased vascular permeability, that IgG and IgM are as important, if not more important, than IgA. I say that to start an argument.

van Furth I do not see the role of the Fc receptor in the herpes infected cells, because at the time that IgG is already bound, it is impossible for the staphylococcus with protein A to bind to that structure because it will not reach it. So how does that argument go?

Wilton That is one of the peculiar things; if you take the infected cells and just simply add DEAE-purified IgG, you can show that there is binding. It is not very good binding until you aggregate your IgG. This, of course, increases the ligand binding affinity enormously, but it does not seem to allow the binding of staphylococci to those cells. But if you take this elastase-digested Fc fragment, allow it to absorb to the cells and then add the staphylococci, the staphylococci stick very well. I cannot explain that.

Quie Do the digestion products of IgG and IgM act as opsonins by themselves or in the presence of complement?

Wilton Let me put it this way: you get an effect above background until you add complement and then you get as good an effect for phagocytosis as if you had the whole, specific antibody.

One other point I would like to make is that IgA will act as an opsonin if you take an organism which itself is capable of activating the alternative pathway. Is it a true opsonin in that sense? You might as well ask "Is IgM a true opsonin in that sense since it can only function through C3?". There is a small increase in the numbers of particles phagocytosed over that which is due to the complement mediated system alone, so it is a small effect but it seems to be a real one.

Peters In relation to the last point, do you know whether there is any distinction between binding and ingestion in these systems, because complement-dependent effects usually produce binding, not binding and ingestion?

Wilton I was hoping that Helgei Valdimarsson would come in there because he and I disagree fairly fundamentally about whether complement does ever, in fact, mediate ingestion at all.

Peters Whether it does or not, if there is a distinction in the system it is of very great interest.

Wilton Yes, I must say I have not separated the two events.

Mogensen I want to turn to examples of viral infections predisposing to bacterial infection in the urinary tract. I recall at least one paper published in the middle of the 1960s in the *Journal of Experimental Medicine* of adenovirus infection predisposing to pyelonephritis caused by *E. coli.* Moreover, it has been shown in a series of papers by Thomsen and co-workers in recent years that mycoplasmas in a rat model predispose to pyelonephritis caused by *E. coli.*

van Furth Is this mycoplasma infection really relevant? Do mycoplasma infections of the kidney occur in humans? Of course you can cause a lesion with mycoplasma and then you can have a secondary bacterial infection. You can also promote pyelonephritis by adding zinc to the bladder. You can have all kinds of models. The point is what is clinically relevant and what clinical infections can predispose to infection in the urinary tract. Is not your model artificial?

Mogensen It is true that both the mycoplasma infection and the bacterial infection were artificially induced, but the same authors have shown that mycoplasmas can be isolated from the upper urinary tract of a proportion of patients with pyelonephritis.

Bacterial Interference with Nonspecific, Nonphagocytic Defences

ABRAHAM I. BRAUDE

Department of Medicine and Pathology,
University of California,
San Diego, California, USA.

Infectious agents must break through four lines of defence before they can establish themselves in the tissues; namely, the body surfaces, the circulating body fluids, the connective tissue matrix and the cells. Resistance to infection depends on the joint activity of the processes which operate at these four levels. This account deals with defence in the circulating body fluids and describes the devices which bacteria use to counteract the nonspecific mechanisms at this level of resistance. These nonspecific mechanisms are the serum bactericidins, complement, transferrin, Eh, and elevated temperature. The bactericidins are regarded as nonspecific because they are present in the absence of any known specific antigenic stimulus.

MECHANISMS OF PROTECTION BY NONSPECIFIC, NONPHAGOCYTIC DEFENCE SYSTEMS

Bactericidal System: The Joint Action of Bactericidins and Complement

Bactericidins are natural antibodies that cause lysis of Gram negative bacteria in the absence of phagocytes. Bacteriolysis by natural antibody results from a reaction between the bacterial surface antigens, IgM and complement. The first step in bacteriolysis of the meningococcus, *Haemophilus influenzae* and certain enteric bacilli is the attachment of the Fab portion of IgM to the capsular polysaccharide antigen. Then the first component of complement (C1) attaches through its subunit C1q to a binding site on the Fc portion of IgM. This interaction with antibody globulin activates C1 and catalyses the assembly of C4 and C2. The $C\overline{42}$ functions as the enzyme C3 convertase, which cleaves C3 into two fragments, C3a and C3b. The C3a fragment is opsonic, but C3b attaches to receptors on the bacterial cell and then combines with neighbouring $C\overline{42}$. This combination apparently modifies the specificity of $C\overline{42}$ so that it can now cleave C5 into C5a and C5b. The large fragment C5b attaches to the bacterial cell membrane, binding in turn C6 and C7 to form the trimolecular complex $C\overline{567}$, which then becomes tetramolecular when C8 is incorporated. The terminal complex of C activation becomes complete when C9 fixes to binding sites on $C\overline{5678}$. The large complex of the five individual terminal C proteins is essential for killing susceptible Gram negative bacteria. The series of reactions just described represents killing via the classical pathway of complement activation and is initiated by union of antigen with antibody (Müller-Eberhard, 1977).

Bactericidal activity can also be generated through the alternative (or properdin) pathway (Gotze and Müller-Eberhard, 1974). The lipopolysaccharide in Gram negative bacteria can activate the alternative pathway by reacting directly with a noncomplement protein, C3 proactivator (properdin B or C3PA). Upon reacting with LPS, C3PA splits into at least two fragments: one has the electrophoretic mobility of gamma globulin (mol. wt 60 000) and the second consists of an acidic peptide (mol. wt 20 000). The larger fragment, known as C3 activator, splits C3 into C3a and C3b (properdin A), and thereby initiates the terminal sequences of complement activation.

In addition to C, lysozyme, calcium and magnesium are important components of extracellular fluids that are required for killing by bactericidins, Ca^{2+} and Mg^{2+} ions are essential for initiation of the classical complement sequence, and lysozyme is needed for disrupting the cell wall peptidoglycan. Lysozyme splits the 1–4 glycosidic linkages between *N*-acetyl muramic acid and *N*-acetylglucosamine in the peptidoglycan so that C might have greater access for attack on the cytoplasmic membrane.

In many Gram negative bacteria, the LPS is the key intermediate in killing because it activates C by either pathway. Each of the three primary structural components of LPS–O antigens, core sugars, and Lipid A–can activate either classical pathway by direct reaction with C1q or the alternative pathway (Morrison and Ulevitch, 1978). The importance of complement in natural resistance to human infection is seen in patients who share a familial deficiency of C6, C7, and C8 and are subject to severe recurrent attacks of bacteraemia due to the *Gonococcus* and *Meningococcus*. Phagocytosis of these bacteria is normal because opsonins can be produced through C3, but the serum of these patients cannot kill pathogenic *Neisseria* because the terminal complex of C is not formed.

Transferrin

The virulence of many bacteria is a function of the amount of iron available in body fluids to stimulate their growth. Staphylococci, clostridia, *Listeria*, mycobacteria, various enteric bacteria, *Pseudomonas*, *Pasteurella*, *Yersinia*, *Vibrio*, and *Aeromonas* are among the genera of bacteria whose members are stimulated by excess iron to grow in body fluids (Weinberg, 1978). This growth stimulation by iron in serum and other body fluids is thought to depend on saturation of transferrin, a nonhaem, iron-binding protein with a molecular weight in the range of 75 000–80 000. It binds reversibly two ferric ions per molecule through tyrosyl and histidyl residues. Under normal conditions human transferrin is 25–35% saturated so that the amount of free ionic iron in plasma is at least 100 million-fold less than that required for bacterial growth (0·4–4·0 μm). If circulating transferrin is saturated by injecting iron intravenously, intraperitoneally, or intramuscularly, there is an increased mortality rate of animals with experimental candidiasis, tuberculosis, staphylococcal infections, meningococcal infections and salmonellosis. By saturating transferrin, the injection of iron makes available enough free iron to meet microbial growth requirements. Impaired resistance to infection is not limited to experimental animals treated with iron, since impaired resistance has been reported in human beings after exposure to excess iron. Thus, the incidence of serious Gram negative infections has increased in newborn infants after intramuscular injection of iron (Barry and Reeve, 1977). It should be noted that transferrin can also be saturated if its concentration falls in relation to iron, as occurs in patients with kwashiorkor who cannot make iron-binding proteins for nutritional reasons. The plasma obtained from kwashiorkor victims supports growth of *S. aureus* and is bacteriostatic upon addition of transferrin.

Redox Potential

The relatively high oxidation–reduction potential (Eh) of the extracellular fluids help prevent infection by anaerobic bacteria. The Eh is a measure (mV) of the tendency to give up electrons or the potential that would exist between the body fluids and a hydrogen half-cell at pH 6. Eh of extracellular fluids is a function not only of their inherent reducing tendency but also of their hydrogen concentration and becomes more negative as hydrogen ion concentration diminishes. The importance of Eh was first brought out in the case of tetanus by Fildes (1929) who showed that tetanus spores will not germinate readily at an Eh more oxidizing than +10 mV at pH 7·0–7·6. In living animal tissues he found the Eh to be approximately 120 mV at the prevailing pH 7·4. If the Eh is kept down by electrical methods, clostridia will grow even if a stream of air is passed through the culture (Hanke and Bailey, 1945) or if the pH is kept in the acid range (6·4–6·8) *Clostridium perfringens* will grow at an Eh of +160 or more. In ischaemic tissues the anoxia lowers the Eh and lactic acid accumulation lowers the pH so that anaerobic bacteria proliferate at Eh levels that are too high for their growth at the normal pH of 7·4. Since acidosis enhances proteolysis and accumulation of amino acids, the pH falls even more. Anaerobic infections do not occur unless the redox potential is lowered by impairment of local blood supply (i.e. arterial occlusion); pressure of foreign bodies (sutures, clotting, dirt, and metal); contamination of wounds with ionized calcium salts commonly present in fertile soil from farm lands, a powerful cause of tissue necrosis; or destruction of tissues by trauma, infection or injection of quinine or epinephrine.

Fever

Fever can protect against bacterial infection in three ways:

(1) *By inhibiting the growth of heat-sensitive bacteria.* Two important species of mycobacteria—*marinum* and *leprae*—grow poorly even at core body temperatures and the infections they cause are usually confined to the cooler parts of the body in the skin, nasopharynx, or superficial nerves. Although *Mycobacterium leprae* cannot be cultured on artificial medium, *M. marinum* is known to grow optimally at 30 °C, but not in primary cultures or infected tissues at 37 °C. *Mycobacterium marinum* is a marine organism that lives normally in the cooler temperatures of sea water, swimming pools, or infected fish tissues; and often causes a chronic skin granuloma of the arms or legs. Most patients give a history of exposure to fish tanks or swimming pools, and some develop a lymphangitis resembling sporotrichosis, a fungus infection also due to an organism (*Sporothrix schenkii*) which is sensitive to heat and seldom infects deep viscera. Two other important pathogenic bacteria with enough heat sensitivity to be affected adversely by fever are the gonococcus and *Treponema pallidum.* Both organisms are injured at temperatures in the range of 40–41 °C. Since these temperatures can be tolerated by man for several hours, patients with neurosyphilis and gonococcal infections have been treated with fever therapy before penicillin was on the market. The inoculation of *Plasmodium vivax* has been used most effectively for fever therapy of neurosyphilis, with good results occurring after eight or ten fever paroxysms (DuBois, 1948).

(2) *By enhancement of phagocytosis.* Phagocytosis by human leukocytes is greatest

between 38°C and 40°C (Ellingson and Clark, 1942). In lizards whose temperature can be regulated by controlling ambient temperatures, allowing them to have fever causes increased migration of leukocytes so that infection is localized.

(3) *By lowering the level of circulating iron.* During fever the reticuloendothelial system in the liver and spleen takes up iron and circulating iron levels fall. In addition, the production of siderophores, the iron binding proteins of bacteria, is suppressed at higher temperatures so that the organisms can take up less iron. When infected lizards are allowed to develop fever, more of them survive (Griger and Kluger, 1978).

MECHANISMS BY WHICH BACTERIA INTERFERE WITH NONSPECIFIC NONPHAGOCYTIC DEFENCES

Bactericidins and Complement: The Bactericidal System

Bacteria can oppose the bactericidal system by interfering with either bactericidins or C. Such interference is perhaps most striking in Gram positive bacteria which are innately resistant to lysis by C. The difference in susceptibility between Gram positive and Gram negative bacteria to serum bacteriolysis is best explained by the concept that the cell wall of Gram positives is a barrier which hinders access of C to the cytoplasmic membrane. This idea is reinforced by the fact that protoplasts of Gram positive bacteria, whose cell wall is removed, are killed by C. The thicker peptidoglycan and the absence of LPS could explain how the cytoplasmic membrane enjoys a sanctuary in Gram positive bacteria from C.

Similar barriers probably explain the resistance to serum-killing in certain Gram negative bacteria. Among enteric bacilli, rough Gram negative organisms are killed by fresh serum, even though their parent, smooth bacteria are resistant to killing. Since only the smooth bacteria are rich in O antigen on their surface, the oligosaccharides in this antigen are probably responsible for resistance to serum. It has been proposed that the enormous excess of superficial O antigen may hinder physically the access of bactericidins to other target antigens such as outer membrane proteins, LPS core sugars, and lipid A (Rowley, 1973), and thus prevent the antigen–antibody reactions that activate the classic pathway. It is also likely that this physical barrier may prevent activated C from reaching the cytoplasmic membrane. In fact there is reason to believe that the O oligosaccharides plus O antibody activate C but resist killing by blocking its penetration to the inner membrane. According to the studies of Reynolds, such resistant organisms became sensitive after incubation in tris buffer because a change occurred in the physical configuration of the

LPS that permitted activated C to penetrate to its membrane target (Reynolds, 1971). This physical barrier would also protect the cytoplasmic membrane after C had been activated through the alternative pathway by LPS in the absence of any bactericidins with specific antibody activity for the surface bacterial antigens.

The neisseria use a different device to escape killing by serum. Gonococci become resistant to killing by normal serum if they have a surface receptor for a blocking antibody. This blocking antibody is present in all human serum and belongs to the IgG class of immunoglobulins (McCutchan *et al.*, 1978). It was discovered when normal human serum was found to block the killing of sensitive gonococci by rabbit serum. Its removal by absorption onto resistant gonococci uncovers the killing power of serum bactericidins in normal serum. Since gonococci invade the blood to produce disseminated gonococcal infection only if they are resistant to killing by bactericidins (Spink and Keefer, 1937), it is clear that the receptor for blocking antibody is an extremely successful bacterial mechanism for interfering with natural resistance.

Meningococci may also have a receptor for an antibody that blocks serum killing, but this blocker is IgA, and its receptor may be the galactose in LPS. The IgA blocker has been found in the acute-phase sera of patients with meningococcal septicaemia or meningitis (Griffis, 1977). Since these acute sera were unable to kill meningococci, it seems that susceptibility to disseminated meningococcal infection may result from blocking the bactericidal IgM by circulating IgA. Thus, both pathogenic neisserial organisms, the gonococcus and meningococcus, use a receptor for blocking antibody to overcome natural bactericidins, the major nonspecific defense against disseminated infection by these organisms.

Entirely different processes are involved in the potential attack by certain bacteria on complement. One of these involves the inactivation of complement by *Proteus* or *Klebsiella* organisms. Their urease splits urea in the kidney and thereby releases ammonia,* which can inactivate complement. Since the normal renal medulla tends to be anticomplementary, *Proteus* infections there would only aggravate a pre-existing condition.

Transferrin

Iron is an essential trace element for bacteria, as it is for all living cells, but in its natural state iron is not available for bacterial use because it forms compounds of extremely low solubility. Bacteria have overcome this problem by developing powerful chelators which are synthesized by the cells under iron-

* Although some argue over whether NH_3 or NH_4OH is anticomplementary in aqueous ammonia solutions, protons transfer rapidly between nitrogen and oxygen atoms that the distinction between NH_3 plus H_2O and NH_4OH is arbitary.

deficient conditions and are excreted into their environment where they can complex and solubilize the available iron. Since iron complexed to a certain ligand may be available only to the species which secretes it, these iron-binding compounds were probably used first to survive the competition between different bacterial species for iron (Rosenberg and Young, 1974). When bacteria became pathogenic they used these chelators to compete for iron in the infected host. The iron carrier produced by all enteric bacteria is enterochelin, a cyclic trimer of 2,3 dehydroxy-*N*-benzoyl-L-serine. Enterochelin solubilizes iron and helps transport it into the cell where iron is released. In Gram positive bacteria other chelating agents are produced for iron transport (Byers, 1974). Mycobacteria, for example, seem to need two chelating agents, one soluble in water, and the other lipophilic. The soluble chelator, salicylic acid, appears to function as an extracellular chelator which brings its iron to the membrane-bound chelator, mycobactin. Mycobactin, which is a hydroxamate soluble in lipid solvents, is the initial receptor of iron for the mycobacterial cell and forms a ferric chelate. The iron is then removed from the chelate by enzymic reduction to ferrous ion, for which the hydroxamate has a low affinity, and releases it into the cell for assimilation.

There is growing evidence that in order for bacteria to be pathogenic, they must possess chelators that can take Fe^{3+} away from transferrin for their own vital processes. This constitutes an attack against a key nonspecific defense system since transferrin can inhibit bacterial growth by keeping the concentration of iron low in the body fluids. When pathogenic organisms first enter an iron-depleted body fluid at the start of infection they can draw upon their own iron stores for initiation of growth. Thereafter they must appropriate the iron from its complex with transferrin and this requires that the bacterial chelators have association constants for Fe^{3+} that are as high as those of the host's iron-binding proteins (Bullen *et al.*, 1974).

In addition to a transfer of iron from transferrin to transport compounds secreted into the body fluids by bacteria, it has also been suggested that bacteria obtain iron when transferrin brings the iron to the bacterial surface. This donation to cells occurs normally when transferrin brings iron to the normoblast surface where it is incorporated into ferritin for subsequent hemoglobin synthesis. It is possible that transferrin might mistake bacterial surfaces for those of normoblasts and release iron to a ferritin-like protein in the outer membrane of bacteria. A more important attack by bacteria on transferrin is a flanking manoeuver that bypasses it. This happens when haemolytic organisms release haemoglobin from red cells during infection. The haem iron can be used by bacteria with no competition by iron-binding proteins of the host because transferrin or lactoferrin can bind only Fe^{3+} and not haem compounds. Haem will stimulate bacterial growth and enhance susceptibility to infection, and sometimes does so more effectively than iron. In experimental gonococcal infections, for example, haem markedly lowers susceptibility to infection in the presence of mucin, but iron has no effect (Corbeil *et al.*, 1979).

On theoretical grounds, it is also possible that bacterial proteases might attack transferrin and release Fe^{3+} by proteolytic destruction of the iron-binding site but there is no evidence to support this possibility (Bullen *et al.*, 1974).

Redox Potential

Bacteria can lower the defensive power of Eh against anaerobes by four mechanisms: (1) Depleting the oxygen supply of tissues; (2) Lowering the pH; (3) Killing tissues; (4) Causing vascular occlusion.

The oxygen supply of tissues is depleted most effectively by facultative bacteria, such as the enteric bacilli, because they can continue to grow even when residual O_2 tension is low enough to create micro-aerophilic conditions. Growth of facultative bacteria such as Group A streptococci can cut the Eh in half, e.g. from 300 mV to 150mV and *E. coli* can lower it to −400 mV when grown in stoppered bottles! Moreover the production of acid by these organisms will lower the pH so that anaerobes will grow at a redox-potential that is too high for their survival at pH 7·0. Mixed infections with streptococci or *E. coli* will thus lower the resistance of tissues by producing abnormal combinations of Eh and pH that allow clostridia to survive and produce tetanus or gas gangrene. *Clostridium perfringens*, for example, will grow at an Eh of 160mV or more if the pH stays in the acid range (6·4–6·8) but cannot grow at 120mV, the normal Eh of living tissues if the normal pH prevails.

Once anaerobes get a foothold and start growing in the tissues they can lower further the Eh by causing thrombosis or killing tissues directly. In either case, the loss of blood supply and, consequently, oxygen supply, and the release of organic acids from dead cells undergoing proteolysis, creates again the simultaneous lowering of Eh and pH that together promote anaerobic infection. The ability of dead tissue to enhance growth of anaerobic bacteria is brought out by the simple observation that chopped meat is a superb anaerobic culture medium. Tissues are killed by the lecithinases of *C. perfringens* and the other gas gangrene clostridia. Thrombosis is especially likely to occur in infections by *Bacteroides fragilis*, perhaps because it elaborates a heparinase (Gesner and Jenkins, 1961).

Fever

Suppression of fever by bacteria which might otherwise be killed by it is most striking in lepromatous leprosy. In this disease delayed hypersensitivity is paralysed not only for *M. leprae* antigens but for other microbial antigens as well (Bullock, 1978). The mechanism for the depression of delayed hypersensitivity (and cell mediated immunity), is not known, but one effect is a loss of the febrile response to the antigens of the infecting organism that is so prominent when patients with tuberculosis, brucellosis, blastomycosis, and other causes of delayed hypersensitivity are given injections of whole cells or antigens of the infecting organism. This absence of fever in lepromatous leprosy probably protects the heat-sensitive cells of *M. leprae* from destruction. The generalized nonspecific anergy in lepromatous leprosy also minimizes the occurrence of fever on exposure to other microbial antigens to which the patient might otherwise be sensitive. In this way the agent of leprosy protects itself not only against the cellular immune response that would destroy it, but also against the broad range of febrile reactions from its own and other microbial antigens that might be harmful to the bacillus. An additional factor for minimizing fever in leprosy might be the failure of the damaged skin to mount the circulatory changes that are needed to raise the body temperature. The generalized reflex vascoconstriction that prevents heat loss in the early stages of fever might very well be impaired because of nerve damage and massive histiocytic infiltration around skin vessels.

CONCLUSIONS

In the past, most thinking about virulence of bacteria has centered around their ability to damage tissues, and less about their facility for eluding defense mechanisms of the host. One reason for this situation is that little was known until lately about the mechanisms of natural resistance, but now that its features are better understood in chemical terms, it is possible to study how pathogenic bacteria deal with them. One of the payoffs from this research is a better insight into how to keep pathogenic bacteria from causing infection. Take the gonococcus, for example: the new information on how serum-resistance occurs makes it clear that vaccines should be prepared only from serum-sensitive strains so that blocking antibody will not be stimulated. Another example is found in anaerobic infections where an appreciation of how aerobic bacteria lower the redox potential calls for drug prophylaxis and therapy against both types of organism. The need for drugs against aerobes, as well, is underscored by the fact that postoperative infections have been found to develop in 71% of surgical patients undergoing abdominal surgery whose wounds contained both aerobes and anaerobes (Kelly, 1980), but only in 22% with anaerobes alone.

One of the most promising developments from applying the new knowledge on bacterial attack on nonspecific defenses comes from work with enterochelin. Rogers *et al.* (1980) postulated that complexes of enterochelin with ions other than Fe^{+} might act as antimetabolites and inhibit bacterial multiplication by interfering with the assimilation of ferric enterochelin. They found that a complex containing scandium was bacteriostatic for *Klebsiella pneumoniae* and a complex with indium increased the generation time. Moreover, the scandum complex of enterochelin was as effective as kanamycin in protecting mice against lethal intraperitoneal *Klebsiella* infections. These exciting results appear to be due to competitive inhibition of ferric enterochelin.

These observations are just the beginning, and further work in the area of nonspecific resistance will continue to produce insights into the practical problems of controlling infectious diseases.

REFERENCES

Barry, D., and Reeve, A. (1977). Increased incidence of gram-negative neonatal sepsis with intramuscular iron administration. *Pediatrics* 60, 908–912.

Bullen, J., Rogers, H., and Griffiths, E. (1974). Bacterial iron metabolism in infection and immunity. In "Microbial Iron Metabolism" (Ed. J. B. Neilands), pp. 518–581. Academic Press, London and New York.

Bullock, W. E. (1978). Leprosy: a model of immunological perturbation in chronic infection. *Journal of Infectious Diseases* 137, 341–354.

Byers, E. R. (1974). Iron transport in gram positive and acid-fast bacilli. *In* "Microbial Iron Metabolism" (Ed. J. B. Neilands), pp. 83–107. Academic Press, London and New York.

DuBois. (1948). "Fever and The Regulation of Body Temperature". Charles C. Thomas, Springfield.

Gesner, B., and Jenkins, S. R. (1961). Production of heparinase by *Bacteroides. Journal of Bacteriology* 81, 595–604.

Götze, O. and Müller-Eberhard, H. (1974). The role of properdin in the alternate pathway of complement activation. *Journal of Experimental Medicine* 139, 44–57.

Griffiss, J. M., and Bertram, M. A. (1977). Immunoepidemiology of meningococcal disease in military recruits II. Blocking of serum bactericidal activity by circulating IgA early in the course of invasive disease. *Journal of Infectious Diseases* 136, 733–739.

Griger, T., and Kluger, M. (1978). Fever and survival: the role of serum iron. *Journal of Physiology (London)* 279, 187–196.

Hanke, M., and Bailey, J. (1945). Oxidation-reduction potential requirements of *C. welchii* and other Clostridia. *Proceedings of the Society for Experimental Biology and Medicine* 59, 163–166.

Kelly, M. J. (1980). Wound infection: a controlled chemical and experimental demonstration of synergy between aerobic (*Escherichia coli*) and anaerobic (*Bacteroides fragilis*) bacteria. *Annals of the Royal College of Surgery England* 62, 52–59.

McCutchan, A., Katzenstein, D., Norquist, D., Chikami, G., Wunderlich, A., and Braude, A. (1978). Role of blocking antibody in disseminated gonococcal infection. *Journal of Immunology* **121**, 1884–1888.

Morrison, D. and Ulevitch, R. (1978). The effects of bacterial endotoxins on host mediation systems: A review. *American Journal of Pathology* **93**, 527–617.

Müller-Eberhard, H. (1977). Chemistry and function of the complement system. *Hospital Practice* **August**, 33–43.

Reynolds, B., and Pruul, H. (1971). Sensitization of complement-resistant smooth gram-negative bacterial strains. *Infection and Immunity* **3**, 365–372.

Rogers, H., Synge, C., and Woods, E. (1980). Antibacterial effect of scandium and indium complexes of Enterochelin on Klebsiella pneumoniae. *Antimicrobial Agents and Chemotherapy* **18**, 63–68.

Rosenberg, H. and Young, I. (1974). Iron Transport in the Enteric Bacteria. *In* "Microbial Iron Metabolism" (Ed. J. B. Neilands), pp. 67–81. Academic Press London and New York.

Rowley, D. (1973). Antibacterial Action of Antibody and Complement. *In* "Bacterial Lipopolysaccharides" (Eds E. Kass and S. Wolff), pp. 162–166. University of Chicago Press, Chicago.

Spink, W., and Keefer, C. (1937). Studies of gonococcal infection. II. The bacteriolytic power of the whole defibrinated blood of patients with gonococcal arthritis. *Journal of Clinical Investigation* **16**, 177–184.

Weinberg, E. (1978). Iron and infection. *Microbiological Reviews* **42**, 45–65.

DISCUSSION

Smith With regard to the gonococcus, you have a stable serum resistance: namely that the organisms retain their resistance on subculture in the laboratory. It is this kind of serum resistance which seems to be mediated by blocking antibody. But there is another type of serum resistance shown by gonococci which both Dr Braude and ourselves, and indeed Alan Glynn at Mary's, have described. It is a phenotypic serum resistance. The gonococci are resistant when they are growing *in vivo* but it is lost on subculture in the laboratory. Could Dr Braude tell us whether or not he thinks the mechanism of this second type of resistance is the same or different from that which he described.

Braude I think there is little doubt that the mechanisms are different. The mechanism of resistance that develops in otherwise serum-sensitive organisms is related to pili. The reason I say this is that it is seen only with type 2 cells and not with the type 4 cells which have no pili.

Mims I should just like to throw out something to stir up a comment on serum resistance. Could I maintain that all antibacterial serum factors are laboratory artefacts and that serum as we usually take it has got nothing to do with the fluid that circulates separately from the blood cells in the animal? It contains all those important substances released from disrupted platelets and white cells and the serum we should be dealing with is the "plasma serum" obtained by separating the cells first and then defibrinating it. I wonder how many of the serum factors so common in bacteriological journals in past years would have to be re-assessed if one did it that way?

Braude I think that I can offer you pretty good evidence that what we see *in vitro* also happens in the patient or in the animal. There are several lines of evidence that I would like to refer to. First of all, one can get exactly the same effect with plasma as with serum, so that the clotting factors that are released are more or less excluded from consideration. Secondly, one can work with purified components, that is with purified immunoglobulins and purified complement components and get exactly the same effect. Thirdly, one can show a very striking correlation between the development of disseminated infections and the presence of serum sensitivity or resistance by the organisms. I referred to one of these, and I think this is a very important example, namely the gonococcus. Among people who have otherwise normal immune systems there is only one exception to the fact that disseminated gonococcal infections occur only with organisms that are resistant to killing by serum. The one exception, and I think that it helps to establish the thesis, is that patients who have congenital deficiencies in C6, 7 and 8 have a curious predisposition to disseminated infections with gonococci or meningococci.

Finally, we made a systematic clinical correlation because we were concerned about this same point; we did not want to waste our time working in this area if it did not mean anything. We made a systematic study of the serum sensitivity and resistance of organisms isolated from the blood of patients. If our premise were correct and yours wrong, then the organisms isolated from the blood should all be serum resistant in contrast to those from other specimens which may or may not be serum resistant. We did, in fact find this. We found that essentially all the Gram negative organisms, the enteric organisms that cause septicaemia were resistant to serum, whereas in the same individual in the urinary tract, for example, we could get a lot of organisms that were sensitive to serum and they never caused bacteraemia. So I think there is a lot of evidence to indicate that the *in vitro* studies on serum killing have clinical significance.

Arbuthnott I should like to support Dr Braude in this, because Dr Gordon Dugan and his colleagues who are working in my department in Trinity College have studied the growth of serum sensitive and serum resistant strains of *E. coli* in chambers implanted in the peritoneum of rabbits which are permeable to host and bacterial factors. They find that serum resistant organisms will grow in the chambers and serum sensitive organisms will not.

Braude We have also done studies on neutropenic animals to eliminate the granulocyte factor and have shown that only serum resistant organisms were able to cause septicaemia.

Jeljaszewicz While the Gram negative story concerning serum resistance seems more or less clear, with some Gram positive bacteria, especially staphylococci, it is quite obscure. For instance, most staphylococci grow easily in normal serum, but there are strains which are inhibited. Why some of them grow and some do not is completely obscure. Some time ago we followed up a claim in the literature that coagulase reverses serum antibacterial activity because it happens that coagulase positive strains grow and coagulase negative strains do not. This proved not to be the case and addition of any protein or even some peptides can reverse serum antistaphylococcal activity.

Braude I am glad you brought up the question of the Gram positives. I did not talk about serum killing of Gram positives because the bactericidin complement system is not involved in the killing of Gram positive organisms. I am not sure that the system that is involved, the β-lysins, is important in resistance to infection in patients or even experimentally.

There are agents that appear in serum that can kill Gram positive organisms and I think the most interesting one was discovered by William Tillett. It is called the "Tillett" factor. I was intrigued with it 30 years ago when it first came out and I have always been disappointed that it has been dropped because it sounds like a very interesting substance. As some of you may remember, he found that patients with acute streptococcal sore throat develop a factor in their serum that could kill Group A streptococci. It was not complement or antibody. He thought this was an important acute phase substance responsible for recovery from streptococcal sore throat before other immune mechanisms could go into operation. I think it is important and it is too bad that nobody has taken it up since Tillett. In his day there were not the very sophisticated biochemical methods that are available now and if someone is interested in what I think is a very important problem, I would urge him to look into the Tillet factor.

Draper What I have to say is definitely to be interpreted as perturbation rather than attack on this matter of fever in leprosy. This is a very nice idea of Dr Braude's, but the fact is that it is not entirely borne out by the observations, which are difficult, mostly because you cannot culture *Mycobacterium leprae*, so you cannot show killing.

I have talked to Dr Stanley Brown, a clinician who worked in leprosy in the days before chemotherapy, which was the only time when the sort of experiment one would want to do could have been done. I asked him whether there was any evidence that diseases which caused fever, from influenza to malaria, did anything to help leprosy, as one might expect if the organism is temperature sensitive. The clinical observations are rather the reverse: by and large any sort of infection tends to make leprosy worse. That does not prove anything: it might be a general effect of debility.

Another point is that heat treatment, I suppose based on the idea that *M. leprae* likes lower temperatures, was actually tried at Carville years ago and was not successful. As far as I can make out, the very drastic treatment that was used from time to time to treat syphilis, namely deliberately producing fever with malaria or endotoxin, never was tried in leprosy. That might have been interesting, if not very ethical.

In fact, it has to be questioned how strong the evidence is that *M. leprae* likes lower temperatures. Though there are suspicious indications from observing where it grows in humans, the footpad infection in mice develops in tropical countries in un-airconditioned animal houses where the temperatures are certainly a good deal higher than the mouse footpads in Mill Hill. In immunologically damaged mice and in *nu/nu* mice ones gets the organism multiplying in the internal organs. I have just been looking at some bone marrow from *nu/nu* mice, where it is clearly multiplying; I think it is unlikely that that tissue is very much below mouse blood temperature.

So, while there are some interesting ideas which should be followed up, I think that the evidence on the whole suggests that the leprosy bacillus really does not care much about the temperature.

Braude If I had heard this before I wrote my talk, I do not think I would have mentioned this theory about fever and leprosy. I am willing to withdraw it.

Peters I think one of the difficulties in analysing the role of specific and nonspecific factors is the lack of, in most instances, a suitable experiment of nature. Where there are experiments of nature, then one or two ideas start to become a little frail, to say the least. For example, the idea of complement activation in the kidney by organisms that have split C4 does not seem to stand up to the admittedly few experiments of nature. So far as I am aware, none of the C3 or C4 deficient subjects have been particularly affected by renal infections. Professor Mims will correct me on this, but I am not sure that any of the *in vitro* work analysing the role of antibody T lymphocytes and NK cells in defence against certain types of virus infections have actually made much greater contribution than observations in patients or animals which are specifically deficient in certain types of immunological defence.

To come on to a more positive suggestion, does anybody know of any examples of particular deficiencies in the various nonimmunologically specific mechanisms—deficiencies in the acute phase response or some other aspects which might be seized upon—which have been shown to produce a generalized or particular type of immunity deficiency?

Braude I referred to one, and I think it is very clear-cut and exciting. This is the deficiency in C6, 7 and 8 that is uniquely associated with disseminated gonococcal and other neisserial infections.

Peters That is a particularly interesting example, because until those deficiencies had been identified in man that role of complement had not been suspected in so far as, for example, C5 deficient mice and C6 deficient rabbits did not seem to be unusually susceptible to infection—at least under laboratory conditions.

Braude One of the reasons it is interesting is because phagocytosis is perfectly normal in these people and therefore bactericidal antibody is the crucial thing for their protection—more than cellular immune mechanisms.

As far as the kidney is concerned, I have always regarded this as an organ that illustrated well the importance of complement in resistance against infection by Gram negative bacteria. The kidney is the only organ I know that is susceptible to infection by Gram negative bacteria in a healthy individual. We see the relatively nonvirulent Gram negatives in the bowel cause disseminated infection in people who have become immunocompromised, but in healthy people infections by them are very rare, except in the gall bladder. But in the kidney this happens all the time. *E. coli* causes practically all pyelonephritis and the reason I have regarded this observation as evidence in favour of the importance of complement is because, as Beeson and Rowley showed, the kidney, to begin with, is anticomplementary. The ammonia generated by normal metabolic activity of the kidney has made kidney slices anticomplementary. It is very easy to demonstrate this. But this is a mild degree of anticomplementary activity. I think it is enough to get *E. coli* started, but usually they are able to recover from it as complement is brought in from the circulation. With *Proteus*, on the other hand, this recovery does not occur. In other words, *Proteus* really goes to town in damaging the kidney. My feeling has been that *Proteus*, in contrast to *E. coli*, not only can gain a foothold because of the primary complement deficiency of the kidney but can actually produce much more severe disease by further inactivating complement through urea breakdown.

Mims To come back to the transferrin story. Is there any evidence that people who have higher than normal levels of circulating iron are more susceptible to infection? If I recall correctly, those with iron-deficiency anaemia and shortage of circulating iron are more susceptible, rather than less susceptible. Would alterations in blood transferrin levels have any effect? I am sure that a patient with kwashiorkor has less circulating transferrin. Is this reflected in increased susceptibilities to bacterial infection or do the patients have too many other host defence defects?

Braude I think that had been a tough question to answer in patients until recently, when reports have been coming out of New Zealand and Australia and several other places which show that the administration of iron intramuscularly to iron-deficient children is associated with a high incidence of intercurrent infections. This was accompanied, of course, by increased iron levels. So the administration of iron to children carries the hazard of increased susceptibility to infection.

Williams May I add an account of what the Murrays found with nomads in Ethiopia who were existing very happily with haemoglobin levels of 8–9 g. They gave one group a large amount of iron to bring their haemoglobins up to 13 g. They had a control group and they managed to produce quite a series of infections in the treated group. These infections were not mild but included disseminated salmenellosis, malaria and tuberculosis. There were quite a few deaths in that treated group. It appears that overloading the transfer system is a good way of producing clinical infection. Furthermore there is a clear association between anaemia and pyelonephritis in pregnancy. This association is made more clear by the administration of large doses of iron which precipitates the pyelonephritis.

The clinical evidence is that the transferrin system is a good defence mechanism, yet in the test tube it seems to be perturbed very easily. The enterochelins of *Klebsiella*, for example, have far more affinity for iron than the transferrin has. Could we hear something about the different mechanisms which different bacteria have for acquiring their iron needs?

Braude I can tell you about some but I do not know whether they apply to your question. I have been interested in the different nature of the chelating substances produced by mycobacteria, for example, as compared with the enteric organisms. Mycobacteria produce two substances that are used for chelating iron. One is soluble and liberated into the fluids and the other is mycobactin. This system is not as effective as enterochelin in capturing iron and transporting it into the cell. There are differences among bacteria and they have different effectiveness. Maybe this explains the phenomenon that you are talking about.

Arbuthnott In Gram negative bacteria, in addition to the enterochelin system, I think I am correct in saying that several cell membrane associated iron binding proteins have now been identified. It is likely that there are several mechanisms by which Gram negative organisms can scavenge iron.

Wilton Did I understand you correctly to say that *E. coli* causes pyelonephritis because the kidney has a natural anticomplementary system such that the normal bactericidal mechanism does not operate there? This to me is further evidence of the importance in resistance to Gram negative infections of the normal bactericidal system involving complement because the one organ that normally inactivates the system—the kidney—is the one organ that gets infected by *E. coli*. The reason I raise the point is that there is a recent paper from a group in New Zealand showing that when they decompelemented mice with cobra venom factor and then induced *E. coli* pyelonephritis, there was no difference in the intensity or progression of the infection nor of the inflammatory infiltrate in the kidney. This was used by them as an argument against complement providing chemotactic factors in these circumstances, but it can also be interpreted in a number of other ways.

Smith With regard to the enterochelins, how do they work? I can understand how a membrane bound iron chelator might be able to do its job. It chelates iron which is then in the membrane and can be transferred to the cell but some of these enterochelins are secreted into the medium to chelate the iron. Why do they go back into the bacteria? I find that mechanism quite intriguing. I do not know whether anyone else has thought about it.

Draper I should like to make a comment about these iron binding compounds which I think is relevant to Professor Smith's question. Bacteria need enterochelin or something like it to get iron—full stop. The reason is that the concentration of ferric iron in an aerobic environment is exceedingly small. I do not know whether transferrin performs the same function for the cells of the host, but clearly there is a competition between the transferrin on the one hand and the enterochelin or mycobacterial factors on the other for an extremely rare substance. Surely the point about putting a soluble iron binding compound out into the medium is that if the bacterium has a specific transport mechanism to get it back in, it has won. Bacteria, on the whole, have not developed a method of getting transferrin in so they put out competing substances.

Wilton May I raise another point which comes back to the earlier discussion? In meningococcal and gonococcal infections there is a strong possibility that there is an antigenaemia of surface structures which is independent of the invading organism. Has any one any information about models where this has been used and where an antigenaemia has been used to try to modify the susceptibility of a host, say by lowering the LD_{50} of an infection?

Braude What you say about meningococcaemia is true. There is both capsular antigen and lipopolysaccharide (LPS) in the circulation. Dr Hoffman demonstrated this very nicely several years ago during an outbreak in San Diego. LPS in sufficient concentration can depress serum complement levels and at the same time lower resistance to infection acutely, as has been well established by a number of investigators. This goes along, I think with the idea that complement is important.

Viral Interference with Nonspecific, Nonphagocytic Defences

C. SWEET

Department of Microbiology,
University of Birmingham,
Birmingham, UK.

Apart from interest in interferon, nonspecific, nonphagocytic host defence against virus infections has received little attention. Furthermore, there have been few investigations of the mechanisms by which virulent viruses, both within and outside infected cells, counteract these defences (Mims, 1972, 1977; Smith, 1972). Here, I summarize these defences and discuss possible mechanisms of resistance to them largely in relation to viruses *per se* rather than to virus-infected cells. Although experiments *in vitro* indicate that infected cells can be destroyed nonspecifically by "natural killer" (NK) cells and by polymorphonuclear (PMN) phagocytes and complement (see later), they appear particularly prone to immunospecific defences (Blanden *et al.*, 1977; Rawls and Tompkins, 1975). Resistance to the latter, like that to phagocytes, is not the subject of this chapter.

NONSPECIFIC DEFENCE MECHANISMS AGAINST VIRUSES

These mechanisms are more effective in adult than young animals and involve humoral, cellular, and environmental factors that are present before infection, or are rapidly induced by it (Mims, 1972, 1977; Smith, 1972). At the beginning of infection and during cell-to-cell transfer, viruses encounter inhibitors or virucidal materials in the tissue fluids. When viruses attack cells, host nucleases may destroy their nucleic acid (Newton, 1970) and interferons may be induced which prevent viral replication. Viral replication induces an inflammatory response and may activate complement (Mims, 1977) and mediators released from damaged tissue cause contraction of vascular endothelial cells with leakage of plasma contents—including virucidal inhibitors and phagocytes—through the resulting gaps. Later, chemotactic factors released from the virus-infected tissue cause active passage of PMN and then mononuclear (MN) phagocytes through the endothelium to the site of infection. Virus–phagocyte interaction can produce more interferon (Finter, 1973) and endogenous pyrogen, the mediator of fever (Bernheim *et al.*, 1979). Inflammatory exudates are generally acidic and this may be antiviral (Mims, 1972). Virus escaping from this primary lodgement site encounters humoral inhibitors as well as PMN and MN phagocytes in the blood and lymph. Also, when virus interacts with fixed MN phagocytes (macrophages) in tissues such as the spleen and liver more interferon and endogenous pyrogen may be released. Although PMN and MN phagocytes form the main nonspecific cellular defence against viruses, lymphocytes may occasionally play a nonspecific role but their main function is in the immune response.

Overcoming these defences depends on the strength of the defences and the viruses' capacities to counteract them. In natural disease, a small infecting dose must increase to a population sufficiently large to cause host damage despite the nonspecific host defence mechanisms that are initially heavily weighted against the few invading virions. Obviously virulent viruses counteract these defences but how they do it and the determinants concerned are largely unknown. There are possibly two reasons for this lack of knowledge. Firstly, it is difficult to determine whether the failure of a virus to replicate in a cell is due to the absence of one or more host cell factors that are required for viral replication, e.g. receptors, or to the presence of factors which destroy the virus or interfere with virion production, e.g. interferon. To distinguish between these two possibilities is an essential step in identifying virion components or virus-induced products of virulent viruses which resist or inactivate host defences. Secondly, few comparisons of the interaction of virulent and attenuated strains with nonspecific defences have been made even though this is a classical approach to investigation of the mechanisms and determinants of virulence.

RESISTANCE TO HUMORAL INHIBITORS

Nonspecific viral inhibitors have been identified in sera, urine and milk of animals and in homogenates of lung and intestinal mucosae (Burrows, 1972). Some, such as the lipid and nonlipid inhibitors of normal sera, inhibit many viruses, while others are fairly specific, e.g. the protein and glycoprotein α, β and δ inhibitors of myxoviruses and the mucoid inhibitors of mumps virus and pneumonia virus of mice (Burrows, 1972). The most studied are the inhibitors of influenza virus which prevent viral attachment to receptors on susceptable cells *in vitro* (Krizanova and Rathova, 1969). Their role in host defence is unclear and little is known of how viruses counteract them. In man, resistance to β inhibitors, which neutralize infectivity, may have allowed Asian strains of influenza virus to infect the lung more readily (Mulder and Hers, 1972). However, although the virulence of influenza virus for mice correlated with resistance to β inhibitors in one study (Briody *et al.*, 1955) it did not in others (Barb and Takatsy, 1972; Hirst, 1947; Raut *et al.*, 1975). If resistance to these inhibitors is important in pathogenicity, then viral neuraminidase could be the virulence determinant since it digests some nonspecific inhibitors.

Although the acid pH of inflammatory exudates may have an adverse effect on some viruses, only rarely has this possibility been investigated, although one group reported that virulent strains of myxoma virus were able to withstand the effect (Ross and Sanders, 1979).

RESISTANCE TO HOST CELL NUCLEASES

Host cell nucleases may be free in the cytoplasm or released into vacuoles by lysosomes (Newton, 1970). Clearly the nucleic acid of viruses that replicate successfully is protected from these nucleases but the mechanisms involved are unclear. The nucleic acid of vaccinia virus remains associated with protein while that of myxoviruses, picornaviruses and reoviruses remains localized to intracellular membranes and these associations may protect the nucleic acids against nuclease attack. Double stranded nucleic acids are not usually degraded by nucleases and this may apply to viruses such as reoviruses (Newton, 1970). Whether modification of nucleic acid with resultant nuclease resistance, evident in some bacteriophages, occurs in viral infections of animal cells is unknown.

DEPRESSION OF COMPLEMENT ACTIVITY

In addition to its role in antibody-dependent lysis of infected cells (Rawls and Tompkins, 1975) complement may act nonspecifically, in the absence of antiviral antibody, to neutralize viruses (Cooper *et al.*, 1976; Bartholomew *et al.*, 1978; Welsh, 1977; Mills and Cooper, 1978) or lyse virus-infected cells (Grewal *et al.*, 1980). During viral infections, complement may be activated by the classical (Welsh, 1977; Mills and Cooper, 1978) or alternate (Hirsch *et al.*, 1980) pathway but the following examples show that the mechanism of its action varies with the virus–host system. Neutralization of vesicular stomatitis virus occurred when complement was activated following attachment of the C1 component to viral glycoprotein; deposition of complement components on the virion probably masked surface components important for infectivity (Mills and Cooper, 1978). Complement inactivation of lymphocytic choriomeningitis virus required natural antibody to normal host cell components incorporated in the viral envelope (Welsh, 1977). Complement may enhance nonspecific killing by phagocytes since mice decomplemented with cobra venom factor showed impaired clearance of virulent and avirulent strains of Sindbis virus from the bloodstream in the absence of antiviral antibody (Hirsch *et al.*, 1980) and PMN phagocytes were cytotoxic for herpes virus-infected cells in the presence of complement (Grewal *et al.*, 1980).

Virulent viruses, or cells infected with them, might fail to activate complement or depress its activity. Although depressed complement levels have been found in dengue haemorrhagic fever and acute viral infectious hepatitis (Minta and Movat, 1979), the mechanisms and virion components concerned are unknown.

INHIBITION OF INTERFERON

Tests *in vitro* show that glycoprotein interferons are induced by virus-infected cells and that they prevent viral replication in further cells (Finter, 1973). Originally interferon was regarded as a single entity but it is now recognized that this is not so (Borden, 1979). Three human interferons have been characterized: two type I interferons produced by leukocytes or fibroblasts respectively, and type II "immune" interferon produced by T lymphocytes (Borden, 1979). These interferons can be distinguished by physicochemical and antigenic criteria. For example, antisera to leukocyte and fibroblast interferons do not neutralize the biological activity of type II interferon and the latter, unlike leukocyte and fibroblast interferons, is labile at pH 2. All three interferons have similar biological properties but type I interferons are more potent antiviral agents while type II interferon is more active as an immunomodulator (see later). Here, I have considered interferon as one entity since all interferons are antiviral and because most of the information was obtained before separate interferons were characterized.

Interferon is produced in virus-infected animals. It has been demonstrated in rabbit skin after infection with vaccinia virus, in the throat washings of patients with influenza and in mouse brain following infection with togavirus (Fenner *et al.*, 1974). Often there is a temporal association between the presence of virus and interferon in different tissues but this is not proof of protection *in vivo* (Gresser *et al.*, 1976a). In influenza of man the quantities of interferon are usually related directly to the degree of replication and the severity of illness (Douglas, 1975). Nevertheless, in some cases interferon is protective. Administration of interferon protected animals against viral infection (Finter, 1973) and anti-interferon immunoglobulin enhanced infections of mice with encephalomyocarditis virus (Gresser *et al.*, 1976a), herpes simplex virus, Maloney sarcoma virus, vesicular stomatitis virus and Newcastle disease virus (Gresser *et al.*, 1976b).

The mechanism by which interferon exerts its antiviral effects *in vivo* is not entirely clear since human interferon, which does not protect monkey cells against vaccinia virus infection *in vitro*, did so *in vivo* (Schellekens *et al.*, 1979). Thus, interferon may not only exert its protective effect by acting directly on infected cells but also through its effects on the immune system, for example, interferon can markedly augment the cytotoxicity of T and NK lymphocytes for appropriate target cells (Borden, 1979; Trinchieri and Santoli, 1978; Zarling *et al.*, 1979).

Viral species and strains within species differ both in the amount of interferon they induce and in their susceptibility to it. In some cases, virulent strains induce less interferon, or are more resistant to it, than attenuated strains suggesting that ability to counteract interferon is important in virulence. In other cases the reverse is true (Finter, 1973; Holland, 1964). However, a strict correlation would not be expected because of the multifactorial nature of virulence. Interferon certainly contributes to host defence against some diseases and a capacity to reduce its production or to resist its action would be advantageous to an invading virus. How could this be achieved?

Early inhibition of host cell mRNA and protein syntheses, as occurs with enteroviruses, may depress interferon production. In experiments *in vitro*, "persistent fractions" of the viral population are often detected which can replicate despite the presence of interferon. The reason for their refractory nature is unknown but such fractions may be important *in vivo* (Finter, 1973). Also, cells infected with vaccinia virus, herpes simplex virus, echovirus or vesicular stomatitis virus at a level greater than one infectious particle/cell were not protected by interferon (Stitz and Schellekens, 1980). The mechanism of viral resistance is unknown but this type of resistance may occur *in vivo* if a local viral population becomes high. Virus-induced interferon antagonists—termed stimulons, enhancers and anti-interferons—have been reported in tissue culture and in infected tissue (Smith, 1972; Mims, 1972). For example, substances of this nature have been detected in the serum of mice infected with encephalomyocarditis virus, Semliki Forest virus, influenza virus, herpes simplex virus type 2 and murine cytomegalovirus (Stringfellow *et al.*, 1977). The nature of these antagonists is unknown. Whether they are virulence determinants is uncertain because substances with similar properties have been found in uninfected tissue (Mims, 1972). Recently, prostaglandins, which could be induced by viruses at inflammatory sites, have been reported to inhibit interferon activity (Trofatter and Daniels, 1980).

INHIBITION OF LYMPHOCYTE FUNCTION

Some viruses such as influenza and coxsackie virus are inactivated nonspecifically by lymphocytes while others, such as herpes simplex virus, vesicular stomatitis virus, yellow fever virus, echovirus, vaccinia virus, ectromelia virus and adenovirus, replicate in lymphocytes (Mims, 1972).

At present we are ignorant of the viral products or mechanisms which determine inactivation, survival or replication in lymphocytes. A virion component may promote intracellular survival and replication of its own virion nucleic acid by directly interfering with cellular inhibitors. However, survival of the invading population of virions may be due to overall inhibition of lymphocyte function by preliminary infection with virions which may or may not replicate fully. Several viruses are cytotoxic for lymphocytes (Smith, 1972; Woodruff and Woodruff, 1975); this may result directly from viral cytopathic effects or indirectly from host components arising as a response to infection. An immunoglobulin-like factor, toxic for lymphocytes, was present in sera from patients with a variety of viral infections (Woodruff and Woodruff, 1975). However, we need to learn more about the biochemical basis of viral cytotoxicity to recognize the determinants of survival and replication of some viruses in lymphocytes.

RESISTANCE OF VIRUS-INFECTED CELLS TO NK CELLS

NK cells, first recognized when normal spleen cells of some strains of mice were found to be cytotoxic *in vitro* for neoplastic cells (Kiessling *et al.*, 1975), are cytotoxic for virus-infected cells without the need for previous sensitization or antibody (Anderson, 1978; Santoli *et al.*, 1978; Fujimiya *et al.*, 1978; Morahan *et al.*, 1980). They are lymphocytes of T cell lineage (Bloom, 1980) but they are not histocompatability (H-2 or HLA) restricted and most, but not all, carry Fc receptors while some carry C3 receptors as well (Blazar *et al.*, 1980). It may well be that NK cell activity is mediated by more than one cell type in different systems.

These cells probably operate *in vivo* as another nonspecific mechanism against viral infection since in some mouse strains resistance and susceptibility to herpes simplex type 1 infection was related to the numbers of NK cells and in human patients suffering from severe herpes infections, antibody levels were not depleted but the number of NK cells were significantly lower than in normal subjects or individuals infected with other viruses (Ching and Lopez, 1979).

How NK cells recognize and kill infected cells and whether host cells infected with virulent strains survive better against them than cells infected with attenuated strains is unknown. However, some viruses kill T lymphocytes (see above) and such cytotoxic T cells circulating in blood and lymph may be directed away from infected cells to be phagocytosed and destroyed by liver macrophages (Woodruff and Woodruff, 1975). If similar effects occurred with NK cells, this could explain the decrease in numbers of NK cells observed in some viral infections. Also, since interferon is a mediator of NK cell activity, a capacity to reduce interferon production or activity could be an important mechanism for depressing NK cell activity.

RESISTANCE TO PYREXIAL TEMPERATURES

Small variations in temperature affect viral replication *in vitro* and viral virulence *in vivo* (Mims, 1972; Fenner *et al.*, 1974). The temperatures of the upper respiratory tract and the extremities are significantly lower than those of internal organs and these differences influence viral behaviour. Thus, the optimal temperature for growth of rhinoviruses is 33 °C and this explains to some extent their localization in the upper respiratory tract (Mims, 1977). Similarly, changes in temperature may occur in normally favourable environments as the result of fever. Based on work with strains of poliovirus differing in neurovirulence for primates, Lwoff (1959, 1969) suggested that fever was a host defence mechanism against viral infections and that differences in virulence between strains might relate to a greater capacity of virulent strains to replicate at pyrexial temperatures. When animals infected with Sindbis, vaccinia, ectromelia, coxsackie B and other viruses were kept at elevated environmental temperatures, viral infection was reduced compared to that at normal temperatures, especially for attenuated strains (Fenner *et al.*, 1974; Roberts, 1979). Thus, fever could be a host defence mechanism but there are few experimental data to relate causally fever and cessation of viral growth *in vivo*. However, reduction of fever with drugs in vaccinia-induced pneumonia of rabbits enhanced virus production in the lungs and increased the percentage mortality (Kirn *et al.*, 1966). Furthermore, investigations into differences in virulence for ferrets of two clones of a recombinant influenza virus showed, for both clones, significant correlations between rise in rectal temperatures and subsequent reduction of viral titres in nasal washes (Sweet and Smith, 1980; Sweet *et al.*, 1980). These effects occurred earlier for the attenuated clone than for the virulent clone and replication of the attenuated clone in organ cultures of nasal turbinates was more restricted than that of the virulent clone at pryexial temperatures. Similar results were obtained with four other strains of differing virulence from the same recombinant series (Matsuyama *et al.*, 1980).

If fever is a host defence mechanism, how do virulent viruses resist it? Lwoff (1969) suggested that the raised temperature inhibited the RNA polymerase activity of attenuated strains of poliovirus and also, with other factors, may have promoted the release of lysosomal nucleases which destroyed the viral nucleic acid. Virulent strains had replicases that worked rapidly at high temperature so that viral replication probably occurred before nucleases were released. Alternatively, proteins other than those of the polymerase complex may have tertiary structures which are relatively thermolabile at elevated temperatures with resultant structural instability and loss of function. Thus, temperature-sensitive mutation in any gene may lead to attenuation (Richman and Murphy, 1979).

In conclusion, while many nonspecific, nonphagocytic defences have been described, little is known of their precise role in host defence against viral infection and even less of the mechanisms and determinants involved.

REFERENCES

Anderson, M. J. (1978). Innate cytotoxicity of CBA mouse spleen cells to Sendai virus-infected L cells. *Infection and Immunity* **20**, 608–612.

Barb, K. and Takatsy, G. (1972). Inhibitor sensitive and inhibitor resistant strains of influenza A_2 virus populations. *Acta Microbiologica Academiae Scientiarum Hungaricae* **19**, 195–205.

Bartholomew, R. M., Esser, A. F. and Müller-Eberhard, H. J. (1978). Lysis of oncornaviruses by human serum. Isolation of the viral complement (C1) receptor and identification as p15E. *Journal of Experimental Medicine* **147**, 844–853.

Bernheim, H. A., Block, L. H. and Atkins, E. (1979). Fever: pathogenesis, pathophysiology, and purpose. *Annals of Internal Medicine* **91**, 261–270.

Blanden, R. V., Pang, T. E. and Dunlop, M. B. C. (1977). T cell recognition of virus-infected cells. *In* "Virus Infection and the Cell Surface". Cell Surface Reviews, pp. 249–290. Vol. 2, North-Holland Oxford.

Blazar, B., Patarroyo, M., Klein, E. and Klein, G. (1980). Increased sensitivity of human lymphoid lines to natural killer cells after induction of the Epstein-Barr viral cycle by superinfection or sodium butyrate. *Journal of Experimental Medicine* **151**, 614–627.

Bloom, B. R. (1980). Interferons and the immune system. *Nature (London)* **280**, 593–595.

Borden, E. C. (1979). Interferons: rationale for clinical trials in neoplastic disease. *Annals of Internal Medicine* **91**, 472–479.

Briody, B. A., Cassel, W. A. and Medill, M. A. (1955). Adaptation of influenza virus to mice. 3. Development of resistance to β inhibitor. *Journal of Immunology* **74**, 41–45.

Burrows, R. (1972). Early stages of virus infection: studies *in vivo* and *in vitro*. *Symposium of the Society for General Microbiology* **22**, 303–332.

Ching, C. and Lopez, C. (1979). Natural killing of herpes simplex virus type 1-infected target cells: normal human responses and influence of antiviral antibody. *Infection and Immunity* **26**, 49–56.

Cooper, N. R., Jensen, F. C., Welsh, R. M. and Oldstone, M. B. A. (1976). Lysis of RNA tumor viruses by human serum: direct antibody-independent triggering of the classical complement pathway. *Journal of Experimental Medicine* **144**, 970–984.

Douglas, R. G. (1975). Influenza in man. *In* "The Influenza Viruses and Influenza", pp. 395–481. Academic Press, London and New York.

Fenner, F., McAuslan, B. R., Mims, C. A., Sambrook, J. and White, D. O. (1974). "The Biology of Animal Viruses". Academic Press, London and New York.

Finter, N. B. (1973). "Interferon and Interferon Inducers". North-Holland, Amsterdam.

Fujimiya, Y., Babiuk, L. H. and Rouse, B. T. (1978). Direct lymphocytotoxicity against herpes simplex virus infected cells. *Canadian Journal of Microbiology* **24**, 1076–1081.

Gresser, I., Tovey, M. G., Bandu, M.-T., Maury, C. and Brouty-Boye, D. (1976a). Role of interferon in the pathogenesis of virus diseases in mice as demonstrated by the use of anti-interferon serum. I. Rapid evolution of encephalomyocarditis virus infection. *Journal of Experimental Medicine* **144**, 1305–1315.

Gresser, I., Tovey, M. G., Maury, C. and Bandu, M.-T. (1976b). Role of interferon in the pathogenesis of virus diseases in mice as demonstrated by the use of anti-interferon serum. II. Studies with *Herpes simplex*, Moloney Sarcoma, Vesicular Stomatitis, Newcastle disease and influenza viruses. *Journal of Experimental Medicine* **144**, 1316–1323.

Grewal, A. S., Rouse, B. T. and Babiuk, L. A. (1980). Mechanisms of recovery from viral infections: destruction of infected cells by neutrophils and complement. *Journal of Immunology* **124**, 312–319.

Hirsch, R. L., Griffin, D. E. and Winkelstein, J. A. (1980). The role of complement in viral infections. II. The clearance of sindbis virus from the bloodstream and central nervous system of mice depleted of complement. *Journal of Infectious Diseases* **141**, 212–217.

Hirst, G. K. (1947). Studies on the mechanism of adaptation of influenza virus to mice. *Journal of Experimental Medicine* **86**, 357–366.

Holland, J. J. (1964). Viruses in animals and in cell culture. *Symposium of the Society for General Microbiology* **14**, 257–86.

Kiessling, R., Klein, E. and Wigzell, H. (1975). "Natural" killer cells in the mouse. I. Cytotoxic cells with specificity for mouse Moloney leukaemia cells. Specificity and distribution according to genotype. *European Journal of Immunology* **5**, 112–117.

Kirn, A., Schieffer, K. and Braunwald, J. (1966). L'Hyperthermie provoquée au cours de l'encéphalite a virus vaccinal de la souris. Mechanisme de son action. *Annales de L'Institut Pasteur* **111**, 645–654.

Krizanova, O. and Rathova, V. (1969). Serum inhibitors of myxoviruses. *Current Topics in Microbiology and Immunology* **47**, 125–151.

Lwoff, A. (1959). Factors influencing the evolution of viral diseases at the cellular level and in the organism. *Bacteriological Reviews* **23**, 109–124.

Lwoff, A. (1969). Death and transfiguration of a problem. *Bacteriological Reviews* **33**, 390–403.

Matsuyama, T., Sweet, C., Collie, M. H. and Smith, H. (1980). Aspects of virulence in ferrets exhibited by influenza virus recombinants of known genetic constitution. *Journal of Infectious Diseases* **141**, 351–361.

Mills, B. J. and Cooper, N. R. (1978). Antibody-independent neutralization of vesicular stomatitis virus by human complement. I. Complement requirements. *Journal of Immunology* **121**, 1549–1557.

Mims, C. A. (1972). Host defences against viruses and the latter's ability to counteract them. *Symposium of the Society of General Microbiology* **22**, 333–358.

Mims, C. A. (1977). "The Pathogenesis of Infectious Disease". Academic Press, London and New York.

Minta, J. O. and Movat, H. Z. (1979). The complement system and inflammation. *Current Topics in Pathology* **68**, 135–178.

Mulder, J. and Hers, J. F. Ph. (1972). "Influenza". Wolters-Noordhoff, Groningen.

Morahan, P. S., Morse, S. S. and McGeorge, M. B. (1980). Macrophage extrinsic antiviral activity during *Herpes simplex* virus infection. *Journal of General Virology* **46**, 291–300.

Newton, A. A. (1970). The requirements of a virus. *Symposium of the Society for General Microbiology* **20**, 323–358.

Raut, S., Hurd, J., Cureton, R. J., Blandford, G. and Heath, R. B. (1975). The pathogenesis of infections of the mouse caused by virulent and avirulent variants of an influenza virus. *Journal of Medical Microbiology* **8**, 127–136.

Rawls, W. E. and Tompkins, W. A. F. (1975). Destruction of virus-infected cells by antibody and complement. *In* "Viral Immunology and Immunopathology", pp. 99–111. Academic Press, London and New York.

Richman, D. D. and Murphy, B. R. (1979). The association of the temperature-sensitive phenotype with viral attenuation in animals and humans: implications for the development and use of live virus vaccines. *Reviews of Infectious Diseases* **1**, 413–433.

Roberts, N. J. (1979). Temperature and host defence. *Microbiological Reviews* 43, 241–259.

Ross, J. and Sanders, M. F. (1979). The effects of temperature and pH variations on plaque production by different virulent types of myxoma virus. *Journal of General Virology* 43, 213–216.

Santoli, D., Trinchieri, G. and Koprowski, H. (1978). Cell-mediated cytotoxicity against virus-infected target cells in humans. II. Interferon induction and activation of natural killer cells. *Journal of Immunology* 121, 532–538.

Schellekens, H., Weimar, W., Cantell, K. and Stitz, L. (1979). Antiviral effect of interferon *in vivo* may be mediated by the host. *Nature* (London) 278, 742.

Smith, H. (1972). Mechanisms of virus pathogenicity. *Bacteriological Reviews* 36, 291–310.

Stitz, L. and Schellekens, H. (1980). Influence of input multiplicity of infection on the antiviral activity of interferon. *Journal of General Virology* 46, 205–210.

Stringfellow, D. A., Kern, E. R., Kelsey, D. K. and Glasgow, L. A. (1977). Suppressed response to interferon induction in mice infected with encephalomyocarditis virus, Semliki Forest virus, influenza A_2 virus, *Herpes virus hominis* type 2, or murine cytomegalovirus. *Journal of Infectious Diseases* 135, 540–551.

Sweet, C., Cavanagh, D., Collie, M. H. and Smith, H. (1980). Fever and the virulence of strains of influenza virus. *In* "Thermoregulatory Mechanisms and their Therapeutic Implications", pp. 113–114. Karger, Basel.

Sweet, C. and Smith, H. (1980). The pathogenicity of influenza virus. *Microbiological Reviews* 44, 303–330.

Trinchieri, G. and Santoli, D. (1978). Anti-viral activity induced by culturing lymphocytes with tumor-derived or virus-transformed cells. Enhancement of human natural killer cell activity by interferon and antagonistic inhibition of susceptibility of target cells to lysis. *Journal of Experimental Medicine* 147, 1314–1333.

Trofatter, K. F. and Daniels, C. A. (1980). Effect of prostaglandins and cyclic adenosine 3′, 5′—monophosphate modulators on *Herpes simplex* virus growth and interferon response in human cells. *Infection and Immunity* 27, 158–167.

Welsh, R. M. (1977). Host cell modification of lymphocytic choriomeningitis virus and Newcastle disease virus altering viral inactivation by human complement. *Journal of Immunology* 118, 348–354.

Woodruff, J. F. and Woodruff, J. J. (1975). The effect of viral infections on the function of the immune system. *In* "Viral Immunology and Immunopathology", pp. 393–418. Academic Press, London and New York.

Zarling, J. M., Eskra, L., Borden, E. C., Horoszewicz, J. and Carter, W. A. (1979). Activation of human natural killer cells cytotoxic for human leukaemia cells by purified interferon. *Journal of Immunology* 123, 63–70.

DISCUSSION

Valdimarsson Can I make a comment on the possible role of complement in nonspecific defence against virus infections? The impression is that patients with primary complement deficiency, including patients who lack C3, are not abnormally susceptible to virus infection. I know there are some animal experiments suggesting that complement may be important in a nonspecific way, but I think the human or clinical experience is contradictory.

Secondly, I think there is evidence that certain viruses do activate complement. It has been demonstrated that C3 activates macrophages, which are certainly directly activated by some of the herpes viruses: for instance the Epstein-Barr virus is certainly capable of doing that.

Sweet Most of the evidence I have presented comes from animal experiments and *in vitro* experiments because we have no experience of what happens in the clinical field. I think the evidence suggests that not only is complement activated by the alternate pathway but it may also be activated by the classical pathway via natural antibody. I agree that the evidence from the clinical side may not support this.

Valdimarsson Measles virus is certainly able to activate complement via the classical pathway in the absence of specific antibody.

van Furth In an indirect way, you questioned complement reductions during viral infection. Where immune complexes fix complement you get a reduction of complement levels in patients. You then have a deficiency of complement. It has been demonstrated that C3 activates macrophages, which are important in defence, so when you have reduced levels of C3 you might also have reduced macrophage activity.

The other point on which I want to comment is interferon which has also been demonstrated to activate macrophages in a rather nonspecific way. With suppression of interferon production this kind of activation may be reduced.

Mims I realize that you are willing to give ground, Dr Sweet, on the fever business, but I thought I should point out that we showed many years ago that animals kept in the cold were more susceptible, not less susceptible, to certain virus infections than animals kept at ordinary temperatures. That was because the animals developed hepatitis and an amount of liver damage which at room temperature was nonlethal, but lethal to the cold animals where metabolic activity was greatly increased. In this instance, this was the mechanism by which cold exacerbated pathogenicity—which only goes to show how difficult the field is.

Anderson I would just like to make one point about the importance of fever. Dr John Oxford has recently isolated several temperature-sensitive mutants from human cases of influenza. I wonder how important fever in the whole body is during infection of the respiratory tract?

Sweet There is certainly a problem in relating pyrexial temperatures to what is happening in the upper respiratory tract. We have tried to measure the temperature in the upper respiratory tract with a thermister probe during fever, but unfortunately with the animal model we have used, the ferret, this has proved difficult. The ferret is not easy to handle and the nose tended to bleed so we are not convinced that we are measuring the temperature of the respiratory tract epithelium.

We have looked at the literature and taken advice from experts in this field. I think the evidence suggests that during inflammation in the upper respiratory tract in man the temperature of the respiratory tissue rises to approach that of the rest of the body. On top of that, if you have a fever then I think this will also be expressed in the upper respiratory tract. So, even for respiratory infections, pyrexia may play some role.

Potter We were concerned that influenza virus strains attenuated for man and laboratory animals had this property because of inability to replicate at relatively high temperatures of the lung and were thus limited to the upper respiratory tract. This is certainly true for all the temperature-sensitive mutants which we have tested. But if one looks at attenuated strains that have been produced by other methods there is not a good correlation between attenuation and temperature sensitivity. Clearly, the question of attenuation for influenza is more complex than a simple parallel with temperature sensitivity.

Mogensen In relation to fever as a host defence mechanism against virus infections, I would like to ask about the possibility that lack of a febrile response or even hypothermia is a cause of increased susceptibility to infection of newborns, especially in premature infants. For instance, neonatal herpes simplex affects a disproportionate number of premature infants who are well known to be poikilothermic and may become hypothermic if precautions are not taken.

Sweet Most of the studies I referred to concerning elevation of body temperature by raising environmental temperature were performed in neonatal or infant animals. The virus infections were lethal for these animals unless the body temperature was raised artificially when the animals recovered. I think the lower temperatures of these animals or their inability to respond with pyrexia may be important in the increased susceptibility of these young animals. It may be pertinent that neonatal ferrets, unlike adult ferrets, die from influenza infection. Although this is probably due to increased lower respiratory tract infection, it is possible that the lower body temperature of these animals may also play a part.

Mogensen In our laboratory it has been shown by Teisner and Haahr that neonatal mice, which are susceptible to coxsackie virus infection, can be protected not by being made hyperthermic but simply by raising their body temperature, which is around 32–35 °C, by putting them with their mothers in an incubator. So, just elevating the temperature to normal reduces mortality.

Beale I have one comment and one question. The comment is about interferon. You referred to three types of interferon. We have recently had evidence from aminoacid sequence analysis, done by Dr Allan and Dr Fantis in our laboratory, of the existence of at least five different types of leukocyte interferon and probably seven, and the genetic manipulators are putting the number at at least nine and maybe more. This could be of considerable importance. These different leukocyte interferons have different aminoacid sequences; they also have different biological activities, at least as shown by their relative antiviral effects on bovine and human cells. Obviously there is scope for looking at their biological activity in other systems.

The question relates to delayed type hypersensitivity and its suppression in virus infections, particularly in influenza. Dr Liew and Dr Russell, working in our laboratory, have shown that there is specific suppression of delayed type hypersensitivity in mice infected with influenza virus. Would anyone comment on the role of delayed type hypersensitivity in defence against influenza?

Potter We were concerned some two years ago with the possibility that cellular immune responses to influenza virus infection may contribute to protection against subsequent disease. To test this, we studied a group of volunteers to measure several parameters of cell-mediated immunity to influenza virus. Infection occurred in many of the volunteers and a variety of cellular immune responses occurred, including the development of macrophage inhibiting factor to virus antigen and delayed hypersensitivity reactions to skin tests. We tried to correlate the ability to infect the volunteers with the presence of cell-mediated immune reactions to the inoculated virus but could find no consistent correlation at all. Our conclusions were that many of these cell-mediated responses are epiphenomenal; they occur, but do not make a significant contribution to protection against disease.

Valdimarsson I think we have to draw a distinction here between protection and eradication. I think the evidence is that cell-mediated mechanisms are important in eradicating established infections by many viruses, but not in preventing the infections.

I want also to comment on the question whether viruses can actually destroy or affect lymphocytes *in vivo*. I think the evidence here in relation to measles is quite good. It is well known that measles infection depresses cell-mediated immunity for many weeks, but a few years ago Professor White's group in Glasgow provided fairly conclusive evidence that this is, at least in part, due to the fact that the infection causes a massive destruction of thymic lymphocytes. In the thymus of children who died accidentally shortly after measles they found autopsy evidence of massive destruction of lymphocytes and characteristic measles cytopathic effects.

Smith May I underline and ask again one of the questions that Dr Sweet asked? We have heard an enormous amount about interferon for many years and are now hearing more and more. In fact, in many viral infections the virulent organism grows quite happily despite the fact that there is a lot of interferon around. Has anyone any ideas as to why and how that happens?

Anderson I would not pretend for a moment to answer the whole of that question but one phenomenon that might bear thinking about concerns natural killer (NK) cells. As Dr Sweet said, interferon activates NK cells or stimulates them to greater activity, but it should also be remembered that interferon protects the potential target cells from the action of NK cells, so in one sense interferon can be seen as a mechanism which the virus uses to protect itself against the host.

Potter I would like to confirm the complexity of this problem. NK cells do not lyse all lymphoma target cells, but they will lyse some insensitive target cells after infection with herpes simplex virus: this is not a general phenomenon, since lymphoma cells infected with other viruses are not lysed by NK cells. Activity is stimulated by interferon but the interaction of NK cells, virus-infected target cells and interferon has not been worked out. This is a very complicated system.

Stuart-Harris We would all agree with that. I wanted to ask Dr Beale a question on multiplicity of interferons. Does this in any way relate to molecular size of the interferon? One of the early problems was that everybody who tried to measure the size of interferon molecules came up with a different answer.

Beale As you say, there is a lot of old evidence of heterogeneity amongst interferon, especially in relation to the isoelectric points of different sorts of interferon. But the molecular weight of interferon really falls into two peaks of activity: one at around 18 molecular weight and the other around 22, but there are also dimers of interferon that appear to give much higher molecular weights.

Mims I think some of the best evidence that interferon really is doing something is the occasionally dramatic effect that you get in experimental animals from the administration of anti-interferon serum. Having said that, interferon has many aspects: it will protect a cell to a greater or lesser extent from infection to a degree which varies from one virus to another and may be related to pathogenicity, but it also is an immunoregulator. This is very important and may contribute to its antiviral activities. Then, of course, we have its influence on NK cells. So it is complex not only in its molecular species but also in its mode of action.

Beale A lot of other materials come out of leucocytes when they have been stimulated to produce interferon. Until we have pure interferons we shall not really know what their biological activities are. A lot of activity may be due to other factors released from leukocytes.

Arbuthnott As a nonvirologist, can I ask a possibly naïve question? If we are going to produce interferon in large amounts, perhaps by recombinant DNA techniques, which interferon amongst so many will we choose?

Beale At the moment we are making interferon at Wellcome from lymphoblastoid cells, which make a mixture of all the varieties. Whether that is going to prove in the long term to be the best I do not think we yet know.

Mims Can I take the discussion in a totally different direction? When I read Dr Sweet's account I thought "Well, surely I can think of some more things than this", and one of the things that occurred to me was that viruses need to attach to cells to infect them and yet the plasma membrane of a cell is normally a very good barrier to virus entry. I would like to suggest that viruses may have exploited the presence of certain substances on the plasma membrane which are there for quite different purposes—maybe they are receptors for hormones or substances involved in transport or in the control of morphology and the virus has "engineered" its surface structure so that it specifically combines with those cell surface factors which now we call receptors. There are large numbers of virus "receptors" on cells and work on HeLa cells has shown that they fall into at least four classes. Receptors of one class, for instance, will mediate the attachment of certain types of rhinovirus or an adenovirus. These receptors are not put there in large numbers for the benefit of the virus, but whatever their function the virus has exploited their presence to attach itself to the cell and get in.

Valdimarsson May I follow this up? A few years ago we were studying binding sites on human lymphocytes for measles virus and subsequently extended the investigation to several other animal species. Broadly, we found that animals susceptible to infection with measles or measles-related viruses had binding sites on the lymphocytes for measles virus, whilst animals who did not suffer from any known measles or measles-related diseases did not. I think that perhaps shows the possible importance of these mechanisms.

Stuart-Harris As far as I recall, Professor Mims, there are not many examples of destruction of a receptor interfering with the penetration of virus particles, but one is the effect of receptor destruction by neuraminidase on infection with influenza virus. That was part of Burnett's original work, was it not?

Mims This is the classical example where a specific substance, *N*-acetyl neuraminic acid, is necessary for binding. It was a well-defined classic case, but since then people have given the name "receptor" to other types of binding substances which often are not quite so specific or so well characterized. I would like to refer to an interesting recent observation from the USA of viruses "using" naturally occurring cell surface components. In this work evidence was produced that H-2 antigens on cells of the mouse acted as the receptor for one of the arthropod-borne viruses. This does not seem to have held up too well recently because H-2 deficient cells adsorb the virus, but it is an example of a substance on the plasma membrane which might be utilized for attachment by the virus as if it were its own special receptor.

Microbial Interference with Inflammation and Phagocyte Function

J. M. A. WILTON

Department of Oral Immunology and Microbiology,
Guy's Hospital Medical and Dental Schools,
London, UK.

In this review of the effects of microbes and their products upon the inflammatory response, I shall attempt to examine one particular aspect of the cellular responses of inflammation, the phagocytic cells. In order to facilitate this, a functional classification of phagocytic cell activity has been used, starting from the formation of the cells in the bone marrow and ending with the killing of the ingested microbe (Table I). Where the information is available both types of phagocytic cell, the polymorphonuclear leukocyte (PMN) and the mononuclear phagocyte (MØ) will be discussed and Table I can be read as though either one or both cell types are involved.

Although the principal aim of this review is to examine those aspects of microbial structure and physiology which are thought ultimately to allow the organism to avoid recognition and subsequent killing by phagocytic cells, it should be remembered that certain microbial products particularly from bacteria may enhance the function of phagocytic cells. The enhancement is not restricted to the inducing microbe but extends to others that may be ingested.

TABLE I.

A functional classification of polymorphonuclear leukocyte (PMN) and mononuclear phagocyte (MØ) activity.

Maturation and release of cells in bone marrow
Adherence to vascular endothelium
Random migration and chemotaxis
Adherence of particles
Phagocytosis
Intracellular killing and digestion
Degranulation

The effect may be directly upon the phagocyte but may also be mediated by other inflammatory cells such as the lymphocyte and upon humoral factors such as complement proteins. Bacterial products can stimulate the phagocytic capacity of both PMN and MØ, may cause enhanced production and extracellular release of lysosomal enzymes and will cause MØ to become activated with enhanced metabolic activity and an increased ability to kill tumour cells.

MATURATION AND RELEASE OF CELLS IN BONE MARROW

To my knowledge there are no microorganisms which depress the maturation of stem cells of either the myeloid or monocyte lines within the bone marrow. The usual consequences of infection are a leukocytosis although some viral diseases may cause a lymphopenia. There will be a discussion later of leukocidins produced by various bacteria but there is no evidence that these substances have any lethal effect on cells whilst they reside in the bone marrow. The documented effects of microbial products on haemopoiesis are mostly concerned with the enhancement of the maturation of PMN and MØ precursor cells with some evidence for a role in the release of mature PMN into the blood. A commensal flora may be important for the proper maturation and release of leukocytes. It is known that specific pathogen free rats and germ free mice have lower peripheral neutrophil counts than conventional animals (Godwin *et al.*, 1964; Boggs *et al.*, 1967). The bone marrow in the mice contained normal numbers of PMN precursors. If the germ free mice were moved to conventional surroundings, the mature bone marrow pool fell rapidly and over the next month the mitotic pool increased. Injection of bacterial lipopolysaccharide into a variety of animal species, including humans, is followed within 4–6 h by a profound peripheral neutropenia. This is caused, not by a toxic effect on the circulating PMN but by an increase in the margination of the cells especially in the lung (Murphy, 1976). One of the factors controlling myelopoiesis is colony stimulating factor (CSF) which will induce progenitor cells to differentiate into mature PMN and monocytes in culture. It is a glycoprotein of mol. wt 45 000 and can be produced by monocytes and MØ by direct stimulation or via the T lymphocyte (Metcalf, 1979). CSF can be induced both *in vivo* and *in vitro* in a number of species including man (Metcalf, 1979). LPS from a number of Gram negative bacteria are able to stimulate monocytes to synthesize and release CSF and both the lipid A and polysaccharide portions of the molecule seem to possess this ability. In the mouse, intravenous injection of *E. coli* K235 LPS, lipid A and a lipid A protein, a polysaccharide from *S. typhimurium* and a peptidoglycan increased the amount of CSF in serum and increased the number of granulocyte precursors in bone marrow (Urbaschek, 1980). Other bacterial substances and products which can initiate CSF production include a lipoprotein and murein from *E. coli* (Staber, 1979).

ADHERENCE TO VASCULAR ENDOTHELIUM

The adherence to vascular endothelium and the emigration of phagocytes between the endothelial cells and into the tissues is essential for an intact and successful immune response. Little is known about this process for the monocytes but we now have an understanding of the process for the PMN. Up to one half of the intravascular pool of PMN are marginated in venules and capillaries and this number increases markedly during inflammation. The adherence of human PMN to nylon wool has been shown to correlate with the adherence to endothelial cell monolayers. Using the nylon wool model, it has been shown that a major determinant of enhanced granulocyte adherence is the binding to the PMN surface of C5a which can be activated in a number of ways for example by zymosan and LPS. Binding of C5a to the PMN surfaces also causes aggregation of the PMN and inhibition of the random migration of the cells due to increased adhesiveness (Gallin, 1980). There does not appear to be any published evidence for bacterial or viral inhibition of phagocyte adherence and studies of such interactions have shown that adhesion is enhanced. LPS causes increased adhesiveness and spreading of monocytes and MØ *in vitro* (Leonard and Skehel, 1980), and *E. coli* LPS and *Staphylococcus pyogenes* culture filtrate have been shown to enhance human neutrophil adhesion to plastic surfaces, both as a direct effect and also mediated by serum components, probably complement (Spagnuolo and Ellner, 1980). Live BCG and water soluble extracts from BCG and *Mycobacterium smegmatis* are also reported to enhance spreading and adherence of peritoneal MØ after injection into mice (Bruley-Rosset *et al.*, 1976). LPS will cause neutropenia after injection into many mammalian species and this is not a toxic effect but is apparently due to increased margination of PMN in capillaries (Morrison and Ulevich, 1978). The neutropenia is followed by a leukocytosis due to increased production of a granulocyte releasing factor which should be distinguished from the CSF already discussed.

The ability of bacteria to suppress the critical early events, for example vascular permeability, in inflammation would confer virulence to the pathogen but there are few studies regarding this process. *Staphylococcus pyogenes* produced a factor which inhibited the initial inflammatory response (Agarwal, 1967). Staphylococci containing this factor suppressed the oedema of the inflammatory response induced by cotton dust and it was later shown by Hill (1968) that mucopeptide and protein from virulent strains would enhance the lesions produced by small doses of virulent staphylococci by inhibiting oedema. The factor was resistant to periodate, trypsin and heating to 100 °C for 10 min but destroyed by lysozyme (muramidase) suggesting that the principal activity resided with the mucopeptide moiety. (Hill, 1969). It is possible that other bacterial or viral products exist which inhibit phagocyte adherence and/or inflammation. Whether the increased adherence of PMN induced by bacterial products is relevant *in vivo* and affects cells within the vessel remains to be determined. The importance of such enhancing factors might be manifest in the tissues by inhibiting the motility of the phagocytes and allowing the accumulation of a sufficient number of competent cells.

CHEMOTAXIS

Chemotaxis is the reaction by which the *direction* of locomotion of phagocytes is determined by substances in their environment. Chemokinesis is the reaction by which the *speed* or *frequency* of locomotion and for the frequency and magnitude of *turning* or orientation of randomly motile cells is determined by environmental factors. Both are examples of directional locomotion with a preference for or avoidance of a particular direction (Keller *et al.*, 1977). There are three recent reviews of leukocyte chemotaxis (Gallin and Wolff, 1975; Klebanoff and Clark, 1978, Wilkinson and Lackie, 1979) and these should be consulted for fuller details than are possible in this review.

A chemotaxin is a substance which promotes chemotaxis without other mediators whilst a chemotaxinogen is a substance which induces the production of a chemotaxin from another biological system for example the complement cascade or the clotting sequence.

The principal chemotaxins in inflammation appear to be derived from the activation of complement and the most important of these is C5a or more precisely C5a des arg which is derived from C5a by a carboxypeptidase B in serum. C3 fragments cleaved during complement activation are not chemotactic but cleavage fragments of C3 obtained by treatment with plasmin and other proteases are chemotactic. Other chemotaxins from serum include fibrinopeptide B, prekalleikrein, prostaglandin E, and fragments of IgG obtained after digestion with a PMN protease. Most of the studies in chemotaxis have been performed with PMN and these cells have receptors for known chemotaxins such as C5a and C3 fragments—presumably receptors also exist for other chemotaxins. Monocytes and MØ are also attracted by C5a. Cells responding to a chemotaxin are refractory to addition of a different chemotaxin and also become more adherent, both to surfaces and to each other. Cells treated with chemotaxin C5a may be damaged (Issekutz *et al.*, 1980) and their phagocytic capacity is reduced (Musson and Becker, 1976). Lysosomes and lysosomal enzymes can be released from C5a stimulated PMN. *In vivo* fewer PMN and MØ are attracted to an inflammatory stimulus if mice are deficient in C5 (Snyderman *et al.*, 1971) and infusion of chemotactic factors causes neutropenia in rabbits (O'Flaherty *et al.*, 1977).

Bacterial Chemotaxins

Bacteria can produce chemotaxins which are able to cause the directed migration of both PMN and MØ *in vitro* without the mediation of host components. Many bacterial species appear to be capable of producing PMN chemotaxins (Harris, 1954) but there do not appear to be many studies relating to the MØ. Culture filtrates from *Staph. epidermidis* and *E. coli* contained chemotaxins for rabbit PMN and active growth of these organisms was necessary to produce the factors (Keller and Sorkin, 1967). Culture filtrates from a variety of bacteria including pneumococci, staphylococci, streptococci and Gram negative organisms were chemotactic for PMN (Ward *et al.*, 1968). It is of interest that an avirulent tubercle bacillus and meningococci produced little or no activity. The molecular weight of the products ranges from 150–1500 for *E. coli* PMN chemotaxin (Schiffman *et al.*, 1975) to 3600 for pneumococci and a *Proteus* sp. (Ward *et al.*, 1968). The exact nature of these substances is not known but *E. coli* produced a lipid which attracted both PMN and MØ and lipid–protein complexes which attracted MØ only (Tainer *et al.*, 1975). A group D streptococcus produced a chemotaxin for human PMN (Spagnuolo and Ellner, 1980). Teleologically speaking, for bacteria to produce substances which attract phagocytes to the site of invasion would appear to ensure that their own survival would be impaired. It is possible, however, that *in vivo* these moieties are either not produced at all or are produced in insufficient quantity to be active.

Bacterial Inhibition of Chemotaxis

Cell wall mucopeptide from virulent staphylococci was inhibitory to PMN migration *in vitro* (Weksler and Hill, 1969) and this activity differed from the oedema-inhibiting properties of mucopeptide from the same organism, being less susceptible to lysozyme treatment. (Hill, 1969) *Clostridium perfringens* θ toxins will inhibit chemotaxis of human PMN but neither phospholipase C or sphingomyelinase C had any effect on PMN; both, however, inhibited monocyte migration which was not affected by θ toxin (Wilkinson, 1975). Streptolysin O and streptolysin S inhibited the *in vitro* migration of human, baboon, rabbit and sheep PMN (Van Epps and Andersen, 1974). *Pseudomonas aeruginosa* produced an inhibitor of rabbit PMN chemotaxis which was not exotoxin A but another protein of mol. wt 65 000 which was inactivated by heat and proteolytic enzymes (Nonoyama *et al.*, 1979). Patients with acute bacterial infection show decreased directional locomotion and random migration of PMN (Althaus *et al.*, 1980) but the mechanism for this is not known. Neutrophils from patients with influenza and herpes simplex virus infections have a decreased chemotactic ability (Rabson *et al.*, 1977).

Bacterial Chemotaxinogens

There are a number of bacterial constituents which are capable of activating the alternative pathway of complement in the absence of antibody. The most studied has been LPS and many Gram negative species have been shown to possess LPS with this property (Morrison and Ulevich, 1978). The activity resides in the lipid A portion of the molecule and there are wide variations in potency between different species and between LPS preparations prepared in different ways. Both PMN and MØ are attracted *in vivo* and *in vitro* (Moeller *et al.*, 1978, Wilton and Almeida, 1980). Other bacterial constituents which activate complement by the alternative pathway include peptidoglycan from *Staph. pyogenes* (Verbrugh *et al.*, 1980) and *Strep. mutans* (Wilton, 1977), and teichoic acid from *Strep. pneumoniae* (Winkelstein *et al.*, 1978). Bacterial cells can also activate this pathway including *Strep. mutans* and *Actinomyces viscosus* (Wilton, 1977).

Although most studies on chemotaxis are performed *in vitro* there is evidence that the complement mediated mechanisms also operate *in vivo*. LPS will cause migration of human PMN into skin windows and skin blisters (Wright and Gallin, 1979) and into the peritoneal cavity of mice (Moeller *et al.*, 1978;

Wilton and Almeida, 1980). There are also experiments where the importance of complement for *in vivo* migration of phagocytes is doubtful. In mice with pyelonephritis due to *E. coli* infection, decomplementation with cobra venom factor revealed no differences between the cellular infiltrates of controls and infected mice (Wilson *et al.*, 1980). The relevance of the bacterial inhibitors of chemotaxis *in vivo* is unclear and more experiments will be needed to clarify the role of these products in the virulence of bacteria. The differences in response also vary with the species studied, and the same chemotaxinogen, casein, can decrease the responses of rabbit PMN and MØ but enhance the response of guinea pig PMN when used at the same dose (Jungi, 1977).

PHAGOCYTOSIS

The ingestion of microorganisms by phagocytes is a critical determinant of resistance to infectious diseases. The mechanisms of phagocytosis will be outlined here and the reader is referred to reviews by Klebanoff and Clark (1978) and Walters and Papadimitrios (1978) for a fuller account of PMN and monocyte MØ phagocytosis. The process can be divided into two stages, attachment and ingestion. The particle to be ingested attaches to the phagocyte surface and this attachment will be affected by a number of factors including the surface charge of the particle, whether it is coated by opsonins and whether the particle is attached to a surface. Bacteria can be phagocytosed if attached to surfaces but free bacteria are less easily phagocytosed. The process is made much more efficient by the attachment to the bacterial surface of the activated third component of complement, C3b, either via the alternative pathway or by activation by immune complexes containing IgG or IgM antibodies. This is because both PMN and MØ from mammals have a receptor for C3b and the Fc portion of IgG. The two receptors are functionally independent and attachment is dependent upon divalent cations such as Ca^{2+} and Mg^{2+}. IgM is opsonic because it can utilize the C3b receptor on human PMN and monocytes but activated immune MØ express a receptor for Fc of IgM. The IgG antibodies can also attach to the phagocyte Fc receptor in the sheep, mouse and guinea pig and enhance phagocytosis in this way. The C3b receptor seems to be most important for the attachment of particles whilst the Fc IgG receptor mediates the internalization. These two receptors are both independent of the receptors for chemotaxins. In the case of the MØ, activation of the cell leads to an increased number of Fc receptors and C3b receptors. Attachment of the particle can be separated from the ingestion process using inhibitors such as cytochalasin B and attachment and phagocytosis is accompanied by lysosomal degranulation. If a particle is too large it is not phagocytosed but phagocytes will attach to the surface and discharge their enzymes.

The evasion of phagocytosis appears to be the principle method by which bacteria escape the host defences and these have been reviewed in detail (Glynn, 1972; Smith, 1977). Microorganisms may evade phagocytosis in a number of different ways. They may produce toxins which by killing the cell make phagocytosis impossible. They may fail to adhere to the phagocyte or if adherent, they may resist ingestion. In doing so they may not escape killing since some of the bactericidal mechanisms of the cells, particularly cationic proteins from PMN, are known to operate extracellularly (Weiss *et al.*, 1978).

Toxin Production

Pseudomonas aeruginosa produces a leukotoxin for bovine PMN (Scharman, 1976) and rabbit PMN (Nonoyama *et al.*, 1979). Lipopolysaccharide from *E. coli* is toxic *in vitro* for murine peritoneal macrophages (Shands *et al.*, 1974), guinea pig peritoneal macrophages (Heilman, 1965) and guinea pig monocytes (Weiner and Levanon, 1968). *Actinobacillus actinomycetemcomitans* strains produced a heat labile protein toxin which was toxic for rabbit and human peripheral blood PMN (Baehni *et al.*, 1979), for human inflammatory PMN (Taichman and Wilton, 1981) and for human peripheral blood monocytes (Taichman *et al.*, 1980). M protein from *Strep. pyogenes* is cytotoxic for human PMN (Beachey and Stollerman, 1971). *Fusobacterium nucleatum* produces a leukocidin for PMN (Roberts, 1967). *Staphylococcus pyogenes* produces a leukotoxin which kills both human and rabbit PMN. The toxic activity is dependent upon two proteins, F (mol. wt 32 000) and S (mol. wt 38 000) and entry of the toxin into the PMN is accompanied by swelling and degranulation (Woodin, 1973). Both streptolysins O and S will cause degranulation of murine (Benheimer and Schwartz, 1960) and rabbit PMN (Hirsh *et al.*, 1963).

Antiphagocytic Surface Components

These will be dealt with in some detail later and only an outline of these mechanisms is presented here. Most bacteria which resist phagocytosis are capsulated and the correlation between the resistance to phagocytosis and possession of a capsule is epitomized by *Streptococcus pneumoniae* (Wood, 1960). Fully capsulated *Strep. pneumonia* smooth (S) strains are virulent, noncapsulated (R) strains are avirulent and removal of the capsule permits phagocytosis of S strains. An additional mechanism of antiphagocytic resistance by pneumococci was suggested by Dhingra *et al* (1977) who showed that purified mucopeptide but not purified capsular polysaccharide inhibited phagocytosis by human PMN. Encapsulated *E. Coli* if attached to human and murine MØ by concanavalin A are not phagocytosed in contrast to a noncapsulated mutant. (Horvitz and Silverstein, 1980). The mechanism suggested for this resistance to phagocytosis was the blocking of complement fixation to the microbial surface components, such as LPS, which can activate the alternative complement pathway. Both PMN and MØ failed to ingest and kill capsulated bacteria unless specific IgG antibody and C3 were present. An alternative explanation was postulated by Wilkinson *et al.* (1979a) for the failure of human PMN to phagocytose encapsulated *Staph. pyogenes* (Wilkinson *et al.*, 1979b). They showed that isolated peptidoglycans could activate both complement pathways and be subsequently phagocytosed and that C3b was bound to the surface of whole bacteria. Election microscopy showed, however, that the C3b was subcapsular and it was suggested that it was not available to bind to the C3b receptors of the PMN.

Many *Staph. pyogenes* strains possess a cell wall component, protein A, which combines with the Fc portion of IgG. It has been demonstrated that protein A is antiphagocytic since it interferes with the binding of opsonic antibodies to the Fc receptor of PMN (Forsgren and Quie, 1974). Strains containing protein A are poorly phagocytosed in the presence of IgG compared with protein A deficient strains (Peterson *et al.*, 1977). In contrast, Dossett *et al.* (1969) showed that although two protein A rich strains were poorly phagocytosed, there was no correlation between protein A content and resistence to phagocytosis in another eight strains. Group A streptococci possess two surface components—M protein and a hyaluronic acid capsule—which are antiphagocytic for PMN. (Foley and Wood, 1959; Domingue and Pierce, 1965). Hyaluronic acid has also been incriminated as the mechanism by which *Treponema pallidum* resists phagocytosis (Krause, 1977).

The structure of the LPS on the surface of Gram negative bacteria may influence the susceptibility of the organisms to phagocytosis by PMN. A strain of *Salmonella typhimurium* with a short surface LPS chain was phagocytosed by rabbit PMN in contrast to organisms with longer side chains which were relatively resistant to phagocytosis (Stendahl and Edebo, 1972). *In vivo* and *in vitro* phagocytosis by murine MØ distinguished between two *S. typhimurium* recombinants differing only in the length of the LPS molecule side chains (Valtonen, 1977). The organism with the shorter side chain was phagocytosed more easily and was less virulent.

Other surface components of bacteria which prevent ingestion by phagocytes include the poly-D-glutamic acid of *Bacillus anthracis*, the acid polysaccharide K antigens of *E. coli* (Howard and Glynn, 1971), enterobacterial common antigen (Makela and Mayer, 1976) and the Vi antigen of *Salmonella typhi* (Bhatnagar, 1935). *Yersinia pestis* may also be pathogenic due in part at least to its resistance to phagocytosis by murine PMN but the exact components responsible for this is not known (Burrows, 1955). The adherence of gonococci to PMN is apparently mediated by a trypsin sensitive, leukocyte associated protein, (LA) (King and Swanson, 1978).

Virulent strains of *Neisseria gonorrhoeae* possess pili which may inhibit phagocytosis (Veale *et al.*, 1977). Gonococci of all colonial morphologies whether LA+ or LA− appear to possess a capsule which also could interfere with phagocytosis (James and Swanson, 1977). The pili do not seem to interfere with attachment of type 1 and 2 to human PMN but, although attached, the cells are not phagocytosed (Densen and Mandell, 1978). PMN oxidative metabolism was stimulated by the attachment but primary lysosomal granule release was inhibited. In contrast, type 1 gonococci attachment to human PMN was not accompanied by an increase in oxidative metabolism but type 4 and killed type 2 organisms were stimulatory (Krieger *et al.*, 1980). It was suggested that the differences between this study and that of Densen and Mandell (1978) might be due to the use of a type 2 strain isolated from a patient with a disseminated infection in contrast to strains from localized infections.

Whilst the above examples of bacterial antiphagocytic activity indicate that specific surface structures may function by preventing attachment of the organism to the Fc or C3b receptor on the phagocytes, other more nonspecific mechanisms may also be operative.

The surface charge of the particle to be ingested, for example Gram negative bacteria with enterobacterial common antigen, may cause mutual electrostatic repulsion of the particle and the phagocyte and the increased interfacial tension shown by encapsulated bacteria could also prevent contact of the organism and the phagocyte. (Van Oss and Gilman, 1972). It is important to study intact bacteria as well as their purified components since the effect of the interactions of the components on the behaviour of the organisms may not be revealed by a study of each individual component. Protein A–IgG complexes activate complement (Stalenheim *et al.*, 1973) so that it might be expected that such complexes would bind to the C3b receptors of the phagocytes, yet protein A is antiphagocytic in pure form. Isolated peptidoglycans can activate complement (Verbrugh *et al.*, 1980) but the studies of Wilkinson *et al.* (1979a) have indicated the importance of studying intact bacteria. More studies of this type using other bacteria will be needed to determine the interactions of the different surface components, serum opsonins such as IgG and C3 and the phagocytic cells. Encapsulated bacteria take up less C3 than strains lacking capsules and will resist subsequent phagocytosis (Verbrugh *et al.*, 1979). More experiments are also needed on the role of surface components such as capsular materials which are shed from the organism *in vivo* and which could bind to phagocytic cells (Sutherland, 1972) and interfere with their function. There are certain other points which must be considered when interpreting the results of experiments where phagocytosis is claimed to be depressed or enhanced. Phagocytosis and killing should be measured as independent events. If only killing is measured and found to be low, this may reflect either a decrease in the number of particles ingested or a defect of killing. Phagocytosis may be normal but killing may be depressed as will be discussed in the next section. In addition, the effect of serum opsonin must always be considered before depressed uptake is ascribed to a defect of the cell. *In vivo* clearance studies do not necessarily measure phagocytosis and could also be a measure of the serum sensitivity of the organism or the efficiency of opsonization.

Viral Interference with Phagocytosis

This topic will be covered in detail by Dr Mogensen but a few examples may be cited here. The Armstrong strains of lymphocytic choriomeningitis virus is not taken up by mouse spleen and liver macrophages after intravenous injection (Tosolini and Mims, 1971). Paradoxically this leads to a failure of infection since the virus normally grows in macrophages. Many viruses will grow in macrophages and the ability to grow in these cells is a virulence marker (Mims, 1972). The influenza viruses seem to possess the ability to interfere with phagocytosis of bacteria by MØ. Influenza virus was inhibitory to guinea pig PMN phagocytosis (Fisher and Ginsberg, 1956) and mumps and influenza viruses decreased leukocyte phagocytosis (Merchant and Morgan, 1950; Sawyer, 1969). Infection of PMN *in vitro* with viruses decreases phagocytic capacity but this is difficult to achieve using the MØ. This depression of phagocytosis does not appear to be a result of the infection of the phagocyte by the virus and the mechanisms are not known at present but could include interference with receptor function or the replacement of functional cells with less competent precursors in the case of the MØ.

KILLING AND DEGRADATION

The enzymes of the PMN and MØ thought to be concerned with microbial killing are contained within lysosomes and these fuse with the phagosome, discharging their contents. Human PMN contain two types of granule: the azurophil (primary) granules are large, round and electron-dense containing myeloperoxidase (MPO), neutral proteases, lysozyme and acid hydrolases; the specific (secondary) granules are more numerous, electron-lucent and contain lysozyme and lactoferrin (LF). Further information may be found in the review by Spitznaegel (1977). Monocytes contain a few MPO containing granules which are the equivalent of the secondary granules of PMN. MØ contain no peroxidases but possess numerous electron-dense granules containing acid hydrolases (for review see Nichols and Bainton, 1975). Although there is much known about microbicidal mechanisms in phagocytes the relative importance of these for the PMN and MØ are still the subject of dispute and more information can be obtained from recent reviews. (Goren, 1977; Klebanoff and Clark, 1978; Walters and Papadimitriou, 1978). They may conveniently be divided into oxygen-independent systems and those requiring oxygen such as the MPO mediated generation of H_2O_2 and production of the superoxide anion. The latter system requires cofactors such as iodide and thiocyanate ions and is inhibited by catalase and organisms producing catalase may have enhanced virulence. There are other oxygen dependent microbicidal systems independent of the MPO system which include H_2O_2, superoxide anion and hydroxyl radicals. The oxygen independent processess are primarily composed of acid, lysozyme, unsaturated lactoferrin, and cationic proteins. Although phagocytes have a significantly reduced microbicidal capacity under anaerobic conditions, killing of ingested organisms does still take place. The susceptibility of organisms under these conditions ranges from very resistant to highly susceptible (Mandell, 1974).

There are some differences between PMN and MØ antimicrobial systems. MØ lack lactoferrin although they can take up exogenous lactoferrin, contain much less MPO and do not possess cationic proteins. Other possible mechanisms possessed by MØ include catalase and lipid peroxidation. MØ killing can also be stimulated by the activation of the cell by products of antigen activated T lymphocytes but the microbicidal mechanism is unknown.

Little is known of the breakdown of microbes during and after phagocytosis and such information as exists has been comprehensively reviewed by Elsbach (1980). As he points out, there is little quantitative information regarding the extent of degradation and the persistance of undigested material. Killing may not take place as a result of direct action of microbicidal systems but may also require autolytic enzymes in the case of bacteria. In PMN only partial digestion may occur and it is a matter for speculation whether MØ synergize to kill organisms damaged by PMN. It is conceivable that the longer lived MØ can kill and degrade more efficiently but no evidence exists that the MØ is better equipped than the PMN for killing. Existing methods for answering these questions are not entirely adequate and new techniques will probably have to be devised. Finally, generalizations about microorganisms with widely different surface structures are unwise and it may be that a variety of killing mechanisms and degradation processes exist.

The ingestion of most bacteria and viruses is followed by fusion of both primary and secondary lysosomal granules with the phagosome. Certain bacteria and viruses can avoid this process and thus escape killing within the cell. Viable *Mycobacterium tuberculosis* inhibited the fusion of phagosome and lysosome in murine macrophages (Armstrong and D'Arcy Hart, 1971). This has been attributed to anionic sulphur-containing glycolipids (sulphatides) obtained from virulent strains (Goren *et al.*, 1976). When yeast cells are coated with a sulphatide the normal phagosome–lysosome fusion induced by the yeast fails to occur. Both viable and nonviable *Nocardia asteroides* cells, harvested at different times of culture and ingested by rabbit alveolar macrophages inhibited phagosome–lysosome fusion to varying degrees (Davis-Scibienski and Beaman, 1980). Organisms from the logarithmic phase of growth were most active; viable organisms harvested later were less active but maintained activity even if killed. The bacterial component (s) responsible are not known at present.

Viruses can also interfere with phagosome lysosome fusion but most studies have dealt with indirect effects of this process such as killing of bacteria in an attempt to account for the increased susceptibility to bacterial infection after viral pneumonia. Sendai virus infected mice yield alveolar MØ which fail to degranulate into the phagosome containing *Candida krusei* ingested *in vitro* (Jakab *et al.*, 1980). The defect was most profound seven days after infection and the cells had returned to normal within 21 days but the killing of the yeasts was not measured. Murine alveolar MØ from animals infected with influenza virus had a decreased capacity to kill *Staph. pyogenes* and lysosomes had not discharged into the phagosome but into the cytoplasm (Silverberg *et al.*, 1979).

Preincubation of human PMN with *E. coli* LPS reduced the bactericidal activity of the phagocytes for *E. coli* and *Staph. pyogenes* whilst simultaneously activating nitro blue tetrazolium reduction and hexose monophosphate shunt activity (Proctor, 1979). The mechanism for this is not known but PMN phagocytosis of bacteria was not depressed. Some bacteria can resist the bactericidal effect of lysosomal enzymes even though these are discharged into the phagocytic vacuole. *Mycobacterium lepramurium* survive in phagolysosomes and this may depend on a capsular peptidoglycolipid "mycoside c" and a similar material is produced by *Myco. avium* (Draper and D'Arcy Hart, 1975). Even if *Myco. tuberculosis* is opsonized by specific antibody so that phagosome lysosome fusion occurs, the microorganisms are not killed, presumably due to a resistance confered by components of the cell wall. The resistance mechanisms of the mycobacteria will be dealt with in more detail by Dr Draper.

DEGRANULATION

It is now known that surface stimulation of phagocytes will cause degranulation of lysosomes without the death of the cell. Many stimuli are capable of this phenomenon and the subect has been comprehensively reviewed by Weissman

(1977). Degranulating stimuli include binding of C5a, C3a and C3b, Fc–IgG, Fc–IgA, chemotaxins, and immune complexes or bacteria when bound to surfaces. Bacteria are also able to cause degranulation directly and *Strep. mutans* and *Actinomyces viscosus* are stimulatory in this manner for rabbit PMN (Taichman and McArthur, 1976). Granule release will also occur during phagocytosis and on the death of the cell (Table II).

Specific granules appear to degranulate more readily than azurophil granules. Both granules discharge rapidly (within 5 s) and MPO and LF appear at the complementary surface of human PMN pseudopodia forming a phagosome (Pryzwansky *et al.*, 1979). In this study, surface LF of PMN stimulated with *E. coli* appeared independent of pseudopodia suggesting specific granule extrusion independent of phagocytosis. This selective release of specific granules was also shown by human PMN incubated with Ca^{2+}, adhering to glass or nylon wool, responding to C5a chemotaxin and in PMN which had emigrated into skin windows or blister fluid (Wright and Gallin, 1979).

Although killing of microorganisms can be achieved by PMN and MØ enzymes acting outside the phagolysosome, the principal mechanism appears to be the fusion of the lysosomes of the phagocyte with the phagosome containing the ingested organism (s). Both types of granule appear to be able to exert a microbicidal effect outside the confines of the phagolysosome on a number of bacterial species. In the case of fungi where the organism is too large for ingestion by a single phagocyte, PMN are able to release granule constituents and oxidative metabolites such as H_2O_2 which damage and kill *Candida albicans* pseudohyphae (Diamond *et al.*, 1978). Some strains of *E. coli* and S. *typhimurium* are killed by cationic proteins isolated from rabbit and human PMN (Weiss *et al.*, 1978). Other strains can resist this bactericidal action and resistance is determined by the possession of long chain LPS (Weiss *et al.*, 1980). Virulent gonococci attach to the surfaces of human PMN which then release specific granule enzymes such as lactoferrin but little primary granule release, as assessed by β glucuronidase levels and the myeloperoxidase-mediated iodination of bacterial protein, and are able to resist killing at this site (Densen and Mandell, 1978). Lactoferrin killed *Strep. mutans* and *E. coli* (Arnold *et al.*, 1977) and the MPO–halide–H_2O_2 system will kill bacteria precoated with MPO (Selvaraj *et al.*, 1978).

The apparently selective release of secondary granule enzymes such as lactoferrin and the growth inhibiting effects of cationic proteins, both of which can function extracellularly at least *in vitro*, raises the intriguing possibility that binding of microorganisms to the phagocyte may be sufficient to inhibit or at least slow down the infectious process. Phacocytosis is obviously important in eliminating pathogens but further research is needed to assess the relative importance of intracellular and extracellular killing. Many pathogens must attach to epithelial surfaces to initiate infection and dental caries is dependent upon attachment of *Strep. mutans* to tooth enamel whilst periodontal disease is due to accumulation of bacteria on tooth surfaces adjacent to the gingivae (Wilton and Lehner, 1980). The inhibition of such colonization would be an important defence mechanism and we have recently been investigating the role of PMN and MØ and their enzymes in the modulation of bacterial attachment. It appears that PMN and MØ degranulate on attachment to bacterial films adherent to glass, plastic and human tooth enamel. Phagocytosis was minimal but killing of bacteria is rapid and is often accompanied by detachment of the bacteria from the surface. Dextran was inhibitory to detachment but not to killing and complement and specific IgG antibodies enhanced the release of phagocyte enzymes. Both Gram positive and Gram negative bacteria were equally susceptible to detachment and killing.

It has been speculated that the release of specific and azurophil granules may be triggered by separate intracellular processes (Bentwood and Henson, 1980) since a variety of agents, both soluble and particulate, cause specific granule release before azurophil granule release. It is possible that the selective early release of specific granule enzymes such as lactoferrin would be important for controlling bacterial colonization, both by bactericidal activity and by detaching bacteria adherent to mucosal surfaces. I am presently investigating whether this process would be important for the control of bacterial attachment to oral epithelial cells. It should also be remembered that both types of granules are eventually released (Table II) and that azurophil enzymes could also affect bacterial colonization.

TABLE II.
Induction of enzyme release by phagocytes.

Granules released	Induction process
S/A[a]	During phagocytosis (regurgitation during feeding)
S/A	By attachment to surface bound immune complexes or nonopsonized bacteria
S/A	As a response to membrane binding of Fc–IgG, Fc–IgA, C3b, C5a, chemotaxins and bacteria whether opsonized or not
S	In the presence of physiological concentrations of Ca^{2+}
S	On adherence to surfaces in the presence of Ca^{2+} and during *in vivo* and *in vitro* migration
S/A	On the death of the cell due to lysis from within or without

[a] S, specific granules; A, azurophil granules.

It is hoped that this review has served to identify some of the areas in which current research on the function of phagocytes has progressed and indicated other areas where further research might be fruitful. The ubiquity of LPS and the wide range of biological effects of this material especially those affecting platelets, PMN and MØ either directly or indirectly via the complement system (Morrison and Ullevich, 1978; Morrison and Ryan, 1979) should be remembered when considering the experimental results presented in this review. LPS can contaminate biological products easily and is active in nanogram amounts so that at least some of the processes ascribed to other bacterial and even viral constituents could be due, at least in part, to LPS.

The reader is urged to consult the reviews which have been cited to obtain more comprehensive knowledge than is possible from a review of this nature. I have not dealt with parasites and these have unique mechanisms of avoidance some of which could apply to bacteria for example antigenic mimicry. In conclusion it would be fair to say that we know much about adherence, migration, phagocytosis and killing of microorganisms by phagocytes but understand little about the mechanisms of interference with these processes *in vivo*.

REFERENCES

Agarwal, D. S. (1967). Subcutaneous staphylococcal infection in mice. II. The inflammatory response to different strains of staphylococci and micrococci. *British Journal of Experimental Pathology* **48**, 468–482.

Althaus, D., Keller, U., Hess, M. W. and Cottier, H. (1980). Impaired neutrophil locomotion during acute bacterial infections. *International Archives of Allergy and Applied Immunology* **61**, 321–328.

Armstrong, J. A. and D'Arcy Hart, P. (1971). Response of cultured macrophages to *Mycobacterium tuberculosis* with observations on fusion of lysosomes with phagosomes. *Journal of Experimental Medicine* **134**, 713–740.

Arnold, R. R., Cole, M. F. and McGhee, J. R. (1977). A bactericidal effect for human lactoferrin. *Science* **197**, 263–265.

Baehni, P., Tsai, C. C., McArthur, W. P., Hammond, B. F., and Taichman N. S. (1979). Interaction of inflammatory cells and oral microorganisms VII Detection of leukotoxic activity of a plaque-derived Gram negative microorganism *Infection and Immunity* **24**, 233–243.

Beachey, E. H., and Stollerman, G. H. (1971). Toxic effects of Streptococcal M protein on platelets and polymorphonuclear leucocytes in human blood. *Journal of Experimental Medicine* **134**, 351–365.

Bentwood, B. J. and Henson, P. M. (1980). The sequential release of granule constituents from human neutrophils. *Journal of Immunology* **124**, 855–862.

Bernheimer, A. W. and Schwartz, L. L. (1960). Leucocidal agents of haemolytic streptococci. *Journal of Pathology and Bacteriology* **79**, 39–46.

Bhatriagar, S. S. (1935). Phagocytosis of *B. typhosus* in relation to its antigenic structure and to the antibody components of the sensitising serum. *The British Journal of Experimental Pathology* **16**, 375–384.

Boggs, D. R., Chevenick, P. A., Marsh, C. A., Pilgrim, H. I., Cartwright, G. E. and Wintrobe, R. R. (1967). Granulocytopoeisis in germ-free mice. *Proceedings of the Society for Experimental Biology and Medicine* **125**, 325–330.

Burrows, T. W. (1955). The basis of virulence for mice of *Pasteurella pestis*. *Symposium of the Society for General Microbiology* **5**, 152–175.

Davis-Scibienski, C. and Beaman, B. L. (1980). Interaction of *Nocardia asteroides* with rabbit alveolar macrophages: effect of growth phase and viability on phagosome lysosome fusion. *Infection and Immunity* **29**, 24–29.

Densen, P. and Mandell, G. L. (1978). Gonococcal interaction with polymorphonuclear neutrophils: importance of the phagosome for bactericidal activity. *Journal of Clinical Investigation* **62**, 1161–1171.

Dhingra, R. K., Williams, R. L. Jr and Reed, W. P. (1977). Effects of pneumococcal mucopeptide and capsular polysaccharide on phagocytosis. *Infection and Immunity* **15**, 169–174.

Diamond, R. D., Kriescki, R. and Jao, W. (1978). Damage to pseudohyphal forms of *Candida albicans* by neutrophils in the presence of serum *in vitro*. *Journal of Clinical Investigation* **61**, 349–359.

Domingue, G. J. and Pearce, W. A. Jr (1965). Effect of partially purified Streptococcal M protein on the *in vitro* phagocytosis of *Streptococcus pyogenes*. *Journal of Bacteriology* **89**, 583–588.

Dossett, J. H., Kronvall, G., Williams, R. C. Jr and Quie, P. G. (1969). Antiphagocytic effects of Staphylococcal Protein A. *Journal of Immunology* **103**, 1405–1410.

Draper, P. and D'Arcy Hart, P. (1975). Phagosomes, Lysosomes and Mycobacteria: cellular and microbial aspects. *In* "Mononuclear Phagocytes" (Ed. R. van Furth), pp. 575–589. Blackwell Scientific, Oxford.

Elsbach, P. (1980). Degradation of microorganisms by phagocytic cells. *Reviews of Infectious Diseases* **2**, 106–128.

Van Epps, D. E. and Anderson B. R. (1974). Streptolysin 0 inhibition of neutrophil chemotaxis and mobility: nonimmune phenomenon with species speficity. *Infection and Immunity* **9**, 27–33.

Fisher, T. N. and Ginsberg, H. S. (1956). The reaction of influenza viruses with guinea pig polymorphonuclear leukocytes. III Studies on the mechanisms by which influenza viruses inhibit phagocytosis. *Virology* **2**, 637–655.

Foley, M. J. and Wood, W. B. Jr (1959). Studies on the pathogenicity of group A Streptococci II. The antiphagocytic effects of M protein and the capsular gel. *Journal of Experimental Medicine* **110**, 603–616.

Forsgren, A. and Quie, P. G. (1974). Effects of Staphylococcal protein A on heat labile opsonins. *Journal of Immunology* **121**, 1177–1180.

Gallin, J. I. (1980). Degranulating stimuli decrease the negative surface charge and increase the adhesiveness on human neutrophils. *Journal of Clinical Investigation* **65**, 298–306.

Gallin, J. I. and Wolff, S. M. (1975). Leucocyte chemotaxis: physiological considerations and abnormalities. *Clinics in Haematology* **4**, 567–607.

Glynn, A. A. (1972). Bacterial factors inhibiting host defence mechanisms. *Symposium of the Society for General Microbiology* **22**, 75–112.

Godwin, K. O., Fraser, F. J. and Ibbotson, R. N. (1964). Haematological observations on healthy (SPF) rats. *British Journal of Experimental Pathology* **45**, 514–524.

Goren, M. B. (1977). Phagocyte lysosomes: interactions with infectious agents, phagosomes and experimental perturbations in function. *Annual Review of Microbiology* **31**, 507–533.

Goren, M. B., D'Arcy Hart, P., Young, M. C., and Armstrong, J. A. (1976). Prevention of phagosome lysosome fusion in cultured macrophages by sulfatides of *Mycobacterium tuberculosis*. *Proceedings of the National Academy of Sciences U.S.A.* **73**, 2510–2514.

Harris, H. (1954). Chemotaxins of granulocytes. *Journal of Pathology and Bacteriology* **66**, 135–146.

Heilman, D. H. (1965). The selective toxicity of endotoxin for phagocytic cells of the reticulo-endothelial system. *International Archives of Allergy and Applied Immunology* **26**, 63–79.

Hill, M. J. (1968). A Staphylococcal aggressin. *Journal of Medical Microbiology* **1**, 33–43.

Hill, M. J. (1969). Protection of mice against infection by *Staphylococcus aureus*. *Journal of Medical Microbiology* **2**, 1–7.

Hirsh, J. G., Bernheimer, A. W. and Weismann, G. (1963). Motion picture study of the toxic actions of Streptolysins on leucocytes. *Journal of Experimental Medicine* **118**, 223–227.

Horwitz, M. A. and Silverstein, S. C. (1980). Influence of *Escherichia coli* capsule on complement fixation and on phagocytosis and killing by human phagocytes. *Journal of Clinical Investigation* **65**, 82–94.

Howard, C. J. and Glynn, A. A. (1971). The virulence for mice of strains of *Escherichia coli* related to the effect of K antigens on their resistance to phagocytosis and killing by complement. *Immunology* **20**, 767–777.

Issekutz, A. C., Movat, K. W. and Movat, H. Z. (1980). Enhanced vascular permeability and haemorrhage inducing activity of rabbit C5a des arg: probable role of polymorphonuclear leucocyte lysosomes. *Clinical and Experimental Immunology* **41**, 512–520.

Jakab, G. J., Warr, G. A. and Sannes, P. C. (1980). Alveolar macrophage ingestion and phagosome lysosome fusion; defect associated with virus pneumonia. *Infection and Immunity* **27**, 960–968.

James, J. F. and Swanson, J. (1977). The capsule of the gonococcus. *Journal of Experimental Medicine* **145**, 1082–1086.

Jungi, T. W. (1977). Different concentrations of chemotactic factors can produce attraction or migration inhibition of leukocytes. *International Archives of Allergy and Applied Immunology* **53**, 29–36.

Keller, H. U. and Sorkin, E. (1967). Studies on chemotaxis. V. on the chemotactic effect of bacteria. *International Archives of Allergy and Applied Immunology* **31**, 505–517.

Keller, H. U., Wilkinson, P. C., Abercrombie, M., Becker, Hirsh, J. G., Miller, M. F., Ramsay, W. W. and Zigmond, S. H. (1977). A proposal for the definition of terms related to the locomotion of leukocytes and other cells. *Clinical and Experimental Immunology* 27, 377–380.

King, G. J. and Swanson, J. (1978). Studies on gonococcus infection. XV. Identification of surface proteins of *Neisseria gonorrhoeae* correlated with leukocyte association. *Infection and Immunity* 21, 575–584.

Klebanoff, S. S. and Clark, R. A. (1978). The Neutrophil: Function and Clinical Disorders". Elsevier/North Holland, Amsterdam.

Krause, R. M. (1972). Workshop on the biology of the Treponemes. *Journal of Infectious Diseases* 125, 332–336.

Krieger, A. G., Schiller, N. C. and Roberts, R. B. (1980). Gonococci–Human PMN interactions: Metabolic studies associated with attachment and ingestion. *Infection and Immunity* 28, 991–100.

Leonard, E. J. and Skenel, A. H. (1980). Enhancement of spreading, phagocytosis and chemotaxis by macrophage stimulating protein (MSP). *In* "Advances in Experimental Medicine and Biology" (Eds M. R. Escobar and H. Friedman), vol. 121B, pp. 181–194. Plenum Press, New York.

Makela, P. H. and Mayer, H. (1976). Enterobacterial common antigen. *Bacteriological Reviews* 40, 591–632.

Mandell, G. L. (1974). Bactericidal activity of aerobic and anaerobic polymorphonuclear neutrophils. *Infection and Immunity* 9, 337–341.

Merchant, D. J. and Morgan, H. R. (1950). Inhibition of the phagocytic action of leukocytes by mumps and influenza viruses *Proceedings of the Society for Experimental Medicine and Biology* 74, 651–653.

Metcalf, D. (1979). Production of colony stimulating factors by lymphoid tissues *In* "Biology of the Lymphokines" (Eds S. Cohen, E. Pick and J. J. Oppenheim), pp. 515–540. Academic Press, New York.

Mims, C. A. (1972). Host defences against viruses and the latters ability to counteract them. *Symposium of the Society of General Microbiology* 22, 333–358.

Moeller, G. R., Terry, L. and Snyderman (1978). The inflammatory response and resistance to endotoxin in mice. *Journal of Immunology* 120, 116–123.

Morrison, D. C. and Ryan, J. L. (1979). Bacterial endotoxins and host immune responses *In* "Advances in Immunology" 28, (Eds F. J. Dixon and H. G. Kunkel), pp. 293–450. Academic Press, New York.

Morrison, D. C. and Ulevich, R. J. (1978). The effects of bacterial endotoxins on host mediation systems. *American Journal of Pathology* 93, 527–617.

Murphy, P. (1976). "The Neutrophil". Plenum Publishing, New York.

Musson, R. A. and Becker, E. L. (1976). The inhibitory effect of chemotactic factors on erythrophagocytosis by human neutrophils. *Journal of Immunology* 117, 433–439.

Nichols, B. A. and Bainton, D. F. (1975). Ultrastructure and cytochemistry of mononuclear phagocytes. *In* "Mononuclear Phagocytes" (Ed. R. van Furth), pp. 17–55. Blackwell Scientific, Oxford.

Nomoyama, J., Kojo, H., Mine, Y., Nishida, M., Got, S. and Kuwahara, S. (1979). Inhibitory effect of *Pseudomonas aeruginosa* on the phagocytic and killing activity of rabbit polymorphonuclear leukocytes: Mechanisms of action of a polymorphonuclear leukocyte inhibitor. *Infection and Immunity* 24, 399–403.

O'Flaherty, J. T., Showell, H. J. and Ward, P. A. (1977). Neutropenia induced by systemic infusion of chemotactic factors. *Journal of Immunology* **118**, 1586–1589.

Peterson, P. K., Verhoef, J., Sabath, L. D. and Quie, P. G. (1977). Effect of protein A on Staphylococcal opsonisation. *Infection and Immunity* **15**, 175–179.

Proctor, R. A. (1979). Endotoxin in vitro interactions with human neutrophils: Depression of chemiluminescence, oxygen consumption, superoxide production and killing. *Infection and Immunity* **25**, 912–921.

Pryzwansky, K. B., MacRae, E. K., Spitznaegel, J. K. and Cooney, M. H. (1979). Early degranulation of human neutrophils: Immunocytochemical studies of surface and intracellular phagocytic events. *Cell* **18**, 1025–1033.

Rabson, A. R., Whiting, D. A., Anderson, R., Glover, A. and Koornhof, H. J. (1977). Depressed neutrophil motility in patients with recurrent herpes simplex infections. *In vitro* restoration with Levamisole. *Journal of Infectious Diseases* **135**, 113.

Roberts, D. S. (1967). The pathogenic synergy of *Fusiformis necrophorus* and *Corynebacterium pyogenes*. I. Influence of the leucocidal exotoxin of *F. necrophorus*. *British Journal of Experimental Pathology* **48**, 665–673.

Bruley-Rosset, M., Florentin, A., Khalil, A. M. and Mathe, G. (1976). Non-specific macrophage activation by systemic adjuvants. *International Archives of Allergy and Applied Immunology* **51**, 594–507.

Sawyer, W. D. (1969). Interaction of influenza virus with leukocytes and its effect on phagocytosis. *Journal of Infectious Diseases* **119**, 541–556.

Shands, J. W., Peavy, D. L., Gormus, B. J. and McGraw, J. (1974). *In vitro* and *In vivo* effects of endotoxins on mouse peritoneal cells. *Infection and Immunity* **9**, 106–112.

Scharman, W. (1976). Interaction of purified leukocidins from *Pseudomonas aeruginosa* with bovine polymorphonuclear leukocytes. *Infection and Immunity* **13**, 1046–1053.

Schiffman, E., Showell, H. J., Corcoran, B. A., Ward, P. A., Smith, E. and Becker, E. L. (1975). The isolation and partial characterisation of neutrophil chemotactic factors from *Escherichia coli*. *Journal of Immunology* **114**, 1831–1837.

Selvaraj, R. J., Paul, B. P., Zgliezynski, J. M. and Sbarra, A. J. (1978). Enhanced killing of myeloperoxidase coated bacteria in the myeloperoxidase–H_2O_2–C1 system. *Journal of Infectious Diseases* **137**, 481–485.

Silverberg, B. A., Jakab, G. J., Thomson, R. G., Warr, G. A. and Boo, K. S. (1979). Ultrastructural alteration in phagocytic function of alveolar macrophages after parainfluenza virus infection. *Journal of the Reticulaendothelial Society* **25**, 405–416.

Smith, H. (1977). Microbial surfaces in relation to pathogenicity. *Bacteriological Reviews* **41**, 475–500.

Snyderman, R., Phillips, J. K. and Mergenhagen, S. E. (1971). Biological activity of complement *in vivo*. Role of C5 in the accumulation of polymorphonuclear leukocytes in inflammatory exudates. *Journal of Experimental Medicine* **134**, 1131–1143.

Spagnuolo, P. J. and Ellner, J. J. (1980). Comparative stimulation of granulocyte adherence and chemotaxis by bacterial products. *Infection and Immunity* **27**, 519–524.

Spitznagel, J. K. (1977). Bactericidal Mechanisms of the Granulocyte. *In* "The Granulocyte Function and Clinical Utilisation" (Eds. T. J. Greenwalt and G. A. Jamieson), pp. 103–131. Alan R. Liss, New York.

Staber, F. G. (1979). Comparative effects in mice of purified bacterial cell wall components on granulocyte macrophage progenitor cells and their regulators. *Journal of Immunology* **122**, 1726–1730.

Stalenheim, G., Gotre, O., Cooper, N. R. Sjoguise, J., and Müller-Eberhardt, H. J. (1978). Consumption of human complement components by complexes of IgG with protein A of *Staphylococcus aureus*. *Immunochemistry* **10**, 501–507.

Stendahl, O. and Edebo, L. (1972). Phagocytosis of mutants of *Salmonella typhimurium* by rabbit polymorphonuclear cells. *Acta Pathologica Microbiologica Scandinavica* **80**, 481–488.

Sutherland, I. W. (1972). Bacterial exopolysaccharides. *Advances in Microbiology* **8**, 142–143.

Taichman, N. S. and McArthur, W. P. (1976). Interaction of inflammatory cells and oral bacteria: release of lysosomal hydrolases from rabbit polymorphonuclear leukocytes exposed to Gram-positive plaque bacteria. *Archives of Oral Biology* **21**, 257–263.

Taichman, N. S., Dean, R. T. and Sanderson, C. J. (1980). Biochemical and morphological characterisation of the killing of human monocytes by a leukotoxin derived from *Actinobacillus actinomycetemcomitans*. *Infection and Immunity* **29**, 258–268.

Taichman, N. S. and Wilton, J. M. A. (1980). Cytotoxicity of *Actinobacillus actinomycetemcomitans* (Y4) leukotoxin for gingival crevice polymorphonuclear leukocytes. *Inflammation*, in press.

Tainer, J. A., Turner, S. R. and Lynn, W. S. (1975). New aspects of chemotaxis: specific target cell attraction by lipid and lipoprotein fractions of *Escherichia coli* chemotactic factor. *American Journal of Pathology* **81**, 401–408.

Tosolini, F. A. and Mims, C. A. (1971). Effect of murine strain and viral strain on the pathogenesis of lymphocytic choriomeningitis infection and a study of footpad responses. *Journal of Infectious Diseases* **123**, 134.

Urbaschek, R. (1980). Effects of bacterial products on granulopoiesis. *In* "Advances in Experimental Medicine and Biology" (Eds M. R. Escobar and H. Friedman), vol. 121B, pp. 51–64. Plenum Press, New York.

Van Oss, C. J. and Gillman, C. F. (1977). Phagocytosis as a surface phenomenon. I. Contact angles and phagocytosis of non-opsonised bacteria. *Journal of the Reticuloendothelial Society* **12**, 283–292.

Valtonen, M. V. (1977). Role of phagocytosis in mouse virulence of Salmonella typimurium recombinants with 0 antigen 6,7, or 4,12. *Infection and Immunity* **18**, 579–582.

Veale, D. C., Penn, C. W. and Smith, H. (1977). The resistance of gonococci to killing by human phagocytes. *In* "Gonorrhoea" (Eds F. A. Skinner, H. Smith and P. D. Walker), pp. 97–115. Academic Press, London and New York.

Verbrugh, H. A., Van Dijk, W. C., Van Erne, M. E., Peters, R., Peterson, P. K. and Verhoef, J. (1979). Quantitation of the third component of human complement attached to the surface of opsonised bacteria: opsonic deficient sera and phagocytosis resistant strains. *Infection and Immunity* **26**, 808–812.

Verbrugh, H. A., Van Dijk, W. C., Peters, R., Van Erne, M. E., Dain, M. R., Peterson, P. K. and Verhoef, J. (1980). Opsonic recognition of Staphylococci mediated by cell wall peptidoglycan: antibody-independent activation of human complement and opsonic activity of peptidoglycan antibodies. *Journal of Immunology* **124**, 1167–1173.

Walters, M. N.-I. and Papadimitriou, J. M. (1978). Phagocytosis: A review. CRC Critical Reviews in Toxicology, pp. 377–421.

Ward, P. A., Lepow, I. H. and Newman, W. (1968). Bacterial factors for polymorphonuclear leukocytes. *American Journal of Pathology* **52**, 725–736.

Warshauer, D., Goldstein, E., Akers, T., Lippers, W. and Kim, M. (1977). Effect of influenza viral infection on the ingestion and killing of bacteria by alveolar macrophages. *American Review of Respiratory Disease* **115**, 269–277.

Weiner, E. and Levanons, D. (1968). The *in vitro* interaction between bacterial lipopolysaccharide and differentiating monocytes. *Laboratory Investigation* **19**, 584–590.

Weiss, J., Elsbach, P., Olsson, I. and Odeberg, H. (1978). Purification and characterisation of a potent bactericidal and membrane active protein from the granules of human polymorphonuclear leukocytes. *Journal of Biological Chemistry* **253**, 2664–2672.

Weiss, J., Beckerdite-Quagliate, S. and Elsbach, P. (1980). Resistance of Gram-negative bacteria to purified bactericidal leukocyte proteins: relation to binding and bacterial lipopolysaccharide structure. *Journal of Clinical Investigation* **65**, 619–628.

Weksler, B. B. and Hill, M. J. (1969). Inhibition of leukocyte migration by a staphylococcal factor. *Journal of Bacteriology* **98**, 1030–1035.

Wilkinson, B. J., Sisson, S. P., Kim, Y. and Peterson, P. K. (1979a). Localisation of the third component of complement on the cell wall of encapsulated *Staphylococcus aureus* M; Implications for the mechanism of resistance to phagocytosis. *Infection and Immunity* **26**, 1159–1163.

Wilkinson, B. J., Peterson, P. K. and Quie, P. G. (1979b). Cryptic peptidoglycan and the antiphagocytic effect of the *Staphylococcus aureus* capsule: Model for the antiphagocytic effect of bacterial cell surface polymers. *Infection and Immunity* **23**, 502–508.

Wilkinson, P. C. (1975). Inhibition of leukocyte locomotion and chemotaxis by lipid specific bacterial toxins *Nature* **255**, 485–487.

Wilkinson, P. C. and Lackie, J. M. (1979). The adhesion, migration and chemotaxis of leucocytes in inflammation. *Current Topics in Pathology* **68**, 47–88.

Wilson, D. M., Ormrod, D. J. and Miller, T. E. (1980). Role of complement in chemotaxis. Study of a localised infection. *Infection and Immunity* **29**, 8–12.

Wilton, J. M. A. (1977). The function of complement in crevicular fluid. *In* "The Borderland between Caries and Periodontal Disease" (Ed. T. Lehner), pp. 223–247. Academic Press, London and New York.

Wilton, J. M. A. and Lehner, T. (1980). Immunological and microbial aspects of periodontal disease. *In* "Recent Advances in Clinical Immunology" (Ed. R. A. Thompson), pp. 145–181. Churchill Livingstone, Edinburgh.

Wilton, J. M. A. and Almeida, O. de P. (1980). The comparative effects of dental plaque, lipopolysaccharide, lipoteichoic acid, dextran and levan on leukocytes in the mouse peritoneal cavity. *In* "The Borderland between Caries and Periodontal Diseases" (Eds T. Lehner and G. Cimasoni), vol. 2, pp. 84–97. Academic Press, London and New York. In press.

Winkelstein, J. A., and Tomasz, A. (1978). Activation of the alternative complement pathway by pneumococcal cell wall teichoic acid. *Journal of Immunology* 120, 174.

Wood, W. B. Jr (1960). Phagocytosis with particular reference to encapsulated bacteria. *Bacteriological Reviews* 24, 41–49.

Woodin, A. M. (1973). The leucocidin treated leucocyte. *In* "Lysosomes in Biology and Pathology" (Ed. Dingle), vol. 3, pp. 395–422. North Holland, Amsterdam.

Yamomotu, S., Yoshinaga, M. and Hayashi, H. (1971). The natural mediator for PMN emigration in inflammation. II. Common antigenicity of leucoegresin with Immunoglobulin G. *Immunology* 20, pp. 803–808.

DISCUSSION

Mims I was especially interested, Dr Wilton, to see all those possibilities nicely lined up so that we can think about them; particularly this influence of different quantities of microbial products. For instance, something that in larger concentrations will kill a phagocyte but in smaller concentration will only interfere with its function; or a substance which in concentrated form inhibits migration, but which further away along a concentration gradient may be chemotatic. I think that this is a very important principle.

Quie Dr Wilton, I was especially interested in that observation that serum from patients with serious periodontal disease inhibits the phagocyte toxin. IgA has an affinity for neutrophils and yet lacks the capacity for opsonizing the microorganisms. Do you suppose IgA acts as a blocking type of structure? Do these patients have a peculiarly large amount of IgA which may compromise phagocytosis?

Wilton I think that is at least possible. I can say, I think with fair confidence, that it has not actually been studied because we are talking about an incredibly rare disease; but it is about the only periodontal disease which seems to have a specific association with one pathogen, and that is the *Actinobacillus*. Of course, the data that I showed are with serum and I know that Norton Taichman has gone further than I showed there. It is apparently an IgG antibody, but there is a paradox in that if you pre-incubate the IgG with the toxin you inhibit the effect. My view is that perhaps it is not working because it stops the toxin binding to the surface. It is at least a possibility that the toxin binds to the Fc receptor, or a closely associated structure. Professor Mims spoke yesterday about viruses taking over structures on the cell for their own purposes. At the moment, I think it is an open question.

With regard to IgA, as you know I have shown myself that IgA interferes with IgG-mediated phagocytosis and opsonization, but we do not know anything about that for this particular disease. It is a possibility.

Jeljaszewicz Can you give us some more information about the toxin you used?

Wilton There is published work, the references to which are in the manuscript. The most recent paper showed that it is a protein, it is heat labile, it is inactivated by trypsin and trypsin-like enzymes. That is all I can remember from a chemical standpoint.

It is interesting as a toxin because it affects only human neutrophils and monocytes; it does not touch animal monocytes or neutrophils and it has no toxic effect on any other human cell that we have tested including epithelial cells, erythrocytes or ciliated epithelial cells. It seems to be specific for the two phagocytes in the human.

van Furth You did not mention the *Capnocytophaga*, a bacterium which has some action on neutrophils and I think also comes from the oral cavity.

Wilton *Capnocytophaga ochraceus*, or *Capnocytophaga oralis*, is a very interesting bacterium because it is an obligate anaerobe which is isolated from most cases of periodontal disease, but also seems to be part of the normal flora of the gingiva in small numbers. Recently there has been a description in the *New England Journal of Medicine* of patients with *Capnocytophaga* bacteraemia who had neutrophils which would not migrate properly. A culture supernatant extract from this organism had an effect on both lysosomes and the cell membrane which interfered with mobility. We have tried to find out whether this is responsible for the diminished chemotaxis that you see if you take inflammatory neutrophils from the site of infection, but so far we have not had any success. It is an interesting toxic effect in that it does not involve lipopolysaccharide, although the organism, being Gram negative, contains lipopolysaccharide. It also produces a fibroblast proliferation inhibitory factor, which is important in terms of the periodontal diseases we are talking about. It is a toxin which not only interferes with mobility but by freezing membrane motility presumably interferes with the emigration of the neutrophil between the endothelial cells and the vascular endothelium and also interferes with the proper delivery of lysosomal enzymes to the phagosome. The organisms are phagocytosed, but lysosomal fusion does not take place. We are trying at the moment to identify the bacteria in neutrophils taken from patients with this periodontal disease to see whether organisms which are phagocytosed but which are not accompanied by this degranulatory stimulus are *Capnocytophaga*—but that is a fairly hairy immunoelectron microscopy.

One other thing about this organism is that it is relatively resistant to phagocytosis. Neutrophils which will perfectly well phagocytose staphylococci or *Candida* or streptococci do not seem to like this organism much and only about 30 or 40% of them phagocytose it.

Smith With regard to the nonstimulation of the inflammatory response, could I describe some experiments that Charles Penn has been doing in Birmingham with treponemes harvested from rabbits and introduced into plastic chambers implanted subcutaneously in guinea-pigs? If gonococci are put into one of these chambers a massive inflammatory response occurs within a few hours. With treponemes there is no inflammatory response, or hardly any. If you introduce a mixture of gonococci and treponemes the inflammatory response occurs, i.e. there is no suppression of the inflammatory response by the treponemes. The surface of the treponeme seems to be masked so that the host defence mechanisms are not stimulated. Could anyone suggest a mechanism for this nonstimulation of the inflammatory response?

Wood I want to ask Dr Wilton whether septicaemia is an essential part of the inhibition of mobility or whether this phenomenon occurred if the organism was localized and whether effects on phagocytes could be shown in peripheral blood distant from the site of infection?

Wilton If my memory is correct, both patients had bone abscesses and the demonstration of the abnormality was shown in circulating neutrophils from the patient; with cure of the infection the abnormality disappeared. The patient's isolate, grown from the peripheral blood, and the supernatant from that culture would similarly inhibit the motility of normal neutrophils.

van Furth Was the abnormality in the leukocytes only during the period when there was bacteraemia or was it also found during localized infection in the oral cavity or elsewhere in the body?

I ask this because so often you see peripheral blood leukocyte abnormalities *in vitro* when the bacteria are localized elsewhere. If that can be confirmed for more diseases there must be a factor released at the site of infection which affects the leukocytes in the circulation. The half-life of polymorphs in the circulation is only 7–9 h, so these cells must be affected there or in the bone marrow. The next step should be to take plasma and do all kinds of cross experiments which are usually not done. This could solve the question whether a humoral factor is involved.

Wilton I do not think I can answer the question about when the abnormalities were present, but I can say that defects in motility in patients with juvenile periodontitis have been described by three separate groups, one of which is Peter Ward's, so I think you can believe that it truly is an effect on chemotaxis and not just a disorder of migration. Patients with this disease have defects of neutrophil chemotaxis but not of monocyte chemotaxis. Whether that is because they are infected with *Capnocytophaga* and the toxin is circulating, nobody has dared to say. I know that there is a group working on a radioassay to try to detect this toxin in these patients to see whether, at the time the chemotactic defect is manifest, there is also a toxaemia. If you treat the patients so that you remove the bacterial load very scrupulously and make sure it does not re-accumulate, the chemotactic defect remains. This suggests that there is a synergic effect in which a susceptible neutrophil is attacked by this particular toxin and the net effect is an inhibition of the chemotaxis. Because there seems to be some evidence of a partial inherited defect of neutrophil function in certain relatives of the presenting case, family studies are just being undertaken. So there is a well described toxic effect on neutrophil motility and lysosomal membrane stability, but it is not necessarily the whole story in these patients. There seems to be a genetic factor as well.

Arbuthnott I would like to pick up Dr Wilton's point about bacterial chemotaxins and chemotaxinogens. A few years ago in Glasgow, working with Peter Wilkinson and other colleagues there, I made a study of the effects of staphylococci and their products on the stimulation and inhibition of the mobility of human leukocytes. We found that supernates from different strains produced different effects. But more interesting in relation to stimulation of chemotaxis, we found that when we incubated the cells directly with supernatant the effect was primarily on monocytes rather than on polymorphonuclear leukocytes. When we used a mixture of supernatant and serum we had a very profound effect on polymorphonuclear leukocytes as well, presumably due to formation of chemotaxinogens.

Wilton Professor Arbuthnott has raised an interesting point. It is rather like the state at one time of migration and inhibition factors produced by lymphocytes for macrophages. Everyone concentrated so hard on the inhibition they threw away all the data that showed stimulation. I was as guilty as anyone. I remember the work that Professor Arbuthnott talked about. I will give a further example of how careful one has to be. Casein is a well-known chemotaxin and by varying the concentration we can make it inhibit, have no effect whatsoever, or markedly stimulate. Change the species from the rabbit to the guinea-pig, and we have the converse effects of different doses. It is no good doing single point doses and no dose response curves; we must define the system. We have too many people working with mixed cells and talking about polymorph migration. It is a great source of irritation, in going through the literature for a meeting such as this, that even on close reading of a paper one still does not know whether it is talking about neutrophils or monocytes. What is needed is a lot more precision in people's experimental systems and a lot more *ad hoc* experimentation *in vivo*. In other words, everyone is obsessed with the idea of purification down to the last amino acid and what it does *in vitro*, whereas we need to get back to the 1930s and do a bit more *in vivo* experimentation and sort it out later when we have some data.

Mims I am delighted to hear a comment such as that, especially because people study macrophages induced in inflammatory exudates, and just as in the natural inflammatory exudate the macrophages are preceded by polymorphs and we know that some so-called macrophage enzymes are just taken up from polymorphs. The whole picture can be very confused.

Easmon With regard to what may be happening in the whole animal, does anyone have any experimental evidence or knowledge of any attempt to try to reproduce the phagocytosis conditions of the inflammatory response in an *in vitro* system? We always set the pH, temperature and so on very carefully, but the conditions *in vitro* may not reflect what is going on in an inflammatory response in the animal.

van Furth One can control pH, temperature and so on, but how does one get the whole story? I think that *in vivo* experimentation is much better.

Wilton A comparison of the numbers of *Candida* taken up by inflammatory neutrophils and blood neutrophils is made and the killing as assessed by methylene blue exclusion. By comparing 30% serum—the figure of 30% is purely arbitrary—with exudate, we find some interesting differences. After 60 min 60% of inflammatory cells incubated in 30% serum have taken up *Candida*, but incubated in their own inflammatory exudate nearly 80% of them take up *Candida* and this difference is statistically significant. Again, the number of particles taken up by the inflammatory exudate cells is greater. If we look at killing the position is even more striking—within one hour—in inflammatory exudate it is almost double that in the careful pH stabilized serum system that Dr Easmon talked about and we all use.

Mims To orient that to Dr Easmon's question, do you know what the pH would be in those inflammatory exudates?

Wilton It is about 6·7 or 6·6; it is not the 7·4 or 7·5 that we use in experiments *in vitro*.

Quie Crevicular washings are pretty dilute, are they not? They may be a little closer to the real life situation than 30% serum but still fairly distant.

Wilton Our estimate of the dilution factor, based on our studies of accumulation in various oral sites of labelled immunoglobulins injected into Rhesus monkeys, would be that the serum concentration in that type of preparation would be nearer 0·2%.

Valdimarsssson I have some information that may be relevant to this discussion from a *Candida albicans* killing system, using a radiometric assay, which will be published in the near future in *Clinical and Experimental Immunology*. We have demonstrated that the killing of *Candida albicans* by human neutrophils is more effective in 2·5–5% serum than in serum concentrations about 5%. So although ingestion is not affected in serum concentrations up to about 30%, killing is usually depressed in serum concentrations above 5%. protein concentration of normal extravascular fluids is in the range corresponding to 2·5–5% serum, but it obviously increases when there is an inflammatory reaction going on.

We have also tested the effect of reducing pH in our system and down to a pH of 5·5 but there is no significant inhibition or stimulation of killing of *Candida albicans* by neutrophils and monocytes.

van Furth We recently studied the killing by monocytes of different kinds of bacteria. For the killing of the catalase-positive ones—*E. coli* and so on—one needs extracellular stimulation of the Fc and complement sector. For this we need a concentration of serum of 5% or more. With about 5% we have optimal intracellular killing in an *in vitro* system. In the case of the catalase-negative organisms we get some extra killing, but the killing capacity of the monocytes is apparently greater because there is no destruction of the hydrogen peroxide. The same has been found for granulocytes. Their killing capacity, in the absence of any serum, is still much higher than that of monocytes which is zero. This makes sense because in exudate we usually have a serum concentration of about 5 or 10%.

Dr Easmon asked about temperature effects. We thought that *in vivo* there might be a temperature of 35–40 °C. We found that killing was not affected in that temperature range. At about 45 °C there is an enormous decrease and at 41 °C the function is impaired. The question is whether there is a difference between 37° and 39 °C. Will everything go faster? Is it more efficient? We could not find any difference.

Easmon Could I press the point a little further and go from the phagocyte cell to the organism? Has anyone done any experiments using organisms grown either *in vivo* or *in vitro* under the conditions in which they would be growing *in vivo*, i.e. with less than ideal redox potential and less than ideal pH or temperature and then tested them against phagocytic cells? I am all in favour of doing *in vivo* work, but *in vitro* work is convenient and I think we should attempt to make it as realistic as possible, from the point of view of both the organism and the cell.

Wilton I can answer that with regard to one organism, *Veillonella alcalescens*, a Gram negative coccus grown from the mouth. We grew these in the mouse peritoneal cavity and then compared their phagocytosis with that of organisms grown in conventional static batch culture. Rather disappointingly, we could not find any difference either in the background nonopsonized phagocytosis or in the opsonization of organisms from either source with normal or infected mouse serum which might contain antibody. In retrospect, I think this particular organism is the worst possible example, because it does not produce a very good immunological response. If I had chosen one which gave us a better opsonization system I might have had different results.

Smith There were two studies where organisms were obtained directly from infected animals and put into phagocytosis tests. Some years ago brucellae obtained directly from infected cow placental tissue were studied *in vitro* in bovine phagocytes. These brucellae were more resistant to killing by the bovine phagocyte than those grown *in vitro*. More recently gonococci, admittedly grown in guinea-pig subcutaneous chambers and not obtained directly from patients, were found more resistant to killing by human phagocytes than the same strain grown *in vitro*. Also, there is the work of Ellwood and Tempest. Using continuous culture they grew a Gram negative organism under limiting growth conditions. This changed the cell wall structure, the toxicity of the lipopolysaccharide and, I think, the serum sensitivity. Thus, growing bacteria under limiting conditions which might occur *in vivo*, can change surface components and this might affect resistance to phagocytes.

Valdimarsson I would like to make two comments in relation to the last points that have been made. First, regarding the possible effects of neutrophils on the phagocytic function of monocytes, I think it was first reported by Robert Lehrer in UCLA that monocytes, in the absence of neutrophils, were very ineffective in killing *Candida albicans*; but in the presence of neutrophils they were more effective in killing *Candida albicans* than were neutrophils, that is to say they killed a higher percentage of ingested Candida than did neutrophils. We have certainly confirmed this observation and I think it bears on *in vivo* reality and perhaps argues against the puristic view that we should use defined populations of purified cells wherever possible. We should do that, but we should also bear in mind the *in vivo* reality.

Regarding resistance of organisms *in vivo* and *ex vivo* compared with *in vitro*, *Candida albicans* is a very good example. The organisms form germinal tubules *in vivo* and these are more resistant than blastospores to phagocytic killing. The new imidazole antifungal drug, ketoconazole, which is orally active, is effective *in vivo* at about 10-fold lower concentration than *in vitro*. Our preliminary experiments suggest that the activity of this drug *in vivo* is mainly to prevent tubule formation by the *Candida*, thereby rendering the organism more susceptible to phagocytic killing.

Arbuthnott Karen Vassli, working in my laboratory in Dublin, has done some experiments similar to those described by Professor Smith. She grew several strains of *Staph. aureus* in chambers in the peritoneum of mice and then compared their susceptibility with that of the organism grown *in vitro* to phagocytosis and killing by human leukocytes. In all cases she noted that the *in vivo* grown organisms were more resistant.

But I would just like to add a rider and perhaps a comment which could be expanded later. I am a little worried about standardization of the test systems which people use for investigating phagocytosis. I am not an expert in this field, but people use different test systems and they use the cells from different animal species. In looking through the literature, it is rather confusing and I think it is something we ought to be rather concerned about.

Mims I think we have drawn attention to a number of important practical points. Cell purity and the reproducibility of test systems is one thing, but as Dr Valdimarsson says, macrophages and polymorphs are usually there together in inflammatory exudates and separation is to some extent artificial.

van Furth Dr Wilton, do you need granule release and lysosome enzyme release for extracellular killing of bacteria? We know, although only from *in vitro* experiments, that all kinds of oxidative metabolic products are found in the surroundings of the cell. Although I always regarded that as very artificial, in your scheme it might well be very active in killing bacteria extracellularly.

Wilton For too long, I think, people have said that the enzyme release by phagocytes is an all or none phenomenon. In other words, we know that what has been called regurgitation during feeding must lack selectivity because both types of granule are released simultaneously. There is a beautiful paper by John Sitznagel's group showing this simultaneity and the rapidity with which the enzyme appears on the cell membrane and particularly on the pseudopodia cupping around the *E. coli* which they use for their studies: five seconds is the figure I remember. But other pieces of work in the more recent literature also suggest that there is some sort of specificity for granule release. John Gallin's group at NIH have been particularly interested in this. They have shown very clearly that neutrophils which are migrating, presumably in response to a normal stimulus, into Rebuck chambers or into human skin blisters release selectively the specific granule enzymes but not the azurophil granule enzymes. This has been done in two ways: by looking at the accumulation of the enzymes extracellularly and by showing electromicroscopically that those granules have diminished numerically within the cells. It is not an artefact of cell death or anything like that. It is possible that the importance of degranulation is two-fold. One is the effect it has on bacteria extracellularly. As I showed in my talk, that might be a combination of lethal effects and either stopping bacteria from adhering to surfaces or removing them from surfaces to which they have already adhered. The second is that enzyme release may have nothing to do with bacterial killing at all. It is said—and I am not a cell physiologist, so I do not know what the evidence is—that the specific granules are not strictly lysosomes. Therefore, their contents are probably designed, teleologically speaking, for function outside the cell. We are only just beginning to appreciate those functions and whether they have anything to do with infectious disease or whether they have possibly more to do with tissue damage is purely speculative. One example is the very rapid and powerful degranulation which is induced by the binding of immune complexes to a surface. I think Helson did some experiments to show that the amount of antibody needed to produce the same enzyme release is substantially less than if it was in suspension, even if it was a relatively insoluble complex.

Membrane-damaging Toxins in Relation to Interference with Host Defence Mechanisms

J. P. ARBUTHNOTT

Department of Microbiology,
Moyne Institute,
Trinity College,
Dublin, Eire

INTRODUCTION

It is now realized that with few exceptions bacterial pathogenicity is multifactorial (Smith, 1977) and is rarely the property of a single determinant. The requirements of a successful pathogen are that it must be able to colonize and/or penetrate the body surfaces of the host. Penetration of host surfaces may be accompanied by spread through the tissues and the symptoms of disease are due to the ability of the pathogen to damage host tissues. It is with this last phase that we classically associate bacterial exotoxins as in the case of tetanus, botulism, diphtheria and many forms of diarrhoeal disease and food poisoning. It is possible, however, that extracellular products of invasive pathogens could play a role at an earlier stage of pathogensis by contributing to the invasiveness of the pathogen or by affecting host defence mechanisms. To establish itself within the tissues of the host such a pathogen must be able to resist the barrage of defences at the disposal of the host and particularly it must be able to resist the onslaught of phagocytic cells delivered to the focus of infection by means of the inflammatory response. This situation is often exacerbated from the point of view of the invading organism due to the direct and indirect production of chemotactic factors by the pathogen.

There are several points at which the extracellular products of the pathogen could modify this response: (i) by inhibiting the inflammatory response at an early stage, (ii) by inhibiting the chemotactic response of the phagocytic cells, (iii) by killing or impairing the function of phagocytic cells that arrive at the focus of infection, (iv) by exerting toxic effects within phagocytic cells after the pathogen has been phagocytozed, (v) indirect toxic effects resulting from the action of bacterial products on mediator cells.

The leukotoxic effects of staphylococci and streptococci have been known for a very long time (Van de Velde, 1884; Levaditi, 1918), and a large number of cytolytic agents have since been isolated from culture filtrates of pathogenic bacteria. Such agents differ in their mode of action from the better known bacterial toxins. They exert direct damaging effects on the membranes of susceptible cells, usually through their action on lipids or phospholipids. These lead to altered permeability properties and ultimately to death of the cell. This contrasts with the action of toxins like diphtheria, cholera, the heat labile enterotoxin of *Escherichia coli*; these toxins are bipartite molecules comprising a fragment that binds to a specific receptor in the membrane of a susceptible cell and a fragment that traverses the membrane to impair a vital cellular activity. Such toxins, unlike the cytolytic or membrane-damaging agents, do not affect the integrity of the cell membrane.

Considerable progress has been made in characterizing the membrane damaging toxins and their modes of action on cell membranes. They have been shown to damage many cell types *in vitro* and to exert various "toxicities" when injected into experimental animals. Indeed recently it has been shown that these agents can perturb cell membranes, including the membranes of phagocytic cells, at sublethal concentrations.

The question remains: to what extent, if any, are such effects of importance in bacterial pathogenesis? Clearly if these toxic factors are produced *in vivo* at the initial site of infection, then by inhibiting chemotaxis or by killing or impairing phagocytic cells they may well enable the pathogen to counteract host defence mechanisms.

To establish that such events occur *in vivo* and to pinpoint the role of individual factors is difficult for several reasons: (i) attempts to produce mutants deficient in individual products have been bedevilled by pleiotropic effects in which production of several extracellular products is affected; (ii) several membrane damaging toxins exhibit a marked species specificity and the host response to infection is not uniform in different species which makes extrapolation from results in one animal model to another difficult; (iii) as yet little progress has been made in studying the production of membrane damaging toxins *in vivo* and their effects on the host response under conditions that mimic infection.

In this contribution I will summarize the properties of some of the best studied membrane damaging toxins and describe their effects on leukocytes. I will also outline animal models that we have developed recently in attempts to analyse the importance of certain staphylococcal toxins in pathogenesis.

SUMMARY OF THE PROPERTIES OF MEMBRANE DAMAGING TOXINS

Phospholipases

Many bacterial species produce phospholipases that are capable of attacking glycerophospholipid and sphingolipid substrates at different points in the molecule. Phospholipids have the unique property of being able to form stable bilayers in aqueous solutions and they, together with cholesterol (at a molar ratio to phospholipid of 0·4–1·0), constitute the hydrophobic region of mammalian cytoplasmic membranes. Hydrolysis of membrane phospholipid can therefore greatly modify the properties of cell membranes.

For the most part phospholipases of the A type are membrane or cell-associated and are probably concerned with the regulation and turnover of membrane phospholipid. However, the possible role of phospholipase A in pathogenesis of *Candida albicans* and *Fusobacterium necrophorum* has been suggested (Pugh and Cawson, 1975, 1977; Abe *et al.*, 1978).

Although phospholipases of type D have been associated mainly with plant tissues several such enzymes have recently been demonstrated in bacteria. One of these, namely, the phospholipase D of *Corynebacterium ovis* is dermonecrotic and lethal for guinea pigs and rabbits (Souček *et al.*, 1971). It exhibits a specificity for sphingomyelin and lysolecithin and has several unusual properties, including the fact that it is not haemolytic and it does not affect the membrane permeability of cells in tissue culture (Součková and Souček, 1972; Möllby, 1978). It is not yet possible to explain how an enzyme that causes little perturbation to cell membrane is demonecrotic and lethal. Two possible mechanisms are thrombocyte aggregation and release of vasoactive factors from mast cells (Möllby, 1978).

It is undoubtedly the phospholipases of type C that have attracted most attention from bacterial toxinologists. The α-toxin of *Clostridium perfringens* has long been known to be a phospholipase C and this toxin holds a special place in the history of bacterial toxins as it was the first toxin that was shown to be an enzyme. The type C phospholipases produced by several species of *Clostridium*, *Staphylococcus aureus*, and *Bacillus cereus* have been relatively well characterized (Möllby, 1978). It is notable that some species produce more than one type of phospholipase and that bacterial phospholipases C show a wide variation in substrate specificity. Phospholipases have been widely used as tools in investigations of the structure and function of biological membranes. However, from the point of view of pathogenicity attention has focussed on the α-toxin of *Cl. perfringens* and the β-toxin of *S. aureus*. The main properties of these toxins are summarized in Tables I and II; more detailed information can be found in the reviews of Freer and Arbuthnott (1976) and Möllby (1978).

Despite the fact that *Cl. perfringens* α-toxin is often cited as the principle lethal toxin in gas gangrene, the role of the toxin in pathogenicity is still unclear (Bullen, 1970). Certain poorly toxinogenic strains are known to be highly virulent and for various reasons, including contradictory results obtained with different experimental models, there is still some doubt as to the precise role of this factor in gas gangrene. The role of *S. aureus* β-toxin

TABLE I.

Summary of the properties of *Cl. perfringens* α-toxin (phospholipase C).

(1) Haemolytic, cytotoxic, dermonecrotic, lethal and phospholipase C activities are properties of a single molecular species

(2) Care must be taken in purification to exclude other membrane-active agents, especially θ-toxin

(3) Mol. wt of purified preparations range from c. 30 000 for gel filtration to c. 54 000 by SDS polyacrylamide electrophoresis. Isoelectric point of main form = 5·5

(4) In erythrocyte ghosts 70% of membrane phosphorus is released by α-toxin (order of susceptibility of phospholipids: phosphatidyl choline > sphingomyelin > phosphatidyl ethanolamine)

(5) Hydrolysis products (diglycerides and possibly ceramide) accumulate in the membrane as pools or droplets known as "black dots"

(6) Release of radiolabelled markers from cells is potentiated by presence of Ca^{2+}, hypertonic stretching and pretreatment with sublytic amounts of detergent

(sphingolyelinase C) in pathogenicity is even less understood. It is considerably less lethal than the α-toxin of *S. aureus* and although it is known to cause intense erythema with an accompanying influx of PMN when injected into rabbit skin, there is no convincing evidence that β-toxin plays a dominant role in pathogenesis (Adlam *et al.*, 1977; Ward *et al.*, 1979).

TABLE II.
Properties of *S. aureus* β-toxin (sphingomyelinase C).

(1) "Hot–cold" haemolysin (sheep, bovine, goat RBCs) requiring Mg^{2+} for activity
(2) Causes erythema and PMN infiltration in skin
(3) Mol. wt = 38 000; pI = 9·4
(4) Substrate range confined to sphingomyelin and lysophospholipids
(5) Hydrolysis product (ceramide) accumulates in pools in membrane
(6) β-toxin treated cells show increased susceptibility to α- and δ-toxins of *S. aureus*

Later I will discuss the effects of these toxins on phagocytic cells but it should be emphasized that the susceptibility of cells to damage or lysis by phospholipases is probably extremely complex and cannot be accounted for simply in terms of the phospholipid composition of the cell membrane (Möllby, 1978). Factors such as the amount of ATP in the cell, the number of disulphide bonds between membrane proteins, the presence of endogenous membrane-associated phospholipases and the maximum lateral surface pressure of the phospholipids can all affect accessibility of phospholipids to their substrates in the membrane.

Oxygen-labile Toxins

The oxygen-labile toxins, also referred to as thiol-activated cytolysins, form a group of membrane-damaging toxins that share certain common properties, and are produced by a number of different organisms. In this article it is only possible to present a brief summary of this important group of membrane-damaging toxins; the reader is referred to the comprehensive review of Smyth and Duncan (1978) for detailed information.

The shared common properties of this group of toxins include the following: (i) they are lethal and cardiotoxic; (ii) activation by thiol reducing agents; (iii) inhibition upon addition of small amounts of cholesterol and certain related steroids; (iv) cross-neutralization occurs with hyperimmune horse antisera; (v) similar pH and temperature optima are required for cell-damaging activity.

The best studied members of this group of toxins are streptolysin O (*Streptococcus pyogenes*), θ-toxin (*Cl. perfringens*); cereolysin (*B. cereus*), pneumolysin (*Streptococcus pneumoniae*) and tetanolysin (*Clostridium tetani*), but at least 12 other oxygen-labile cytolysins have been described. Molecular weight values for the group range from 45 000–75 000 and they exhibit charge heterogeneity with most of the multiple forms having pI's in the range pH 6·0–7·0. They are haemolytic for the erythrocytes of a range of species in nanogram amounts and microgram quantities are lethal for mice and rabbits.

In terms of explaining the biochemical basis for the mode of action oxygen-labile toxins, the most important observations relate to the interactions with cholesterol. Smyth and Duncan (1978) have reviewed recent findings relating to the stereospecificity and the stoichiometry of the reaction between oxygen-labile toxins and cholesterol dispersions and current views of the mode of action on cell membranes. Several lines of evidence support the view that cholesterol is the binding site for these agents in the membranes of susceptible cells: only cells that contain cholesterol in the membrane are sensitive; bacterial protoplasts and spheroplasts that lack cholesterol are insensitive to lysis; certain strains of *Mycoplasma* containing cholesterol in the membrane were lysed by streptolysin O whereas saprophytic strains that lack cholesterol were insensitive. Also incubation of oxygen-labile toxins with erythrocyte membranes abolishes their haemolytic activity and the evidence indicates that cholesterol is the membrane lipid component responsible for this inhibition, (see review of Smyth and Duncan, 1978).

An interesting feature of the morphological changes seen in toxin treated erythrocyte membranes is the formation on the membrane of characteristic ring or arc-shaped structures having a border thickness of c. 5–8 nm and an external diameter of 30–60 nm; again cholesterol has been shown to be involved in the formation of these structures although the relationship between the appearance of rings and arcs and lysis is uncertain at present. Recent evidence from freeze-etching studies however indicates that these structures do not penetrate the membrane; in other words they do not form holes through the membrane (Cowell *et al.*, 1978; Mitsui *et al.*, 1979).

The detailed molecular events involved in membrane damage are still not known. It seems likely, however, that after binding to cholesterol in the membrane, toxin–cholesterol complexes then aggregate in the horizontal plane of the membrane, causing increased membrane disorganization due to sequestering of cholesterol which is no longer available to interact with membrane phospholipids (Bernheimer, 1974; Rottem *et al.*, 1976). A similar hypothesis has been proposed for the cholesterol-specific polyene antibiotic filipin (Verkleij *et al.*, 1973; De Kruiff and Demel, 1974).

In no case is the contribution of oxygen-labile toxins to pathogenicity clearly established but the known tissue damaging properties of θ-toxin and streptolysin O are likely to be important in infections caused by *Cl. perfringens* and *St. pyogenes* (see below).

Other Membrane-damaging Toxins

There are many membrane damaging toxins other than phospholipases and oxygen-labile toxins. In most cases however the mode of action of these agents is still poorly understood by comparison with the toxins described above. Limitations of space precludes comprehensive coverage of this diverse group of agents and I have selected only three examples: streptolysin S, staphylococcal α-toxin and staphylococcal leukocidin. In each case the role in pathogenesis is not understood; but each of these entities has a potent effect on leukocytes and therefore may contribute to the establishment of infection.

Streptolysin S

Streptolysin S (SLS) is probably the most potent of all the membrane damaging toxins, having a specific activity of c. $1{\cdot}0 \times 10^7$ haemolytic units mg $^{-1}$ (Lai *et al.*, 1978). Although most work has been done using streptococci belonging to Lancefield Group A it is worth noting that production of SLS by Groups C, G, E, H and L has been reported. It has a wide and relatively nonspecific cytolytic activity, and is capable of damaging many cell types and subcellular organelles. It can be extracted from streptococcal cells by a number of different "carrier" substances—serum albumin, α-liptoprotein, RNA, ribonuclease resistant core RNA, and some nonionic detergents. The best characterized material has been prepared using resistant core RNA (Koyoma, 1963; Lai *et al.*, 1978). SLS also exists in a cell bound form (CBH) in which it appears to be associated with the external surface of the streptococcal surfaces (Ginsburg and Grossowicz, 1958), and in an intracellular form (Callandra and Oginsky, 1975). The biochemical and biological properties of SLS have been the subject of several reviews (Ginsburg, 1970; Bernheimer, 1972; Ginsburg, 1972; Jeljaszewicz *et al.*, 1978). The main properties of SLS are summarized briefly in Table III.

TABLE III.
Properties of streptolysin S.

(1) Exists as a cell bound haemolysin (CBH) and can be extracted by various carriers (e.g. yeast RNA, BSA)
(2) Polypeptide portion consists of approximately 30 amino acids which is active only in carrier-bound state, and is nonantigenic
(3) Cytotoxic for many eukaryotic cell types and for bacterial protoplasts
(4) CBH is responsible for leukotoxic activity of streptococci
(5) Mode of action is unknown but phospholipids inhibit SLS and haemolysis involves a colloid osmotic process

Staphylococcal α-toxin

The α-toxin is the most potent of the four membrane damaging toxins produced by *S. aureus*, being lethal in small doses for mice and rabbits. Highly purified preparations of α-toxin became available from the mid 1960s onwards and its physiochemical and biological properties have been studied in detail and have been the subject of several reviews (Arbuthnott, 1970; Bernheimer, 1974; Wiseman, 1975; Freer and Arbuthnott, 1976; McCartney and Arbuthnott, 1978). The properties of α-toxin are summarized in Table IV.

TABLE IV.
Properties of the staphylococcal α-toxin.

(1) Mol. wt = 26–39 000; Sw_{20} = 3·0 S (polymeric form = 12 S) Electrophoretically heterogeneous; isoelectric point of main form = 8·55
(2) Lethal (10^3) LD_{50} mg^{-1}, dermonecrotic and haemolytic (2×10^4 HU mg^{-1}—rabbit RBC)
(3) Causes increased permeability of small blood vessels and spastic contraction of smooth muscle
(4) Cytotoxic for many cell types *in vitro*
(5) Mode of action: binds to susceptible cells and causes perturbation of the hydrophobic region of the membrane

In the 1960s most work on α-toxin was concerned with its range of cytotoxic and pharmacological effects *in vivo* and *in vitro*. In the past 10–12 years, however, research has focussed on the molecular basis of its membrane damaging action. In particular, four aspects have been examined in some detail (see review of McCartney and Arbuthnott, 1978); (a) interaction of α-toxin with isolated mammalian cell membranes (mainly erythrocyte membranes) and with liposomes and aqueous dispersions of individual lipids; (b) the possible enzymatic action of α-toxin; (c) the release of intracellular markers from cells in tissue culture; (d) the existence of a specific receptor in erythrocyte membranes.

It is clear from this work that α-toxin can bind to cell membranes and can cause disorganization of the hydrophobic regions of cell membranes, resulting in permeability changes. However the precise molecular basis of these changes is still not known.

Staphylococcal α-toxin affects many cells and tissues (Jeljaszewicz *et al.*, 1978) and it has long been thought of as one of the most important factors in staphylococcal pathogenicity. Its necrotizing effects together with its action on blood vessels and leukocytes could be important in initiation of infection. Clear evidence of the role of α-toxin in a spreading gangrenous form of mastitis in rabbits has been established recently (Adlam *et al.*, 1977) and mutants deficient in α-toxin were found to be less virulent than parental strains (Van der Vijver *et al.*, 1975; Kinsman *et al.*, 1980) (see below).

Staphylococcal leucocidin

The most striking features of the Panton–Valentine leukocidin of *S. aureus* are its remarkable specificity of action (it acts only on polymorphonuclear cells (Gladstone and Van Heyningen, 1957), macrophages (Woodin, 1959) and mast cells (Kwarecki *et al.*, 1968) of human and rabbit) and the fact that it consists of two protein components designated F and S (Woodin, 1959, 1960) which act synergistically to generate leukotoxic activity; neither F or S by itself is toxic.

The biological activities and mode of action of leukocidin have been reviewed recently (Jeljaszewicz *et al.*, 1978; McCartney and Arbuthnott, 1978) and will be summarized briefly here. Much of our knowledge of this interesting but complex factor is due to the work of Woodin and his co-workers who studied leukocidin intensively over a period of about 12 years between 1959 and 1972.

Leukocytes exposed to leukocidin *in vitro* become immobilized, the pseudopodia disappear and cytoplasmic degranulation and rupture of the nucleus follows; at high concentrations the cells undergo complete lysis. The mechanism of cytotoxicity appears to be extremely complex. Woodin (1970) proposed that the synergistic action of the F and S components on the membranes of susceptible cells produces a channel permeable to cations. Triphosphoinositide, a minor phospholipid component of membranes, plays a key role in this process and may account for the specificity of the toxin. This perturbation of the membrane by leukocidin results in stimulation of K^{+}-sensitive acylphosphatase and adenylate cyclase which in turn leads to impairment of the sodium–potassium pump. In the presence of a high concentration of Ca^{2+} ions these events trigger a series of secondary effects.

Leukocidin is not lethal for experimental animals but when injected into rabbits it does cause significant changes in the kinetics and the functional state of granulocytes in the peripheral blood (Szmigielski *et al.*, 1973). Its role in pathogenesis is far from clear, although it is produced *in vivo* during staphylococcal infection as antibodies to this toxin are frequently found in the sera of patients with chronic infection.

EFFECTS OF MEMBRANE-DAMAGING TOXINS ON LEUKOCYTES

Until recently, evidence of membrane damage in leukocytes and other cells was assessed by various criteria such as cell lysis, degranulation, cytopathic effects and the development of cytoplasmic extrusions, the release of intracellular markers such as protein or methionine labelled with ^{35}S, and metabolic changes such as inhibition of enzymes involved in carbohydrate metabolism. More direct evidence relating to perturbation of the cell membrane has come from measurement of the release of K^+ ions from leukocytes exposed to staphylococcal leukocidin (Woodin, and Wieneki, 1968). More recently the elegant work of the Karolinska group (Thelestam and Möllby, 1975) showed clearly that certain toxins induced membrane lesions at doses of toxin lower than those required to induce damage as assessed by morphological observations and trypan blue staining.

The ability of several of the membrane damaging toxins described above to kill polymorphonuclear cells and macrophages is well known. In the case of SLS and SLO these toxic effects were studied in some detail during the 1960s (Bernheimer and Schwartz, 1960; Hirsch *et al.*, 1963; Zucher-Franklin, 1965; Fauve *et al.*, 1966). Both streptolysins were shown to induce degranulation of rabbit leukocyte suspensions following derangement of subcellular organization. In the case of SLS, Ofek, *et al.* (1970; 1972), working with mouse leukocytes, demonstrated interesting differences between the different carrier-bound forms of SLS (see above). While all forms of SLS killed mouse leukocyte monolayers at a concentration of 100 HU ml^{-1}, the cell bound haemolysin (CBH) acted more rapidly than either RNA-SLS or serum SLS. Also it was found that the leukotoxic activity of CBH did not require uptake of CBH by leukocytes; leukotoxicity could be demonstrated in the presence of the phagocytosis inhibitor iodoacetamide. These observations point to direct transfer of SLS from the streptococcal cell surface to its target site on the leukocyte. Similar observations were made previously by Ginsburg and Harris (1965) in studies of the interaction between SLS and Ehrlich ascites tumour cells.

From the point of view of the perturbation of host defences, it is perhaps more interesting to note that subtoxic doses of SLS and SLO impair both the phagocytic activity and the mobility of leukocytes. Ofek *et al.*, (1972) in their work with mouse leukocytes, showed that sublethal concentrations of SLS and SLO markedly inhibited phagocytosis of heat killed streptococci and suggested that such an effect might modify host response at an early stage of infection. In a related series of studies, Andersen and Van Epps (Andersen and Van Epps, 1972; Van Epps and Andersen, 1974) demonstrated that doses of SLO incapable of causing cell lysis or morphological changes inhibited chemotaxis and random mobility of human neutrophils. They also highlighted interesting differences in the response of leukocytes from different species; human neutrophils were markedly suppressed, baboon and sheep neutrophils were partially affected while rabbit neutrophils were unaffected. Such differences in the behaviour of cells from different species could be related to differences in the response of different species to experimental infections. The specificity of staphylococcal leucocidin for rabbit and human leukocytes has already been referred to. Much is known about the structural and metabolic changes that precede death of leukocytes exposed to leukocidin but it appears that perturbation of leukocytes by sublethal amounts of this toxin have not been studied in any detail, although Woodin (1971) emphasized the action of leukocidin as an inhibitor of various neutrophil functions including chemotaxis.

As an extension of his studies on chemotaxis, Wilkinson (1975; 1977) showed that while proteases and glycosidases had no effect on the locomotion of human neutrophils or monocytes towards casein or alkali-denatured human serum albumin (HSA) the three membrane damaging toxins tested (at sub-toxic doses) namely, *Cl. perfringens*, α-toxin, *S. aureus* β-toxin and *Cl. perfringenes* θ-toxin, had interesting effects. In the case of human leukocytes, both *Cl. perfringens* α-toxin and *S. aureus* β-toxin impaired the chemotaxis of monocytes but not neutrophils, whereas *Cl. perfringens* θ-toxin affected neutrophils but not monocytes. Again however, species differences were found, the chemotaxis of rabbit neutrophils being inhibited by all three membrane damaging toxins. Wilkinson's group (Wilkinson *et al.*, 1976) also drew attention to the fact that lymphocytes migrating chemotactically towards phytohaemagglutinin (PHA) exhibited a different pattern of results. Here the chemoattractant is a ligand known to bind to a glycoprotein receptor and treatment of lymphocytes with proteases or glycosidases reduced locomotion whereas membrane damaging toxins had no effect. In a detailed study of the binding of denatured HSA to human and rabbit neutrophils Wilkinson and Allan (1978) presented evidence that the binding of denatured HSA was specific and was impaired by prior treatment with *Cl. perfringens* θ-toxin and *S. aureus* β-toxin which are known to damage the hydrophobic lipid regions of cell membranes. On this basis they argue that the interaction sites of certain chemoattractants lie within the phospholipid bilayer.

There is therefore a considerable volume of evidence to show that sublethal amounts of membrane damaging toxins can perturb the membranes of leukocytes in such a way as to modify functions that we associate with the normal host response to infection.

In an attempt to obtain an overall view of the capacity of staphylococcal extracellular factors to affect the locomotion of human leukocytes Russell *et al* (1976) examined whole cells, culture supernates and fractions prepared by isoelectric focussing of nine strains of *S. aureus*. This revealed a complex pattern of both stimulatory and inhibitory activities.

The major direct chemotactic activity was for monocytes rather than neutrophils although staphylococci and their fractions also showed indirect chemotactic activity for neutrophils, generating chemotactic factors in the presence of plasma.

The pattern of inhibitory activity was also complex. Many fractions inhibited neutrophil locomotion while fewer fractions inhibited monocytes. Some of the inhibitory fractions could be presumptively identified: purified α-toxin inhibited both neutrophils and monocytes while the β-toxin acted preferentially on monocytes; leukocidin-rich preparations were strongly inhibitory for neutrophils but less inhibitory for monocytes. Mouse virulent strains of *S. aureus* are known to produce a cell-associated mucopeptide–protein complex, that exerts an anti-inflammatory effect and inhibits chemotaxis of neutrophils (Weksler and Hill, 1969). The extent to which extracellular inhibitory factors interact with this material *in vivo* to determine the outcome of infection is not yet understood.

ANIMAL MODELS

Knowledge of the chemical and biological properties of membrane damaging toxins and their effects on host defence cells provides certain clues as to the ways in which such factors might be involved in pathogenic mechanisms. Such studies, however, can be criticized on the grounds that *in vitro* effects bear little relation to the situation that pertains within a focus of infection *in vivo*. For this reason, we recently attempted to assess certain experimental animal models that might allow us to determine the *in vivo* role of staphylococcal membrane damaging toxins in pathogenesis.

Following on the successful use of newborn mice to study the pathogenesis of the staphylococcal scalded skin syndrome, McKay and Arbuthnott (1979) investigated the virulence of six strains of staphylococci of varying toxin and enzyme patterns in different age groups of mice from newborn to weanling. This revealed an age-related susceptibility to infection, in that newborn mice were more susceptible than older mice to death and lesion formation. Resistance to challenge, i.e. the ability to survive challenge to 10^7 cfu developed at about 5 days of age. On subcutaneous infection at low challenge dose, one of the six strains tested (SM9), which produced leukocidin but not detectable amounts of the α- or β- toxins *in vitro*, gave rise to an abcess type of lesion. Histopathological examination of excised skin showed a localized lesion under the dermis containing numerous staphylococci and a marked infiltration of leukocytes. This contrasted with the action of the toxinogenic strain (SM10) tested which produced spreading necrotic lesions in which the organisms spread extensively in the horizontal plane of subcutaneous tissue.

A relationship between virulence and inhibition of weight gain in neonatal mice was demonstrated (Kinsman and Arbuthnott, 1980) and clinical isolates could be ranked according to their effect on weight gain of newborn mice. These findings suggested that the weight gain test could be used to compare the virulence of mutants defective in individual virulence factors. Kinsman *et al.* (1980) prepared a small number of mutants that were defective in only α-toxin or coagulase production. These mutants, when tested in the weight gain test were found to be of reduced virulence, providing direct evidence for the involvement of α-toxin and coagulase in the newborn mouse model.

Convincing evidence for the role of α-toxin also came from the studies of experimental rabbit mastitis by Adlam *et al.* (1977). They showed that the introduction of low numbers of certain strains into mammary tissue caused a spreading lesion in which the mammary tissue became oedematous and haemorrhagic while other strains induced the formation of pus-filled abscesses. In rabbits immunized with highly purified α-toxin the lethal haemorrhagic oedematous form of the disease was reduced to a localized abscess form. No such protection was achieved by immunization with purified β-toxin. These results indicate that α-toxin is a key antigen in the haemorrhagic disease but the staphylococcal factors responsible for the localized abscess lesion are not yet known.

From this work it became clear that there was a need to devise a system which would allow us to study the growth of staphylococci *in vivo* and to monitor the response of the host to the production of virulence factors *in vivo*. We have found that chambers constructed from short lengths of plastic syringe barrels having both ends sealed with membrane filters, when implanted intraperitoneally in mice, can be used to study *in vivo* growth of staphylococci and the host response (Day *et al.*, 1980): larger chambers of the same design can be used in rabbits. This system permits a dynamic interchange of diffusible host and staphylococcal factors and the *in vivo* grown bacteria can be easily recovered for subsequent examination *in vitro*. Staphylococci remained viable in such chambers for up to 9 months.

Chambers containing staphylococci became encapsulated with fibrin and granulation tissue. This was first evident at two days after implantation as a thin mat adhering to the micropore filters. By six days chambers were totally encased; thick cream coloured mats covered the filters and semi-transparent material enveloped the whole chamber. The interior surface of the capsule adhering to the filter consisted mainly of polymorphonuclear cells while the external surface showed both polymorphonuclear and mononuclear cells. Control chambers containing saline did not become encapsulated and it was notable that over a period of 19 days the leukocyte counts in the peritoneal fluid of control and test animals was similar.

The formation of granulation tissue in response to the implantation of three staphylococcal strains was studied by removing chambers at time intervals over a period of 12 weeks and carefully dissecting and weighing the adherent material (Fig.). This revealed interesting strain differences; strain SM9, the non-toxinogenic strain mentioned earlier, induced the accumulation of considerably more capsulation material than either strain Wood 46, an α-toxinogenic strain or AW269 (*S. epidermidis*). The amount of granulation tissue formed could reflect the production of chemotactic factors, membrane damaging toxins and/or coagulase.

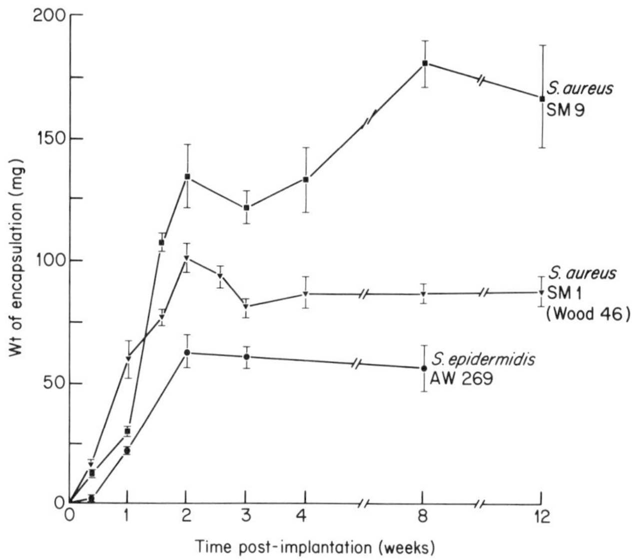

Fig. 1 Formation of granulation tissue by different strains of staphylococci. Mice were implanted each with 2 chambers containing 0·1 ml bacterial suspension, in 0·15 M NaCl, (10^4 cfu ml^{-1}). The mice were killed at different times postimplantation, and the inflammatory tissue encapsulating the chambers dissected out and weighed. For each time-point on the graph, encapsulation weights were averaged from 8 chambers (bars denote standard error).

That α-toxin is produced in such a system and diffuses from the chamber was shown by following the increase in anti α-toxin titre following implantation of strain Wood 46. In rabbits, serum levels of antitoxin began to rise 10 days after implantation and reached a maximum at 24–28 days. The response was slower in mice, beginning at 18 days and again reached a maximum at about 28 days.

This approach is still at a preliminary stage and so far has been restricted to staphylococci. Clearly, however, the chamber system is capable of being exploited to provide more detailed information on host–pathogen interactions and along with the application of modern genetic approaches is likely to play an important part in tackling this important problem.

SUMMARY

In this contribution I have attempted to give an overview of membrane damaging toxins in relation to perturbation of host defences. The availability of highly purified toxins has enabled detailed studies to be made of the mechanisms by which these toxins exert their cytolytic effect. This work has revealed that impairment of membrane functions can occur at subtoxic doses and that such subtle membrane changes profoundly affect the behaviour of the cells of the host defence system. I have outlined the principle effects on the phagocytic and chemotactic activities of polymorphonuclear and mononuclear cells. There are however, many other effects that are likely to mediate the inflammatory response. For instance several membrane damaging toxins act on mast cells and lymphocytes and the responses of these cell types may well be important in the outcome of host/pathogen interaction. Other mediators such as prostaglandins may also be generated as a result of the action of these toxins.

We have begun a series of studies with *in vivo* grown organisms aimed at evaluating which *in vitro* effects predominate *in vivo*. Preliminary results are encouraging but much work remains to be done in this field.

I am grateful to Dr R. J. Russell for his helpful discussions and for reading the manuscript and to Sarah Day for permission to include unpublished data.

REFERENCES

Abe, P. M., Kendall, Carol, J. and Stauffer, L. R. (1979). Haemolytic activity of *Fusobacterium necrophorum* supernatants due to presence of phospholipase A and lysophospholipase. *American Journal of Veterinary Research* 20, 92–96.

Adlam, C., Ward, P. D., McCartney, A. Christine, Arbuthnott, J. P. and Thorley, C. M. (1977). Effect of immunization with highly purified alpha- and beta- toxins on staphylococcal mastitis in rabbits. *Infection and Immunity* 17, 250–256.

Andersen, B. R. and Van Epps, D. E. (1972). Suppression of chemotactic activity of human neutrophils by streptolysin O. *Journal of Infectious Diseases* 125, 353–359.

Arbuthnott, J. P. (1970). Staphylococcal α-toxin. *In* "Microbiol Toxins" (Eds T. C. Montie, S. Kadis and S. J. Ajl), Vol. 3, pp. 189–236. Academic Press, New York.

Bernheimer, A. W. (1972). Haemolysins of streptococci: characterization and effects on biological membranes. *In* "Streptococci and Streptococcal Diseases" (Eds L. W. Wannamaker and J. M. Matsen), pp. 19–31. Academic Press, New York.

Bernheimer, A. W. (1974). Interactions between membranes and cytolytic bacterial toxins. *Biochemica et Biophysica Acta* 344, 27–50.

Bernheimer, A. and Schwartz, L. (1960). Leukocidal agents of haemolytic streptococci. *Journal of Pathology and Bacteriology* 79, 37–46.

Bullen, J. J. (1970). Role of toxins in host–parasite relationships. *In* "Microbial Toxins (Eds S. J. Ajl, S. Kadis and T. C. Montie), Vol. 1, pp. 233–276. Academic Press, London.

Calandra, G. B. and Oginsky, E. L. (1975). Cellular Streptolysin S-Related Hemolysins of Group A Streptococcus C203S. *Infection and Immunity* **12**, 13–28.

Cowell, J. L., Kim, K.-S. and Bernheimer, A. W. (1978). Alteration by cereolysin of the structure of cholesterol-containing membranes. *Biochemica et Biophysica Acta* **507**, 230–241.

Day, S. E. J., Vasli, K. K., Russell, R. J. and Arbuthnott, J. P. (1980). A simple method for the study *in vivo* of bacterial growth and accompanying host response. *Journal of Infection* **2**, 39–51.

De Kruiff, B. and Demel, R. A. (1974). Polyene antibiotic-sterol interactions in membranes of *Acholeplasma laidlawii* cells and lecithin liposomes. III Molecular structure of the polyene antibiotic-cholesterol complexes. *Biochemica et Biophysica Acta* **339**, 57–70.

Fauve, R., Alouf, J., Delauny, A. and Raynaud, M. (1966). Cytotoxic effects in vitro of highly purified streptolysin O on mouse macrophages. *Journal of Bacteriology* **92**, 1150–1153.

Freer, J. H. and Arbuthnott, J. P. (1976). Biochemical and morphologic alterations of membranes by bacterial toxins. *In* "Mechanisms in Bacterial Toxinology" (Ed. A. W. Bernheimer), pp. 169–194. John Wiley, New York.

Gladstone, G. P. and Van Heyningen, W. E. (1957). Staphylococcal leucocidins. *British Journal of Experimental Pathology* **38**, 123–137.

Ginsburg, I. (1970). Streptolysin S. *In* "Microbial Toxins" (Eds T. C. Montie, S. Kadis and S. J. Ajl), Vol. 3, pp. 100–171. Academic Press, New York.

Ginsburg, I. (1972). Mechanisms of cell and tissue injury induced by group A Streptococci; relation to post-Streptococcal sequelae. *Journal of Infectious Diseases* **126**, 294–340.

Ginsburg, I. and Grossowicz, N. (1958). A cell bound hemolysin of group A streptococci. *Bulletin of the Research Council of Israel* **7A**, 237–246.

Ginsburg, I. and Harris, T. N. (1965). Oxygen-stable haemolysins of group A streptococci IV. Studies on the mechanisms of lysis by cell bound haemolysin of red blood cells and Ehrlich ascites tumor cells. *Journal of Experimental Medicine* **121**, 647–656.

Hirsch, J., Bernheimer, A. and Weismann, G. (1963). Motion picture study of the toxic action of streptolysins on leukocytes. *Journal of Experimental Medicine* **118**, 223–228.

Jeljaszewicz, J., Szmigielski, S. and Hryniewicz, W. (1978). Biological effects of staphylococcal and streptococcal toxins. *In* "Bacterial Toxins and Cell Membranes". (Eds J. Jeljaszewicz and T. Wadstrom), pp. 185–227. Academic Press, London.

Kinsman, O. and Arbuthnott, J. P. (1980). Experimental staphylococcal infections in newborn mice: inhibition of weight gain as an index of virulence. *Journal of Medical Microbiology* **13**, 281–290.

Kinsman, O., Jonsson, P., Haraldson, I., Lindberg, M., Arbuthnott, J. P. and Wadstrom, T. (1980). Decreased virulence of alpha-haemolysin negative and coagulase negative mutants of *S. aureus* in experimental infections in mice. *In* "Proceedings of IVth International Symposium on Staphylococci and Staphylococcal Infections". Gustav Fischer Verlag, Stuttgart. In press.

Kojama, J. (1963). Biochemical studies of streptolysin S. II Properties of a polypeptide component and its role in the toxin activity. *Journal of Biochemistry* (Tokyo) **54**, 146–151.

Kwarecki, K., Szmigielski, S., Jeljaszewicz, J. and Zak, C. (1968). Injury of rat peritoneal mast cells in vivo by staphylococcal alpha hemolysin and leukocidin. *Journal of Infectious Diseases* **118**, 361–364.

Lai, C. Y., Wang, M.-T., deFaria, J. B. and Akao, T. (1978). Streptolysin S: improved purification and characterization. *Archives of Biochemistry and Biophysics* **191**, 804–812.

Levaditi, C. (1918). Action leucotoxique du streptocoque perplais de guerre; considerations sur le mécanisme de la phagocytose. *Comptes rendus des séarces de la Société de biologie* **81**, 1064–1067.

McCartney, A. C. and Arbuthnott, J. P. (1978). Mode of action of membrane-damaging toxins produced by staphylococci. *In* "Bacterial Toxins and Cell Membranes" (Eds J. Jeljaszewicz and T. Wadstrom), pp. 89–127. Academic Press, London and New York.

McKay, S. E. and Arbuthnott, J. P. (1979). Age-related susceptibility of mice to staphylococcal infection. *Journal of Medical Microbiology* **12**, 99–105.

Möllby, R. (1978). Bacterial phospholipases. *In* "Bacterial Toxins and Cell Membranes" (Eds J. Jeljaszewicz and T. Wadstrom), pp. 367–424. Academic Press, London and New York.

Mitsui, K., Sekiya, T., Nogawa, Y. and Hase, J. (1979). Alteration of human erythrocyte plasma membranes by perfringiolysin O as revealed by freeze-fracture electron microscopy. Studies on *Clostridum perfringins* exotoxins V. *Biochimica et Biophysica Acta* **554**, 68–75.

Ofek, I., Bergner-Rabinowitz, S. and Ginsburg, I. (1970). Oxygen-stable haemolysins of group A streptococci. VII The relation of the leukotoxic factor to streptolysins. *Journal of Infectious Diseases* **122**, 517–522.

Ofek, I., Bergner-Rabinowitz, S. and Ginsburg, I. (1972). Oxygen stable haemolysins of group A streptococci. VIII Leukotoxic and antiphagocytic effects of streptolysins S and O. *Infection and Immunity* **6**, 459–464.

Pugh, D. and Cawson, R. A. (1975). The cytochemical localization of phospholipase A and lysophospholipase in *Candida ablicans. Sabouraudia* **13**, 110–115.

Pugh, D. and Cawson, R. A. (1977). The cytochemical localization of phospholipase in *Candida albicans* infecting the chick chorio-allantoic membrane. *Sabouraudia* **15**, 29–35.

Rottem, S., Hardegree, M. C., Gabrowski, M. W., Fornwald, R. and Barile, M. F. (1976). Interaction between tetanolysin and mycoplasma cell membrane. *Biochemica et Biophisica Acta* **455**, 876–888.

Russell, R. J., Wilkinson, P. C., McInroy, R. J., McKay, S., McCartney, A. C. and Arbuthnott, J. P. (1976). Effects of staphylococcal products on locomotion and chemotaxis of human blood neutrophils and monocytes. *Journal of Medical Microbiology* **8**, 433–449.

Smith, H. (1977). Microbial surfaces in relation to pathogenicity. *Bacteriological Reviews* **45**, 475–500.

Smyth, C. J. and Duncan, J. L. (1978). Thiol activated (oxygen-labile) cytolysins. *In* "Bacterial Toxins and Cell Membranes" (Eds J. Jeljaszewicz and T. Wadstrom), pp. 129–183. Academic Press, London and New York.

Souček, A., Michalec, C. and Součková, A. (1971). Identification and characterization of a new enzyme of the group "phospholipase D" isolated from *Corynebacterium ovis*. *Biochemica et Biophysica Acta* **227**, 116–128.

Součková, A., and Souček, A. (1972). Inhibition of the haemolytic action of α- and β-lysins of *Staphylococcus pyogenes* by *Corynebacterium haemolyticum, C. ovis* and *C. ulcerans*. *Toxicon* **10**, 501–509.

Szmigielski, S., Kwarecki, K., Jeljaszewicz, J., Möllby, R. and Wadstrom, T. (1973). Alpha-toxin and leukocidin effects on granulopoiesis. *In* "Staphylococci and Staphylococcal Infections" (Ed. J. Jeljaszewicz), pp. 202–208. S. Karger, Basel.

Thelestam, M. and Möllby, R. (1975). A sensitive assay for detection of toxin induced damage to the cytoplasmic membrane of human diploid fibroblasts. *Infection and Immunity* **12**, 225–232.

Van de Velde, H. (1894). Etude sur le mécanisme de la virulence du Staphylocoque pyogene. *La Cellule* **10**, 401–460.

Van der Vijver, J. C. M., Van Es-Boon, M. M. and Michel, M. F. (1975). A study of virulence factors with induced mutants of *Staph. aureus*. *Journal of Medical Microbiology* **8**, 279–287.

Van Epps, D. E. and Anderson, B. R. (1974). Streptolysin O inhibition of neutrophil chemotaxis and mobility: non immune phenomonon with species specificity. *Infection and Immunity* **9**, 27–33.

Verkleij, A. J., De Kruiff, B., Gerritsen, W. F., Demel, R. A., Van Deenan, L. L. M. and Ververgaert, P. H. J. (1973). Freeze-etch electron microscopy of erythrocytes, *Acholeplasma laidlawii* cells and liposomal membranes after the action of filipin and amphotericin B. *Biochimica et Biophysica Acta* **291**, 577–581.

Ward, P. D., Adlam, C., McCartney, A. C., Arbuthnott, J. P. and Thorley, C. M. (1979). A histopathological study of the effects of highly purified staphylococcal alpha- and beta- toxins on the lactating mammary gland and skin of the rabbit. *Journal of Comparative Pathology* **89**, 169–177.

Weksler, B. B. and Hill, M. J. (1969). Inhibition of leukocyte migration by a staphyloccal factor. *Journal of Bacteriology* **98**, 1030–1035.

Wilkinson, P. C. (1975). Inhibition of leukocyte locomotion and chemotaxis by specific bacterial toxins. *Nature (London)* **255**, 485–487.

Wilkinson, P. C. (1977). Action of sphingomyelinase C and other lipid specific agents as inhibitors of Fc binding and locomotion in human leucocytes. *Immunology* **33**, 407–412.

Wilkinson, P. C. and Allan, R. B. (1978). Binding of protein chemotactic factors to the surfaces of neutrophil leucocytes and its modification with lipid-specific bacterial toxins. *Molecular and Cellular Biochemistry* **20**, 25–40.

Wilkinson, P. C., Roberts, J. A., Russell, R. J. and McLoughlin, M. (1976). Chemotaxis of mitogen-activated human lymphocytes and the effects of membrane-active enzymes. *Clinical and Experimental Immunology* **25**, 280–287.

Wiseman, G. M. (1975). The Haemolysins of *Staphylococcus aureus. Bacteriological Reviews* **39**, 317–344.

Woodin, A. M. (1959). Fractionation of the two components of leukocidin from *Staphylococcus aureus. Biochemical Journal* **73**, 225–237.

Woodin, A. M. (1960). Purification of the two components of leukocidin from *Staphylococcus aureus. Biochemical Journal* **75**, 158–165.

Woodin, A. M. (1970). Staphylococcal leukocidin. *In* "Microbial Toxins" (Eds T. C. Montie, S. Kadis and S. J. Ajl), Vol. 3, pp. 327–356. Academic Press, New York.

Woodin, A. M. (1971). Leucocidin, DFP, the leucocyte pump and inhibition of chemotaxis. *In* "The Reticuloendothelial System and Immune Phenomena" (Eds N. R. di Luzio and K. Fleming), p. 71. *Advances in Experimental Medicine and Biology*, Vol. **15**. Plenum, New York.

Woodin, A. M. and Wieneke, A. A. (1968). Role of leucocidin and triphosphoinositide in the control of potassium permeability. *Nature (London)* **220**, 283–286.

Zucher-Franklin, D. (1965). Electron microscope study of the degranulation of polymorphonuclear leukocytes following treatment with streptolysin. *American Journal of Pathology* **47**, 419–434.

DISCUSSION

Mims It is nice to hear about 1930-type experiments as long as we don't do them like 1930-type people.

van Furth Do you think that the site of toxin attack on phagocytic cells is the outer membrane?

Arbuthnott In the case of the toxins which I talked about I think it is the outer membrane of the phagocytic cell. These toxins have very well defined actions on the cytoplasmic membrane of many cell types, as I tried to indicate, and they are all specific for certain membrane components. I think that the action is principally on the outer membrane of the cell.

van Furth I ask the question because I wondered whether anybody had considered the possibility that when ingested bacteria remain in the phagosome and are not killed, they still produce these toxins. Then there might also be an intracellular action of toxins, although phagosomes are in reality extracellular space. Would there be a difference when serum is present or not? It might well be that it is important to have the interaction of the toxins and serum opsonins around the injected bacteria and this could counteract any intracellular action.

Arbuthnott I think that is a most interesting suggestion, but I do not know of any specific information about the production of these factors intracellularly. One of the important things for future work in this field is the development of sensitive methods of toxin detection, both in tissues and in the kind of situation which you have indicated inside the phagocytic cell. If we had these methods of detection we would be able to answer these questions.

Jeljaszewicz I want to spend a little while on a group of toxins which Professor Arbuthnott could not talk about in a short presentation. These are the substances which interfere with blood clotting and fibrinolysis. There are many more than the staphylocoagulase which is usually recognized. It is well known that staphylocoagulase, in contrast to physiological clotting, forms a direct complex with prothrombin stoichiometrically, which then exerts a direct polymerizing effect on fibrinogen, thus producing fibrin, without activation of the fibrinolytic system.

Coagulase is a typical example of a blood clotting substance produced by bacteria, but we have recently shown that staphylocoagulase action may be simulated by a protease which has been isolated by Drapeau in Canada in a pure form. This metalloprotease produces the same clot as staphylocoagulase. We are therefore proposing a modified test for coagulase which contains an inhibitor of protease, so the end result can be attributed to coagulase and not to any metalloprotease present.

However, there are other enzymes or substances which produce fibrin. One which has been isolated by us in collaboration with a Swedish group is identical to staphylocoagulase but is produced by *Peptococcus indolicus*. Also, as I mentioned yesterday, there are several, as yet unidentified, substances of a proteolytic nature produced by *Pseudomonas* and others produced by *Bacteroides melaniogenicus*. We suspect that *Candida albicans* also produces "activators" of clotting and/or fibrinolysis. Probably there are many more and old reports in the literature, which have been neglected or rejected, concerning clotting-like effects by bacteria, and need to be re-investigated.

There are also substances which produce so-called "paracoagulation", such as protamine sulphate which do not polymerize fibrinogen, like thrombin, staphylocoagulase or peptocoagulase, but just precipitate fibrinogen. The best known example is the clumping factor of *Staphylococcus*, but M and T proteins of *Streptococcus pyogenes* also exert the same effect. The protein T of streptococci which has recently been purified by two groups (ours and one in California) can produce a Shwartzman-like reaction through fibrinoid formation in the kidneys.

In my opinion these substances should be taken into consideration when thinking about colonization and the pathogensis of infection and when listing substances which can interfere with many natural mechanisms. This is because during the process of clotting there is a chain of events, including platelet involvement. We know that the release from platelets of many substances of very high biological activity can be of tremendous importance and may perhaps mediate attachment to surfaces including the vascular wall and other surfaces.

If I may slightly disagree with you on one point, Professor Arbuthnott, there is no single staphylococcal product, whether cellular or extracellular which determines staphylococcal infection. I am still not convinced about α-toxin. I think that we still have to have a host factor which significantly influences infection with staphylococci; there must exist a predisposing factor because, by themselves, staphylococci are not pathogenic. They require a defect of some sort in the host and we can speculate that this might influence the fastest activity of staphylococci: clumping. This may prevent phagocytosis and occurs within seconds in the presence of host fibrinogen, which is present not only in blood but other biological fluids. Then protein A may exert the effect which is well known and was discussed yesterday. Later, when the *Staphylococcus* is established, exotoxin production, which takes a few hours at least, can exert all the damaging effects you mention.

Arbuthnott I am not in disagreement with Professor Jeljaszewicz in his views on staphylococcal pathogenicity. I would not claim that α-toxin is the only or even the main factor involved in staphylococcal infection, it is just one of many factors. But there are some situations in which I think we can say that specific tissue-damaging effects are due to that toxin. I think that gangrenous mastitis is one. It is interesting to pursue that a little further because Chris Adlem and his colleagues showed that if you immunize rabbits against α-toxin, you prevent this widespread gangrenous effect. The organism becomes localized and you get a characteristic purulent type of lesion. You do not eliminate or prevent the *Staphylococcus* from establishing itself. So I would agree α-toxin is only one of several factors involved.

Mims It is likely, of course that something important for a *Staphylococcus* infecting a hair follicle might not be so important for a *Staphylococcus* producing gangrene in some central organ.

Arbuthnott I think that is an important point. *Staphylococcus aureus* produces many types of disease. In some of these we can see the role of toxins: for example, in food poisoning or in the scalded skin syndrome where the epidermis is separated from the underlying tissue and you get very extensive blistered lesions appearing. It is an extracellular toxin, epidermolytic toxin, which is responsible for that manifestation of the disease. But the question of what is the factor or what are the factors which allow the organism to become established in this very important initial period which Professor Jeljaszewicz was talking about are still unknown.

Easmon I would like to come back to this initial period after infection. If these membrane-active toxins are going to be effective they have got to be present in the right concentration within two or three hours of the initiation of infection, particularly if they are going to inhibit chemotaxis in a useful way. Is it known how quickly organisms put into the tissues will produce these toxins and what concentrations they will achieve in this very short time?

Arbuthnott That is a difficult question. Frank Kapral has used an intraperitoneal model to study experimental staphylococcal infections. He has used a variety of toxinogenic or nontoxinogenic and encapsulated or nonencapsulated strains. He has shown that once the cells have clumped and begin to form a focus of infection toxin production occurs. When the lesion becomes walled off and surrounded by inflammatory cells in granulation tissue, the level of toxin increases quite substantially and fairly large amounts are produced. I cannot remember offhand just how long it takes for detectable amounts of toxin to be produced. This comes back to the problem I outlined earlier that our methods of detection of small concentrations of toxin *in vivo* are not adequate at present and I would like to emphasize that these toxins perturb cell membranes at sublethal or subtoxic doses. I do not think we should necessarily be thinking in terms of large amounts of toxins being involved in this initial period. Very small concentration of toxin may suffice, but we do not know anything about the kinetics of that at present and we should try to devise ways of tackling the problem.

Jeljaszewicz I would just like to say that before Kapral, Gladstone demonstrated that small amounts of α-toxin are produced in peritoneal chambers.

Smith One way in which we may in the future anlyse the situation may be to combine the sort of animal model that Professor Arbuthnott has described with the use of specific antibody—dare I mention monoclonal antibodies? If you had specific antibodies against all the various toxins their influence on the early stages of infection could be studied in the animal models described. This might tell which of the toxins were important in the early infective stages, but it will be a long time before we have all the antibodies to do the job.

Arbuthnott I think that is a very good approach to the problem, but another way of tackling it is by genetic manipulation of the organism. In that regard we are now entering a phase when we certainly can begin to do quite sophisticated experiments.

Wilton Professor Arbuthnott has shown very clearly that *in vitro* sublethal doses of certain staphylococcal toxins have an inhibitory effect on chemotaxis and yet in his pictures those lesions are absolutely stuffed with cells. I think we want to revise the idea that chemotaxis *in vivo* is just operating to increase cells migrating to an area, but possibly turn the thing on its head and say it is also keeping them there once they arrive. The range over which these molecules can exert their effect is really very small and I do not think that, except in cases of massive or disseminated infection, those moieties which have been shown to inhibit chemotaxis are going to operate on the other side of the blood vessel. That is the first point I want to make.

The second refers to Professor Smith's point about monoclonal antibodies. You would have to be very careful about the interpretation of that sort of experiment because you would have effects due to immune complexes which might have nothing to do with the initial toxin effects. That might be what is happening in the immune host with antibodies to these toxins, but I think you want to remember in designing that sort of experiment what happens when you inject very small amounts of immune complexes and the cutaneous lesions you can get.

Arbuthnott My remit was to deal with the inhibitory effects of toxins, which I tried to summarize, but I would just like to re-emphasize the comment I made earlier that staphylococci produce a number of chemotaxins and chemotaxinogens and clearly interactions *in vivo* are complex. It seems that in our chamber model the chemotactic response is dominant because these chambers are surrounded by very large numbers of cells although, as I indicated, strains vary in the amount of encapsulation material produced.

Beale Chris Adlam's α-toxoid has now been tried against gangrenous mastitis in sheep and will prevent death and gangrenous disease although, as we already know from the rabbit experiments, it does not prevent infection and the development of pustules. However, it does prevent death and it does prevent the loss of a mammary gland.

Campa I have a very simple question. Do we know anything about differences in species susceptibility of cells in relation to receptors and if so, whether the expression of these receptors is under genetic control?

Arbuthnott I mentioned briefly that many of the cytolytic or membrane-damaging toxins exhibit species specificity. This can be seen in various ways. For instance, the α-toxin of *Staphylococcus aureus* is very haemolytic for rabbit erythrocytes, moderately haemolytic for sheep erythrocytes and almost totally inactive against human erythrocytes. Sydney Harshmann in America claims that there is a receptor in the rabbit erythrocyte membrane and not in the human erythrocyte membrane and that is the reason for the specificity. In other cases the specificity can quite simply be demonstrated in terms of phospholipid composition. This is the case for the β-toxin of *Staph. aureus*; cells which are rich in sphingomyelin, like bovine cells, are very susceptible to the action of the toxin; cells which are not so rich are less sensitive. So we do have some clues, but I do not think we have much information about specificity in relation to the membranes of phagocytic cells.

Perhaps I could ask the people who know more about phagocytic cells than I do, what is known about differences in the membranes and in the receptors of these cells in different species.

Wilton The only difference I know relates to the Fc–IgG receptor and that is in the human. Goat IgG does not bind, so it is a very useful species of antibody to get over nonspecific effects of binding to Fc receptors if you are seeking rather more specific effects. As far as I am aware there is enormous cross-species binding of all classes of IgG on to all phagocytes, but nevertheless there are differences in affinity. I think Graham Leslie's work from Nottingham shows very nicely the differences within subclasses of IgG in their affinity for the receptors on the guinea-pig monocyte.

Valdimarsson I want to ask one question and make one comment. The question is about phospholipase A that may or may not be associated with Candida. Is it cell-bound or released into the environment?

Arbuthnott So far as I know, it is cell-bound.

Valdimarsson As I am not a microbiologist, I have some conceptual difficulties in relation to the definition of toxins. As I understand it, they are defined either as something which is lethal to the animal or tissue damaging. The tissue damage could be due to direct toxic effect on cells or to the activation of a clotting system, or to the activation of other inflammatory mechanisms.

I feel that some of the so-called toxins could be substances which would stimulate rather than perturb the defence mechanism by inducing phlogistic responses. It might be worth reassessing the factors that are released by the bacteria in terms of their ability to perturb the immune or defence responses. Perhaps we could talk about toxins on the one hand and perturbants—for lack of a better word—on the other hand in relation to defence mechanisms. There may be a lot of factors released from microorganisms that without being tissue damaging could have an important depressive influence on the inflammatory and defence response and this would sometimes be quite different from any directly toxic activities.

Arbuthnott Dr Valdimarsson is not alone in being confused in relation to what is a toxin. This question concerns toxinologists at almost every meeting and we have some strongly held views. The best definition of a toxin that I can find is a substance which produces harmful effects when introduced in small doses. That definition is very weak. What is a harmful effect and what is a small dose? Dick Finkelstein, who has done much work with cholera toxin and *E. coli* enterotoxins, takes a very strict line. He maintains that we should not give agents the name "toxin" unless they have been proved to have a pathological effect in the disease process.

I think that that is too strict a definition, but many years ago Professor Oakley attempted to remove the word "toxin" from papers which were submitted to the *Journal of Pathology and Bacteriology*. He later commented that his attempts failed because the word was so widely used and imbued with so much mystery that he could not find a suitable substitute.

Bacterial Mechanisms for Inhibition of Ingestion by Phagocytic Cells

PAUL G. QUIE, G. SCOTT GIEBINK
and PHILLIP K. PETERSON

Departments of Pediatrics, Microbiology and Internal Medicine,
University of Minnesota Medical School,
Minneapolis, Minnesota, USA.

INTRODUCTION

Bacteria associated with human hosts possess surface properties which allow attachment to cell surfaces and capacity for multiplication (colonization). When bacteria invade the environmental barriers of their host and multiply and become successful parasites in tissue they often possess capacity to resist attachment to scavenging phagocytic cells. Therefore, attachment may be an advantage for the microbe in one situation, i.e. on mucosal surfaces, but a disadvantage in tissue.

Most species rely on surface structures and other properties to prevent phagocytosis. Much has been learned about the physiochemical characteristics of these surface structures of bacteria which interact with the microenvironment of the host, such as surface charge or hydrophobicity. Other factors are also involved. For example, lipopolysaccharide is a bacterial surface component of many Gram negative bacteria which may damage phagocytic cells. The lipid A component of lipopolysaccharide is believed to be responsible for many of the biologic activities of these Gram negative bacteria including cytotoxicity, activation of the coagulation system, and pyrogenicity.

The cell walls of most Gram positive bacteria consist of a "backbone" of peptidoglycan which is interlaced with other components such as lipoteichoic acid or autolytic enzymes. These structures are antiphagocytic, i.e. resist phagocytosis by phagocytic cells since surface factors resist attachment of bacteria to cells. Fortunately for the host, however, cell wall surfaces of most bacteria favour the association of a serum alternative complement pathway protein factor B with actively opsonic C3b in serum. When this happens a C3 convertase is activated on the bacterial surface. The presence of this C3 convertase amplifies the deposition of C3b on the bacteria and they attach to phagocytic cells, are phagocytized and killed without specific antibacterial antibodies.

Bacterial species with capsules (usually polysaccharide) have "nonactivating" surfaces which do not support alternative pathway complement activation. These organisms need specific antibody against capsular surface antigens for opsonization. Antibody associated with bacterial surface antigens activate C1q, a serum recognition protein and the classical pathway C3 convertase is activated on the capsule surface. This stimulates C3b deposition on the surface of bacteria. Opsonization, therefore, is a major host defence mechanism which is activated by the alternative pathway in nonencapsulated organisms and after specific antibodies are formed by the classical pathway in encapsulated organisms.

Understanding of the physical structure and chemical composition of the surface of microbes and receptors on host phagocytic cells as well as function of humoral factors which increase efficiency of attachment is necessary for increased understanding of microbial virulence and host resistance. This report will review recent investigation of microbial–phagocyte interactions with emphasis on observations from the authors' laboratory.

HYDROPHOBIC SURFACE PROPERTIES OF BACTERIA

Physical forces involved in bacterial–host cell interactions include hydrophobic attraction between bacteria and host cells. A pili-related attachment site has been identified (Smyth *et al.*, 1978). There is strong evidence that hydrophobic bonds are involved in attachment of piliated *E. coli* to intestinal mucosal epithelium. Similar findings have also been reported for *Streptococcus pyogenes* (Tylewska *et al.*, 1979). These authors have shown that *S. pyogenes* with M protein have higher surface hydrophobicity and attachment to epithelial cells than M-negative strains. *Salmonella typhimurium* species which are encapsulated and rough mutants of these strains (nonencapsulated) have been compared for properties of adherence to polymorphonuclear leukocytes (Edebo *et al.*, 1979). The encapsulated bacteria are less hydrophobic and adhere less well to epithelial and phagocytic cells than the nonencapsulated or rough strains. An interesting contrast has been found in the properties of specific anticapsular antibodies of the IgA class and the IgG class. IgA antibodies decreased the hydrophobicity of the bacteria and reduced adherence to epithelial and phagocytic cells, therefore, prevented adherence. Anticapsular IgG antibodies, on the other hand, increased hydrophobicity and greatly increased adherence between bacteria and phagocytic cells. Bacteria which have high adherence to epithelial and mucosal cells, i.e. rough strains may have little virulence when they cross natural anatomical barriers. They adhere to phagocytic cells and are quickly eliminated. An exception to this rule of course is bacterial endocarditis where adherent organisms (primarily streptococcal species) reach the blood stream, adhere to surfaces on heart valves and because of fibrin deposition and other factors are sequestered from phagocytic cells. Successful parasites have surface properties which colonize mucosal surface and when invasion of tissue occurs are capable of resisting phagocytosis until specific antibacterial antibodies develop.

STAPHYLOCOCCUS AUREUS

Staphylococci are not killed by serum, therefore, phagocytosis by polymorphonuclear neutrophils or macrophages is necessary for host defence against staphylococcal disease. Our laboratory has concentrated on investigation of the interaction of staphylococci with phagocytic cells and serum factors which influence this interaction.

Protein A is a surface factor on nearly all strains of *Staphylococcus aureus* which binds to immunoglobulins in serum without immune specificity. Protein A binds to the Fc part of the immunoglobulin molecule so that antibodies may not be effective as opsonin. Furthermore, protein A released from the organisms activates complement in the fluid phase and complement, therefore, is no longer available to attach to the bacterial surface and serve its function as an opsonic amplifying mechanism (Dossett *et al.*, 1969). Evidence from our laboratory suggests that protein A may play a role in the severity of staphylococcal infection. For example, protein A rich strains are phagocytized poorly when serum has a high concentration of IgG and, in addition, there is reduced amplification of opsonic effect by complement. Protein A enhanced phagocytosis when immunoglobulins were deficient in serum which suggests that complement is directly activated on the surface of bacteria without immunologically specific antigen–antibody in the presence of protein A (Peterson *et al.*, 1977). Another bacterial species which may survive because of a direct effect of a virulence factor on the complement system is *Pseudomonas aeruginosa.* It has been shown that *P. aeruginosa* elastase acts on complement opsonic factor C3b and complement chemotactic factor C5a and these critical humoral factors are inactivated (Schultz *et al.*, 1974).

The cell wall of *Staphylococcus aureus* contains peptidoglycan (mucopeptide) which consists of peptide units connected to pentaglycine bridges and it is this structure which gives the cell wall its rigid structure. Staphylococcal cell walls also contain teichoic acids, either ribitol or glycerol and patients with prolonged staphylococcal disease develop high titres of antibody to teichoic acid which is useful as a serologic diagnostic tool (Crowder and White, 1972). Both cell wall peptidoglycan and teichoic acid are antiphagocytic factors and staphylococci may also possess a capsular structure which is antiphagocytic.

Opsonization is necessary for efficient phagocytosis of *Staphylococcus aureus.* Patients develop heat stable serum opsonins after severe staphylococcal infections, i.e. patients with staphylococcal endocarditis have high titres of heat stable opsonic antibodies which belonged to the IgG class of immunoglobulins (Messner *et al.*, 1968). Although patients with endocarditis have high titres of opsonic activity against their infecting organisms, in heated serum equal opsonic activity is present in fresh serum from patients and from controls suggesting that complement is a primary opsonin for *Staphylococcus aureus.*

When factors which block the Fc fragment of IgG, such as antigammaglobulin factors and protein A are present in serum or when antibody molecules are altered by pepsin or ε-aminocaproic acid, opsonic activity is depressed which suggest that opsonic antibodies, in addition to neutralizing antiphagocytic factors on the surface of bacteria also act as ligands binding bacteria to the surface of phagocytic cells. The Fab part of antibody molecule attaches with immunologic specificity to the surface of the bacteria and the Fc portion attaches to receptors on the phagocyte. The host determinants that are required for efficient opsonization and phagocytosis include antibodies, both specific and cross-reacting, and complement factors which are activated by either classical or alternative pathways.

A method has been established in our laboratory using [^{3}H] thymidine labelled bacteria which allows simultaneous, independent evaluation of the process of opsonization, attachment, ingestion, and killing of staphylococci (Verhoef *et al.*, 1977). The bacteria are opsonized in serum from a variety of sources, i.e. with and without complement factors and with and without immunoglobulin. Uptake of the labelled bacteria by phagocytes was determined at several time points during incubation to determine kinetics of phagocytosis. Using this method with chelated serum or C2 deficient serum as reagents allows measurement of the alternative pathway of complement activation. *Staphylococcus aureus* are slowly opsonized via the alternative pathway, i.e. opsonization via the classical pathway was complete within five minutes while 60 minutes are necessary for opsonization via the alternative pathway. Once complement (presumably C3b) is attached to the bacterial surface, either by the alternative or the classical pathway, organisms were efficiently phagocytized. Bacteria opsonized without complement were not only less efficiently attached to the phagocyte but more slowly engulfed.

Peptidoglycan, a major component of the cell wall of *Staphylococcus aureus* appears to be a scaffold to which peptides, lipids, and teichoic acids are attached. A variety of opsonins were used to determine opsonic requirements of these surface factors of staphylococci. Peptidoglycan in the absence of teichoic acid and teichoic acid deficient mutants of *S. aureus* are opsonized and engulfed as rapidly as staphylococci with teichoic acid using different opsonin sources. *Staphylococcus aureus* peptidoglycan is a potent activator of complement, and there is a direct parallel between kinetics of complement activation and kinetics of opsonization. Staphylococcal cell wall peptidoglycan, therefore, by its property of associating with immunoglobulin and by activating complement plays a significant role in the recognition of staphylococci by phagocytic cells (Verhoef *et al.*, 1977).

Not all strains of staphylococci are opsonized and phagocytized efficiently by normal human serum. *S. aureus* which possess a polysaccharide capsule are not phagocytized efficiently without antibody (Peterson *et al.*, 1978). The capsular polysaccharide acts as a barrier to phagocytosis unless specific antibodies are present. We found that encapsulated variants of two strains of staphylococci were poorly opsonized in a variety of serum sources (fresh, chelated and immunoglobulin-depleted) which effectively opsonized nonencapsulated strains. The capsule, therefore, appears to interfere with phagocytic cell recognition of bacteria that have been opsonized with either IgG and C3B. When rabbits are immunized with capsulated staphylococci, capsulated strains of staphylococci are opsonized by specific anticapsular antibodies. These antibodies opsonized the surface of the capsule and provided recognition sites or ligands for phagocytic cells.

We found that encapsulated staphylococci activated complement in chelated serum (via the alternative pathway) and there was fixation on the bacterial cell wall of the encapsulated staphylococci (Peterson, 1977). Capsular material, therefore, does not interfere with complement activation by peptidoglycan or association of C3b to the bacterial cell wall. The capsule does, however, prevent recognition and attachment of staphylococci to phagocytic cell surfaces. The capsule masks the opsonic ligands on the bacterial cell walls. When specific anticapsular antibodies are present, however, opsonic ligands are present on the surface and efficient phagocytosis takes place.

There is marked hetrogeneity in opsonic requirements among strains of staphylococci (Verhoef *et al.*, 1977). Using radiolabelled bacteria and a variety of serum sources two of the three strains of *S. aureus* (502 and Cowan I) required activation of the classical complement pathway for opsonization. Protein A rich strains are efficiently opsonized in immunoglobulin deficient serum but not in MgEGTA chelated serum, i.e. they are opsonized via the classical pathway but without requirement for immunoglobulin. *Staphylococcus aureus* Wood 46 could opsonize efficiently in MgEGTA serum but IgG was required. Two of three *S. epidermidis* strains required complement for efficient opsonization while a third strain did not.

STREPTOCOCCUS PNEUMONIAE

Streptococcus pneumoniae has a polysaccharide capsule which is antiphagocytic. The capsule is a major virulence factor of *S. pneumoniae* since these organisms do not release extracellular toxin, they are rapidly killed after phagocytosis by granulocytes and monocytes. Efficient killing of pneumococci requires the participation of serum opsonic factors including complement and immunoglobulin. Most strains of pneumococci require specific anticapsular antibodies and complement for efficient opsonization and phagocytosis but there is marked heterogeneity of opsonic requirements among pneumococcal serotypes (Giebink *et al.*, 1977). The kinetics of uptake of four different serotypes of *S. pneumoniae* by human granulocytes was measured in our laboratory using radiolabelled bacteria and a variety of serum sources including normal serum, heat-inactivated serum, IgG deficient serum, C2 deficient serum, and MgEGTA chelated serum. All four serotypes were opsonized by the alternative pathway of complement activation but there were striking differences in the quantity of serum necessary for effective opsonization. These differences in opsonic requirements may be related to the propensity of certain serotypes to be prominent sources of human disease while other serotypes are rarely recovered from pathologic lesions. The rather specific opsonic requirements of pneumococcal strains may also explain the predisposition of patients with antibody or complement deficiencies to suffer severe pneumococcal disease. Patients with overwhelming pneumococcal bacteraemia may have complement depletion because of activation in the circulation via the alternative pathway.

Complement activation products have profound biologic activities including activation of the clotting system and aggregation of leukocytes leading to pulmonary dysfunction. In order to study the possible effect of complement activation on the pathogenesis of pneumococcal disease, the levels of complement components, complement breakdown products, and opsonic activity was measured in patients with pneumococcal bacteremia (Giebink *et al.*, 1980). In one patient there was evidence of C3 breakdown products, depressed levels of serum C3 and depressed serum opsonic activity. The patient died. Surviving patients had depressed C3 and C4 serum levels but opsonic activity was normal. All had normal complement levels during convalescence. Depression of opsonically active serum complement components by the polysaccharide of *S. pneumoniae* may be important in the pathogenesis of disease in certain patients with defective host defences such as postsplenectomy patients. Absence of splenic function may allow replication of pneumococci with large numbers of circulating organisms. Complement activation may take place in serum and bacteria are not cleared from the blood-stream due to a deficient reticulo-endothelial system. This may lead to further depletion of opsonic capacity and result in overwhelming sepsis. We tested this hypothesis by incubating pneumococcal organisms and polysaccharide in human serum (Giebink *et al.*, 1978). Serum was incubated with suspensions of whole *S. pneumoniae* types 6, 7, 18, or 23 or with purified capsular polysaccharide from each of these types, and residual complement activity and opsonic capacity were measured. Haemolytic C3–9 complement activity and opsonic capacity for ^{3}H-thymidine labelled *Salmonella typhimurium*, a species effectively opsonized via the alternative pathway, were reduced in serum following incubation. Polysaccharide concentrations as low as 1 μg ml^{-1} inhibited serum opsonic capacity for *Salmonella.* Whole pneumococci and pneumococcal capsular polysaccharide also inhibited the opsonic activity of human C2 deficient serum for *Salmonella*, further evidence for activation of complement via the alternative pathway. Pneumococcal capsular polysaccharide markedly inhibited the opsonic capacity of normal serum for the homologous pneumococcal type. Thus, amount of pneumococcal capsular polysaccharide is similar to that found in the serum of patients with pneumococcal disease. Decomplementation of serum via activation of the alternative pathway inhibits pneumococcal opsonization. Evidence has been presented recently which suggests that antibody response to bacterial polysaccharide antigens may be of a single immunoglobulin subclass IgG2 (Siber *et al.*, 1980). These investigators found a direct correlation between IgG2 concentrations in serum an antibody response to 11 pneumococcal polysaccharides and *Haemophilus influenzae* type B antigen. There was no correlation between IgG2 and antibody response to protein antigens. Patients with Hodgkins' disease did not respond to pneumococcal polysaccharide antigens and had profoundly depressed levels of IgG2 subclass immunoglobulin in their serum. The antibodies that develop after polysaccharide immunization are restricted to a subclass of antibodies suggesting that there is a subclass specific regulating mechanism for response to polysaccharide antigen. This highly specialized antibody response control system may be the reason why normal immunoglobulin levels and antibody responses to protein antigen but poor antibody responses to polysaccharide antigens are found in patients with Wiskott-Aldrich syndrome, Hodgkins' Disease, recurrent sinopulmonary infections, and infants less than 18 months of age.

ESCHERICHIA COLI

Escherichia coli strains with K-1 polysaccharide capsule have been identified in 84% of neonates with *E. coli* meningitis (Robbins *et al.*, 1974). Most strains of K-1 *E. coli* are not killed by humoral factors; therefore, killing requires phagocytosis of the organisms and opsonic factors in serum are necessary for host defence. We compared the opsonic requirements of 28 strains of *E. coli* in our laboratory including 18 strains of K-1 *E. coli* that had been isolated from the spinal fluid of infants with meningitis (Bjorksten *et al.*, 1976). The opsonic requirements of *E. coli* were determined by evaluating uptake and killing by normal human polymorphonuclear leukocytes with normal serum or MgEGTA chelated serum as opsonic sources in the phagocytosis system. Our findings were similar to those described earlier by Glynn *et al.* (1971), i.e. that strains recovered from patients with disease were opsonized poorly in normal serum when compared with strains isolated from the faecal flora.

There was a qualitative as well as quantitative variation in opsonic requirements of different strains of *E. coli*. Strains with K-1 antigen were poorly opsonized and phagocytized. Preliminary data showed that sera from normal newborn infants had lower opsonic activity for *E. coli* strains which activated the alternative pathway, whereas opsonization of strains requiring classical pathway components were equal in mothers and newborns. This contrasts with high opsonic activity in pooled adult serum for strains that activate the alternative pathway and suggest alternative pathway deficiency in newborn sera. Although these laboratory data may not be directly applied to clinical situations, they suggest that susceptibility to *E. coli* septicaemia in the neonatal period may be a consequence of defective opsonic capacity of neonatal sera for strains of *E. coli* which have varying requirements.

The K-1 capsular polysaccharide antigen is a polymer of sialic acid which is immunologically identical to the capsular polysaccharide of *N. meningitidis* group B. There is evidence that the K-1 capsule resists opsonization by the alternative complement pathway and that *E. coli* strains which do not activate complement via the alternative pathway are more virulent for infant rats than *E. coli* strains which do activate the alternative pathway (Bortolussi *et al.*, 1979). Furthermore, strains with a high content of cell-associated K-1 polysaccharide are more resistant to phagocytosis and more virulent in newborn rats than K-1 strains with less K-1 capsular polysaccharide. Passive administration of K-1 antibody protects newborn rats against death from experimental *E. coli* infection by providing specific opsonic antibodies.

BACTEROIDES spp.

Bjornson and Bjornson, 1978 studied opsonic requirements for two species of *Bacteroides* and concluded that the alternative complement pathway was a major mechanism of opsonization. Immunoglobulin was required for the alternative pathway activity at least under the anerobic conditions that were used. We studied the opsonic requirement for four species of *Bacteroides* (Tofte *et al.*, 1980)—*B. fragilis, B. melaninogenicus, B. thetaiotaomicron, and B. vulgatis.* Contribution of the alternative pathway was tested using ethylene glycol-bis (β-aminoethylether)-*N*, *N*-tetracetic acid with added magnesium MgEGTA and C2 deficient serum. There was little uptake of any strain of *Bacteroides* in heated serum so that the object of this study was to determine the relative importance of the classical and alternative complement pathways for opsonization of *Bacteroides.*

All strains were opsonized in the absence of the classical complement pathway; however, kinetic studies revealed that opsonization proceeded at significantly faster rates when the classical complement pathway was intact. Although two strains were opsonized in immunoglobulin-deficient sera, opsonization was less efficient and appeared to occur via the alternative complement pathway. Unexpectedly, all strains were well opsonized by the classical complement pathway in 10% serum which had been effectively chelated with EGTA or EDTA. The explanation for this finding is unknown; however, it is possible that cell wall cations of *Bacteroides* spp. may participate in the activation of complement in chelated serum, resulting in effective opsonization. It was also found that *Bacteroides*, when incubated with an *E. coli* strain in normal serum, could compete for opsonins and thereby reduce phagocytosis of *E. coli.* It is possible that competition for opsonins among bacterial species contributes to the synergistic role these organisms share in mixed floral infections.

Ingham *et al.* (1977) recently described several patients with polymicrobial brain abscesses who responded to an antimicrobial agent effective primarily against anaerobic bacteria with little demonstrable *in vitro* activity against aerobic organisms. To investigate possible mechanisms for this clinical response, they incubated each of three aerobic organisms with either *B. fragilis* or *B. melaninogenicus* in human serum and found that the anaerobic bacteria inhibited phagocytosis and killing of the aerobic organisms. The mechanism for the decreased phagocytosis was not determined; however, it was postulated that *Bacteroides* spp. acted synergistically with the aerobic bacteria. Onderdink *et al.*, 1978 found that mixed fecal organisms, when implanted into rat peritoneal cavities in gelatin capsules, act synergistically to produce abscesses in those animals surviving the initial period of Gram negative bacillary peritonitis and sepsis. Based on the results of these investigations, we postulated that the bacterial synergism may in part be due to competition for opsonins among bacterial species.

To test the hypothesis that competition for opsonins may occur when two or more bacterial species are present, *E. coli* ON2 was incubated in 10% normal serum individually, and with *B. fragilis* and *B. melaninogenicus*. There was a significant reduction in the opsonization of *E. coli* ON2 in the presence of either *Bacteroides* species; however, opsonization of *Bacteroides* was not influenced by the presence of *E. coli* ON2. This suggests that bacterial species which are more efficiently or rapidly opsonized than others present in a given inoculum may actually deprive the remaining organisms of sufficient opsonins. That competition for opsonins occurs *in vivo* is currently speculative. Since opsonins may be present in limited quantities in extravascular spaces, it is possible that in the process of competition for available opsonins, some bacterial species are poorly opsonized. Singly or in combination, these organisms are not opsonically recognized and are therefore able to escape phagocytosis while continuing to multiply unimpeded by normal host defence mechanisms.

STREPTOCOCCUS PYOGENES

We recently examined the role of M protein as an antiphagocytic factor in *Streptococcus pyogenes* (Peterson *et al.*, 1979). Opsonization of an M+ strain and a M− variant of this strain was studied using sera from several sources and control human PMN. A sensitive method was utilized using radiolabelled bacteria and separation of the steps of opsonization and phagocytosis. Phagocytosis was measured by recording leukocyte-associated radioactivity after various times of incubation of opsonized streptococci and PMN. The M strain of streptococci was rapidly phagocytized in the absence of immunoglobulin and in MgEGTA chelated serum M-negative streptococci were efficiently opsonized via the alternative complement pathway. The M+ streptococcal strains were poorly opsonized in chelated or in fresh serum. Specific anti-M protein antibodies are needed for efficient opsonization of streptococci with M protein.

In the absence of specific antibody, the alternative complement pathway plays a major role in promoting phagocytosis of at least some group A streptococci. It also appears that cell surface M protein may interfere with phagocytosis of these same strains by inhibiting opsonization by the alternative complement pathway.

PSEUDOMONAS AERUGINOSA

The opportunistic nature of *Pseudomonas* organisms in producing infection suggests that normal serum and phagocytic cells should be capable of efficient opsonization, phagocytosis and killing. This proved to be the case using six strains of *P. aeruginosa* recovered from blood of patients at the University of Minnesota (Peterson *et al.*, 1978). Complement deficient serum and immunoglobulin deficient serum as well as normal human sera were used as sources of opsonins. There was efficient opsonization in normal serum but a great hetrogeneity of opsonic requirements was found when complement-deficient or immunoglobulin deficient serum was used. Most of the strains were opsonized by complement via the alternative complement pathway but there was more rapid uptake by granulocytes when fresh serum, i.e. classical pathway opsonins were present. Assays with immunoglobulin deficient serum suggested that immunoglobulins were necessary for alternative pathway opsonization of most strains of *P. aeruginosa*. Two strains were opsonized in immunoglobulin-deficient sera and in *Pseudomonas* absorbed sera but not in heated sera so that immunoglobulin was not a requisite for complement activation. There may have been direct activation of complement on the surface of these organisms by structures such as lipopolysaccharide in a fashion similar to that observed with protein A on the surface of *Staphylococcus aureus*.

COMPLEMENT

The bacterial surface sialic acid appears to be a significant factor in the ability of complement to be activated on the surface and act as a ligand between organism and phagocytic cell (Fearon *et al.*, 1980). When the surface of bacteria is "activating" there is an affinity for C3b which is spontaneously produced in the fluid phase. Factor B binds to C3b on the surface and is cleared by a proteolytic enzyme term factor D. When this occurs the bacterial surface has an active C3 convertase on its surface. This C3 convertase is stabilized by properdin and C3b is rapidly generated from C3 where it is most effective on the surface of the bacteria. When specific antibody is associated with antigens on bacterial surfaces the classical pathway of complement is activated and the classical pathway C3 convertase is present on the bacterial surface. The activity of this convertase C42 also generates C3b from C3.

There are inhibitors of C3b which have increased affinity for C3b in the presence of sialic acid; hence bacterial surfaces rich in sialic such as K-1 *E. coli* and group B streptococci are poorly opsonized via the alternative pathway.

The nonimmune host depends on the alternative pathway for opsonization of invading bacteria until specific antibodies are formed. This is usually a highly effective host defence mechanism unless the bacterial species that invade have surface characteristics that do not favour deposition of C3b or formation of C3 convertase on their surface. K-1 *E. coli* and group B streptococci are examples of such bacterial invaders.

The age specificity of K-1 *E. coli* and group B streptococcal disease is evidence for the role the alternative pathway during the neonatal period. Infants born to mothers without antibodies to these microbes are at greatly increased risk and older infants (presumably after cross reacting IgM antibodies have developed) are not at increased risk. Activation of complement via the classical pathway and opsonization by antibodies does not appear to be compromised by bacterial surface sialic acid.

The bactericidal activity of serum is dependent upon activation of the entire complement sequence with formation of the "membrane attack complex", C5b–C9. Immunoglobulins are important in initiating the complement-mediated killing of many, but there appear to be several determinants of serum sensitivity of Gram negative bacteria including lypopolysaccharide. Bacterial killing is attended by the disruption of the outer membrane, and in the presence of serum lysozyme, the peptidoglycan layer is degraded and the bacterial wall is lysed (Schriber *et al.*, 1979).

Serum bactericidal activity seems especially important for host defence against pathogenic *Neisseria* species (Schoolnik *et al.*, 1976). Gonococcal strains that disseminate from the genital tract are serum-resistant, and McCutchan *et al.* (1978) have proposed that the surface of these organisms possess "receptors" for IgG antibodies that block "natural" bactericidal antibodies found in normal human serum. Also, some patients with severe or recurrent neisserial infections have been found to have selective deficiencies of C5, C6, C7, or C8.

Chemotaxis, the directed migration of phagocytic cells along a chemical gradient, is potentially influenced by numerous bacterial surface components capable of activating the complement system with production of the chemotaxin C5a. Chemotaxigenesis by cell surface fractions of *S. aureus*, for example, has been shown to be mediated by protein A, peptidoglycan, teichoic acid, and cell membrane fragments (Schmeling *et al.*, 1979).

SUMMARY

Phagocytosis of bacteria is generally dependent upon the process of bacterial opsonization. Opsonization is usually mediated by the serum complement system with binding of the opsonically active complement fragment C3b to bacterial surfaces. C3b and the Fc fragment of immunoglobulin may both function as ligands between the bacterial surface and specific receptors within the plasma membrane of the phagocyte. The bacterial surface components which initiate or influence the process of opsonization vary with the bacterial species. The heterogeneity of opsonic requirements found among different species and among strains of the same species most likely reflects differences in their cell surface composition.

Peptidoglycan is a key cell wall component in mediating the opsonization. Given the immunologic cross-reactivity of bacterial peptidoglycans, it is postulated that antibodies against this surface component are important determinants of "natural immunity".

Resistance to phagocytosis is associated with the presence of cell surface capsular polysaccharides and encapsulation is an important virulence factor of many species of pathogenic bacteria. The antiphagocytic characteristics of the bacterial capsules may be its interference with opsonization via the alternative pathway or a masking effect on opsonized wall constituents. Patients with immunoglobulin deficiency diseases have difficulty primarily with infections due to encapsulated bacteria since effective opsonization of encapsulated bacteria requires specific anticapsular antibodies. Once opsonization has occurred there is recognition by and attachment to phagocytic cells and most bacterial species are rapidly killed within phagocytes by oxidative and other mechanisms.

REFERENCES

Bjorksten, B., Bortolussi, R., Gothefors, L. and Quie, P. G. (1976). Interaction of *E. coli* strains with human serum: Lack of relationship to K-1 antigen. *Journal of Pediatrics* **89(6)**, 892–897.

Bjornson, A. B. and Bjornson, H. S. (1978). Participation of immunoglobulin and the alternative complement pathway in opsonization of *Bacteroides fragilis* and *Bacteroides thetaiotaomicron*. *Journal of Infectious Diseases* **138**, 351–357.

Bortolussi, R., Ferrieri, P., Bjorksten, B. and Quie, P. G. (1979). Capsular K-1 polysaccharide of *Escherichia coli:* Relationship to virulence in newborn rats and resistance to phagocytosis. *Infection and Immunity* **25**, 293–298.

Crowder, J. G. and White, A. (1972). Teichoic acid antibodies in staphylococcal and non-staphylococcal endocarditis. *Annals Internal Medicine* **77**, 87–90.

Dossett, J. H., Kronvall, G., Williams, R. C., Jr and Quie, P. G. (1969). Antiphagocytic effects of staphylococcal protein A. *Journal of Immunology* **103,** 1405–1410.

Edebo, L. H. E., Kihlstrom, E., Magnusson, K. E. and Stendahl, O. (1979). The adhesion of enterobacteria and the effect of antibodies of different immunoglobulin classes. *In* "Proceedings of Symposium Host-Parasite Interactions, Umea, Sweden, June, 1979", p. 21.

Fearon, D. T. and Austen, K. F. (1980). The alternative pathway of complement: A system for host resistance to microbial infection. *New England Journal of Medicine* **303(5),** 259–262.

Giebink, G. S., Dee, T. H., Kim, Y. and Quie, P. G. (1980). Alterations in serum opsonic activity and complement levels in pneumococcal disease. *Infection and Immunity*, in press.

Giebink, G. S., Grebner, J. V., Kim, Y. and Quie. P. G. (1978). Serum opsonic deficiency produced by *Streptococcus pneumoniae* and by capsular polysaccharide antigens. Yale J. *Biology and Medicine* **51,** 527–538.

Giebink, G. S., Verhoef, J., Peterson, P. K. and Quie, P. G. (1977). Opsonic requirements for phagocytosis of *Streptococcus pneumoniae* types VI, XVIII, XXIII, and XXV. *Infection and Immunity* **18,** 291–297.

Glynn, A. A., Brunfitt, W. and Howard, C. J. (1971). K antigensss of *Escherichia coli* and renal involvement in urinary tract infections. *Lancet* **i,** 514.

Ingham, H. R., Tharagonnet, D., Sisson, P. R., Selkon, J. B. and Codd, A. A. (1977). Inhibition of phagocytosis in vitro by obligate anaerobes. *Lancet* **i,** 1252–1252.

McCutchan, J. A., Katzenstein, D., Norquist, D., Chikami, G., Wunderlich, A. and Braude, A. I. (1978). Role of blocking antibody in disseminated gonococcal infection. *Journal of Immunology* **121,** 1884–1888.

Messner, R. P., Laxdal, T., Quie, P. G. and Williams, R. C., Jr (1968). Serum opsonin, bacteria and polymorphonuclear leukocyte interactions in subacute bacterial endocarditis. *Journal of Clinical Investigation* **47,** 1109–1120.

Onderdonk, A. B., Kasper, D. L., Mansheim, B. J., Louie, T. J., Gorbach, S. L. and Bartlett, J. G. (1979). Experimental animal models for anaerobic infections. *Review of Infectious Diseases* **1,** 291–301.

Peterson, P. K., Kim, Y., Schmeling, D., Lindemann, M., Verhoef, J. and Quie, P. G. Complement-mediated phagocytosis of *Pseudomonas aeruginosa*. *Journal of Laboratory and Clinical Medicine* **92(6),** 883–894.

Peterson, P. K., Schmeling, D., Cleary, P. P., Wilkinson, B. J., Kim, Y. and Quie, P. G. (1979). Inhibition of alternative complement pathway opsonization by group A streptococcal M protein. *Journal of Infectious Diseases* **139(5),** 575–585.

Peterson, P. K., Verhoef, J., Sabath, L. D. and Quie, P. G. (1977). Effect of protein A on staphylococcal opsonization. *Infection and Immunity* **15,** 760–764.

Peterson, P. K., Wilkinson, B. J., Kim, Y., Schmeling, D. and Quie, P. G. (1978). Influence of encapsulation on staphylococcal opsonization and phagocytosis by human polymorphonuclear leukocytes. *Infection and Immunity* **19,** 943–949.

Robbins, J. B., McCracken, G. H., Jr, Gotschlich, E. C., Orskov, F., Orskov, I. and Hanson, L. A. (1974). *Escherichia coli* K-1 capsular polysaccharide associated with neonatal meningitis. *New England Journal of Medicine* **290,** 1216.

Schmeling, D. J., Peterson, P. K., Hammerschmidt, D. E., Kim, Y., Verhoef, J., Wilkinson, B. J. and Quie, P. G. (1979). Chemotaxigenesis by cell surface components of *Staphylococcus aureus*. *Infection and Immunity* **26**, 57–63.

Schoolnik, G. K., Buchanan, T. M. and Holmes, K. K. (1976). Gonococci causing disseminated gonococcal infection are resistant to the bactericidal action of normal human sera. *Journal of Clinical Investigation* **58**, 1163–1173.

Schrieber, R. D., Morrison, D. C., Podack, E. R. and Müller-Eberhard, H. J. (1979). Bactericidal activity of the alternative complement pathway generation from 11 isolated plasma proteins. *Journal of Experimental Medicine* **149**, 870–882.

Schultz, D. R. and Miller, K. D. (1974). Elastase of *Pseudomonas aeruginosa*: Inactivation of complement components and complement-derived chemotactic and phagocytic factors. *Infection and Immunity* **10**, 128–135.

Siber, G. R., Schur, P. H., Aisenberg, A. C., Weitzman, S. A. and Schiffman, G. (1980). Correlation between serum IgG-2 concentrations and the antibody response to bacterial polysaccharide antigens. *New England Journal of Medicine*, 178–182.

Smyth, C. J., Jonsson, P., Olsson, E., Soderland, O., Rosengren, J., Hjerten, S. and Wadstrom, T. (1978). Differences in hydrophobic surface characteristics of porcine enteropathogenic *Escherichia coli* with or without K88 antigen as revealed byhydrophobic interaction chromatography. *Infection and Immunity* **22**, 462–472.

Tofte, R. W., Peterson, P. K., Schmeling, D., Bracke, J., Kim, Y. and Quie, P. G. (1980). Opsonization of four bacteroides species: Role of the classical complement pathway and immunoglobulin. *Infection and Immunity* 27(3), 784–792.

Tylewska, S., Hjerten, S., and Wadstrom, T. (1979). Hydrophobic properties of S. pyogenes related to M. protein. *In* "Proceedings of Symposium on Host-Parasite Interactions, Umea, Sweden, June, 1979", p. 33.

Verhoef, J., Peterson, P. K., Kim, Y., Sabath, L. D. and Quie, P. G. (1977). Opsonic requirements for staphylococcal phagocytosis: Hetrogeneity among strains. *Immunology* **33**, 191–197.

Verhoef, J., Peterson, P. K. and Quie, P. G. (1977). Human polymorphonuclear leukocyte receptors for staphylococcal opsonins. *Immunology* **33**, 231–240.

Verhoef, J., Peterson, P. K. and Quie, P. G. (1977). Kinetics of staphylococcal opsonization, attachment, ingestion, and killing by human polymorphonuclear leukocytes: A quantitative assay using (^{3}H) thymidine labeled bacteria. *Journal of Immunological Methods* 14, 303–311.

DISCUSSION

Smith I am glad that you brought up the possibility that the anaerobes have some antiphagocytic mechanisms. I think that low oxygen tension is very important in pathogenicity but that other factors come into it. There is the experiment of Bartlett's group at Boston. In the gelatine capsule abscess model in rats, they used the actual capsular material of *Bacteroides fragilis*—not the live organism itself—and produced the abscess. However I do not know whether anyone has shown this capsular material to be antiphagocytic in the same way as for pneumococcal polysaccharide.

Quie In stockholm the week before last Dennis Kasper brought me up to date on the speciation of *Bacteroides. Bacteroides fragilis* has been divided into a number of different species and *Bacteroides fragilis* var. *fragilis* is encapsulated. This capsule has been shown to be antiphagocytic, so pathogenic mechanisms of anaerobes may be similar to those of aerobes.

Braude It is true that there are many subspecies of *B. fragilis.* However, I think that one of the weak points in the argument—I do not think that it negates it by any means—is that *B. oralis*, which is a relatively nonpathogenic species of *Bacteroides*, also has a pretty good capsule. I do not know whether any others here have noticed this but we have been impressed in a number of strains that they are very mucoid in their gross cultural characteristics.

I think the most impressive part of the evidence is Dennis Kasper's ability to protect against *B. fragilis* infection with anticapsular antiserum.

Quie I neglected to say that there may be a great deal more to the role of capsules in resisting phagacytosis than masking opsonin ligands. Capsules are so different in their biochemical composition that there may be different antiphagocytic effects involving charge or hydrophobicity as well as distance.

Draper Does anyone know what property of the capsule activates complement or prevents phagocytosis? I have in mind some work which tried to explain the effects in terms of simple physical chemistry, namely contact angle, that is the extent to which it is or is not wetted by water. They investigated the outer surface of a whole range of *Salmonella* mutants where one can modify the surface at will and showed that the more easily they were wetted by water the less easily the bacteria were phagacytosed. That seems a very simple, school chemistry explanation. Is there anything in it or is the chemistry much more subtle?

Quie The work you are referring to is by von Oss and his team at Buffalo, New York, which has been followed up and enhanced by Lars Edebo and his group in Sweden. The organisms' hydrophobicity or hydrophilia may influence attachment and phagocytosis. Lars Edebo has shown that adding IgA antibody to the capsular material from *E. coli* increases hydrophilia. In other words, the organisms like the stream and not the shore. When he incubates *E. coli* with IgG they are much more hydrophobic and attach to surfaces. That is a beautiful story, if it is true, because it explains why IgA prevents attachment to mucosal surfaces and IgG enhances attachment to phagocytic cells.

Mims Can you go any further with the mechanisms of the interaction of complement with the capsule?

Quie My concept has been that many of the surface properties of microbes are associated with attachment or repulsion, but that firm attachment necessary for efficient phagocytosis of encapsulated microbes requires specific antibodies against capsular surface antigens. Once you have specific antibody there may be more of a lock-key type receptor and firm attachment.

Jeljaszewicz I would like to provoke Dr Quie into saying a little more about staphylococcal capsules, because there are mixed views about them. First, how frequently do they occur? Secondly, as the capsular material isolated in various centres has differed greatly, has the staphylococcal capsule been finally analyzed and identified? Thirdly, is there anything in the idea that perhaps this is not a capsule but a sort of slime or cloud of substances easily detached from the surface of the *Staphylococcus*?

Quie The strains we were fortunate enough to work with provided reproducible capsular material, but I would not like to extrapolate information from the M strain to *Staph. aureus* in general. Even the biochemical structures of *Staph. aureus* capsules are different. Talking about capsules brings up the problem about how many strains recovered from clinical material have capsular or antiphagocytic surface structures for which there is specific antibody. I just do not know: the literature will give you any answer you want, from 30% to a rare occurrence.

Jeljaszewicz In our experience, which I do not claim as being the only valid one, using every technique described in the literature, we could find capsular material in no more than 3–4% of strains isolated from clinical specimens.

Draper Could I go back to the question of surface tension? What I was really trying to get Dr Quie to say, which perhaps he does not want to say, is that it is this property which governs whether or not the surface will activate complement. Would he like to comment on that?

Quie The picture is changing rapidly, but it appears that sialic acid on the surface of group B streptococci somehow interferes with activation of complement. The mechanism of action appears to be that sialic acid-rich factor B surfaces favour the association of an inhibitor with C3b rather than association with an alternative pathway component. I doubt if that is related to hydrophobicity but rather a chemical composition which favours one kind of association more than another—and there are a variety of different surfaces which are favourable or antagonistic to alternative pathway activation.

Williams If one is looking for examples of where capsules are important in influencing whether infection occurs, one has only to look at *Haemophilus influenzae* where the noncapsulated strains show no ability to cause severe infection, whereas the capsulated strains are invasive and give rise to meningitis and septicaemia. The capsule is quite likely to be of some importance in perturbing the host defence mechanisms because the critical period of initiation of infection is very short, something like five hours, when a few organisms can lodge and there is a brief period before they can establish themselves. When there are few organisms, they must be producing very minute amounts of toxin or any other factor possibly intefering with host defences. Therefore it must be some anatomical feature, e.g. a capsule, which prevents the macrophage from intervening in the initiation of infection.

Easmon The difficulty with using *Haemophilus influenzae* to illustrate whether capsules necessarily play a part in pathogenicity is that *Haemophilus influenzae* type B is associated with serious disease, but there are five other capsular types of this organism which are rarely associated with serious disease. So even with *Haemophilus* there are about six capsules of which only one seems to have a marked association with common disease processes in man. So why is one capsular type particularly pathogenic and the other five rarely so?

Smith I think we are skirting around the fact that in this area we have to move on to a connection between chemical structure and biological function. At present there have been very few moves. Helena Makela's group in Finland have used mutants of the salmonellae to relate the chemical structure of the lipopolysaccharide to whether the organism is phagocytosed or not. Changing a couple of sugars in the side chain of the LPS can render phagocytosis-resistant organisms phagocytosis-sensitive. This tends to fit in with Dr Quie's idea. I cannot imagine that this kind of change effects hydrophobicity very much. It is more a question of a chemical lock-and-key arrangement. There is similar work on phagocytosis of resistant and sensitive *E. coli*. With our greater knowledge of the chemistry of some bacterial capsular materials, for example, the meningococcal polysaccharides, inhibition studies could be done with various monosaccharides, dissacharides, etc. to indicate a connection between structure and function in resistance to phagocytosis. I go along with Dr Quie: I think phagocytosis in the main is mediated by interaction with chemical receptors—not by degrees of hydrophobicity.

Wilton I would make one comment: that galactosamine is a very good inhibitor of C3b opsonized particle binding.

Braude Tufsin is a tetrapeptide which can be a very effective anti-pneumococcal opsonic factor. Do you know anything about the way it acts that might help explain why the capsule is antiphagocytic?

Quie I really do not know much about tufsin, Dr Braude. It is believed to increase the efficiency of phagocytosis by associating with the leukocyte rather than with the microorganism. As I understand it, the peptide is a little bit of the Fc part of the immunoglobulin molecule which has an affinity for the surface of leukocytes. It is believed that somehow it makes phagocytosis more efficient, but I have no experience of the phenomenon and hesitate to speculate further.

Arbuthnott One of the things we should bear in mind in considering the interaction between the surface of the pathogen and the host defence system is that the organism surface is not a series of onion layers—and this came out nicely when Dr Quie was talking about encapsulated staphylococci—but a mosaic. I think the other important thing we have to remember is that when organisms are growing *in vivo* in a lesion they do not present a pure bacterial surface; there are host derived factors, proteins and other substances, perhaps lipids and glycolipids absorbed on to that surface, so that the interaction may be a good deal more complex than we think at the moment.

Mims I have always been unclear about the role of sialic acid. You mentioned it, I think, Dr Quie. What is the message now? Is there really a reliable relationship between sialic acid content and antiphagocytic activities?

Quie I think that concept is holding up pretty well. The evidence shows that microbes with sialic acid-rich surfaces such as the type 3 group B streptococci are opsonized efficiently if sialic acid is removed by neurominidase. It is believed that there is circulating C3b which on an "activating" surface associates with factor b and becomes C3 convertase.

van Furth Are you saying there is free C3b in the circulation? I wonder? I think it is all split off into C3c and C3d. It is such a rapid process. The most sensitive test of complement activation *in vivo* is to determine circulating C3d.

Wilton Perhaps I could to some extent support Dr Quie. My memory of the complement literature is that the C3b that is bound to membranes is more resistant to the action of C3b inhibitor. It is possible, therefore, that very small amounts of bound C3b, or their absence, could have fairly profound effects one way or the other, either initiating opsonization or not allowing it to proceed.

Draper I have a technical worry about capsules. If one supposes that synthesizing a capsule is a metabolic burden on a bacterium and that having a capsule confers no advantage in the sort of medium that bacteriologists use to grow bacteria, then one will select uncapsulated mutants. Is it conceivable that all the pathogenic Gram positive organisms we have been talking about are encapsulated *in vivo*, but this gets lost when they are grown *in vitro*? Perhaps somebody can reassure me. There is some evidence that wild mycobacteria always have capsules but these are lost in culture—certainly in the culture collections.

Arbuthnott We have grown Dr Quie's M strain in our chambers in the peritoneum of mice and there is no question that the capsule is produced *in vivo*. I can also say something which must be considered to be very preliminary. We have examined the capsular material by staining the cells with cationic ferritin and compared the *in vitro* and *in vivo* grown organisms. In the *in vitro* grown organisms the capsular material appears—and I think Dr Quie would agree—to have a very regular kind of substructure but is not evenly distributed around the cell, so that some of the cell surface might be exposed to the exterior. The *in vivo* grown organisms also possess capsular material which stains with cationic ferritin, but the substructure seems to be quite different in that it has a less ordered appearance. So with this strain the capsule is produced *in vivo*, but perhaps because it reacts with host-derived factors, or for some other reason, it has a different arrangement.

Smith I think we must remember that there are capsules and capsules. Some have a structure with constituents which will prevent the organism from being phagocytosed, but other capsules lack a constituent with the required structure and will not prevent ingestion. That probably explains why many capsulated strains of *Haemophilus* are not pathogenic. The other point is that the bacteria may need another factor in addition to the capsule to be pathogenic. If I go back to my old love, *Bacillus anthracis*, the HM strain has a big capsule composed of poly-D-glutamic acid, just as any virulent strain. However, the HM strain is not virulent because it cannot produce the necessary virulence factor, toxin.

Braude I have always been impressed in patients with meningitis, for example, how easily virulent strains that invade the central nervous system can be demonstrated to have a capsule simply by looking at the spinal fluid and adding antibody. When Hattie Alexander used antiserum for the treatment of *Haemophilus influenzae* meningitis, she gave enough to produce capsular swelling of the *Haemophilus* in the spinal fluid. You could see it; there was no argument about it. I cannot think of a better way to prove capsular production *in vivo* than to show capsular swelling with antibody. We make the diagnosis of pneumococcal meningitis by adding antiserum to spinal fluid and showing capsular swelling. We can give many examples of this. I think that this is such an obvious and well established point that there should be no question about it.

Mims I think it is obvious and well established for certain bacteria, but perhaps less well for others. I am sure Professor Smith put his finger on the point: we need to know more about the relation between the biochemistry and function of capsules.

Williams Can I mention another clinical example of the importance of capsules. In cystic fibrosis many children seem to live quite happily with the feathery type of *Pseudomonas aeruginosa* which does not seem to do any harm, but if the same serotype of *Pseudomonas* develops a capsule and large mucoid forms are recovered in culture, the disease seems to advance very much more rapidly.

Easmon If an organism is an efficient parasite it is living in virtual harmony with its host. I cannot understand why it should be to the advantage of an organism such as the *Meningococcus* to have a capsule which enables it to resist host defence mechanisms once it has invaded, when it can probably exist quite happily colonizing mucosal epithelium without invasion. What is the advantage of a capsule in the absence of invasion? Why should the *Meningococcus* invade and kill the host? It does not seem to be very efficient from the point of view of evolutionary development and the ultimate survival of the organism. As hosts, we look at all these virulence factors as potentially harmful to us, but bacteria, I am sure, do not develop virulence factors primarily to kill or damage their hosts unless there is some evolutionary advantage for their survival in this process.

Mims I like this teleology, but I do not think you need talk in terms of evolutionary advantage. Amongst the meningococci colonizing the nose, some will arise that produce a capsule and may invade, but that has nothing to do with the ultimate success of meningococci in man, because carriage is what matters. In any case, capsules are produced by free living bacteria where they have a lot of functions other than merely resisting host defences.

Anderson I should like to make a comment about evolutionary significance and whether or not it is important for any parasite to damage its host. It seems to me that the most significant part of any organism's life is to reproduce itself. It does not seem, on the face of it, to be important whether or not the host dies. What matters is whether the parasite can transmit itself to a further host before it is eradicated by, or from, the host in which it is already living. Perhaps we should be looking for effects on the success of transmission when thinking about factors such as capsules.

Mycobacterial Inhibition of Intracellular Killing

PHILIP DRAPER

National Institute for Medical Research,
Mill Hill,
London, UK.

Pathogenic mycobacteria

Students of human nature may ponder why leprosy is universally abhorred while tuberculosis has sometimes been regarded as desirably romantic. For microbiologists among them the paradox is sharpened by the knowledge that both are caused by chronic parasitism by mycobacteria able to survive inside phagocytic cells. Pathogenic mycobacteria also cause some economically important diseases of animals and here too the pathogens are able to survive intracellularly. The extent to which each species is found intracellularly or extracellularly varies among the diseases; for instance *Mycobacterium leprae* and *M. lepraemurium* are invariably intracellular, but *M. tuberculosis* occurs extracellularly in severe human pulmonary tuberculosis but not in tuberculosis in mice.

These pathogenic mycobacteria occur inside macrophages by which they are phagocytosed and in which they multiply. The bacterial population may achieve remarkably high levels in the cells, and macrophages accumulate in various sorts of granulomatous tissue formed of more-or-less heavily infected cells. Macrophages are normally considered to function by phagocytosing and eliminating foreign particles including microorganisms. In the case of the pathogenic bacteria the function of elimination seems ineffective; the cells are exploited as a protected environment by the bacteria. Two general properties of the bacteria seem to be adaptations to this way of life: slow growth and low cytoxicity. *Mycobacterium leprae* and *M. lepraemurium* seem almost without toxicity, though *M. tuberculosis* does damage its host cell *in vitro* when the numbers are sufficiently high and cell damage in the tissues is a feature of the human disease.

INTRACELLULAR KILLING

The mechanisms by which macrophages kill phagocytosed microorganisms are not fully understood, though such killing occurs both *in vivo* and *in vitro* and is especially effective if the macrophages are stimulated either nonspecifically (e.g. "elicited" macrophages) or by specific immunological mechanisms ("activated" macrophages). Mechanisms favoured at present mostly involve oxygen derivatives (peroxide, superoxide, hydroxyl radicals, or singlet oxygen) thought to be produced as a result of the burst of oxidative metabolism that accompanies phagocytosis. Reviews of aspects of these mechanisms will be found in van Furth (1980). Cohn and his colleagues (Murray and Cohn, 1979; Murray *et al.*, 1979) have shown that oxygen intermediates may kill *Toxoplasma gondii* in macrophages.

Pathogenic mycobacteria are not killed by macrophages *in vitro*, though recovery of animals and people from mycobacterial disease shows that killing mechanisms must exist. Presumably the tissue culture systems so far investigated are in some way defective. Lowrie and his colleagues have made considerable progress in defining which potential killing mechanisms might be active against *M. tuberculosis* having various degrees of virulence. The organisms were resistant to superoxide irrespective of virulence. Some (but not all) strains of low virulence were sensitive to hydrogen peroxide, especially at low pH (Jackett *et al.*, 1978a).

An important killing mechanism in polymorphs is the myeloperoxidase–peroxide–halide system (Sbarra *et al.*, 1979) and this system is active against *M. tuberculosis* (Jackett *et al.*, 1978b). Myeloperoxidase does not occur in mature macrophages but it is believed that catalase may behave in the same way as peroxidase (Klebanoff, 1969). Catalase is present in macrophages (though not necessarily in the right site) and a catalase–peroxide–halide system is able to kill *M. tuberculosis* in specified conditions (Jackett *et al.*, 1980).

Whether the enzyme is available and the physicochemical environment is such that the system can operate in the intact macrophage remains to be seen.

Meanwhile one may speculate that killing mechanisms may operate during two separate stages of the normal phagocytic process. Exposure to peroxide and related oxygen derivatives may occur in the phagocytic vacuole after ingestion while exposure to lysosomal enzymes requires phagosome–lysosome fusion. It is possible that fusion with nonlysosomal vacuoles with bactericidal contents may also occur (drawing an analogy with the specific granules of neutrophils). Candidate vacuoles remain to be identified in macrophages.

INTRACELLULAR BEHAVIOUR OF PATHOGENIC MYCOBACTERIA

The pathogenic mycobacteria occur in three sites in the host cell:

phagosome
phagolysosome
cytoplasm.

The sites may be interpreted as indicating three different ways of avoiding intracellular killing: inhibition of killing processes, resistance to killing processes, and removal to a site where killing processes cannot operate, respectively. The sites are discussed below in terms of three species each characteristically occurring in one site. Examples are known in each case of other bacteria or protozoa which occur in these sites. The merit of mycobacteria as subjects for investigation is that they are related chemically and biologically. It should (in principle) be simpler to find out which of the relatively few differences between *M. tuberculosis* and *M. lepraemurium* determine whether phagosome–lysosome fusion occurs in an infected macrophage than to obtain that information by comparing *Toxoplasma gondii* (Jones and Hirsch, 1972) with *Salmonella typhimurium* (Carrol *et al.*, 1979).

Survival in Phagolysosomes—*Mycobacterium lepraemurium*

Mycobacterium lepraemurium seems to be indifferent to the effects of phagocytosis and phagosome–lysosome fusion. It may be found multiplying in phagolysosomes of fibroblasts and macrophages *in vitro* (Brown and Draper, 1970; Hart *et al.*, 1972) and of macrophages *in vivo* (Brown and Draper, 1976).

A problem that applies to studies of all intracellular microorganisms *in vivo* is that of determining whether a phagosome has fused with a lysosome. One cannot readily introduce electron-dense markers for lysosomes as is usually done *in vitro*, while histochemical techniques for detecting lysomal enzymes cannot be relied on to stain *every* lysosome (Dr P. d'Arcy Hart, pers. comm.). The bone marrow macrophage of the mouse has naturally electron-dense (secondary) lysosomes, so that fusion is easily observed. It seems important to show that the mycobacteria behave identically *in vivo* and *in vitro*, since it is not clear that cultured macrophages—at least mouse peritoneal macrophages—can develop *in vitro* the full potentiality of such cells for killing or inhibiting mycobacteria *in vivo*.

Presumably intracellular *M. lepraemurium* uses a technique of passive resistance—its surface structures are unaffected by lysosomal enzymes and impermeable to potentially bactericidal chemicals. Dr Rees and I, and independently Dr Nishiura and his colleagues, have identified a capsule of a characteristic peptidoglycolipid as a possible protective mechanism (Draper and Rees, 1970; Nishiura *et al.*, 1972; Draper and Rees, 1973; Nishiura *et al.*, 1977). Such a capsule is also produced by other organisms of the *M. avium* group of mycobacteria (Draper, 1974; Kim *et al.*, 1976). The situation of these organisms inside cells is, however, not well studied.

There is some evidence that *M. lepraemurium* goes beyond mere resistance in its relations with macrophages. If a sufficiently large intravenous dose (10^9 bacteria) is used in mice a small proportion of the bacteria are phagocytosed by the bone-marrow macrophages and multiply unusually rapidly; multiplication in the liver and the spleen, which eventually contain the majority of the organisms in the animal, is slower (Brown and Krenzien, 1976). During the first 8 weeks the doubling times are 15, 7·6 and 4·8 days in liver, spleen and bone-marrow, respectively. In both the liver and the bone marrow the infected cells are "fixed" macrophages. Multiplication in the marrow is accompanied by striking changes in the morphology of the macrophages which become converted to huge cells resembling epithelioid cells in their ultrastructrue but containing many bacteria. It seems possible that some bacterial product is converting the phagocytic and potentially bactericidal macrophage to a primarily "metabolic" cell (with many mitochondria and much endoplasmic reticulum) whose products support the growth of the bacteria. On the other hand the mechanism may be indirect and involve the immunological system; formation of the "granuloma" might be an expression of cell-mediated immunity. In fact an immunological explanation, at least involving cell-mediated immunity, seems unlikely. The large intravenous inoculum used completely suppresses the ability of mice to develop a local cell-mediated immunological reaction to a small dose of *M. lepraemurium* given into the footpad, whether the intravenous infection occurs before (Closs, 1975) or at the same time as (Lefford and Mackaness, 1977) local infection.

Inhibition of Phagosome–Lysosome Fusion—*Mycobacterium tuberculosis*

Mycobacterium tuberculosis and the closely related *M. microti* are phagocytosed by macrophages but the normal phagosome–lysosome fusion process does not occur (Armstrong and Hart, 1971; Hart *et al.*, 1972; Lowrie *et al.*, 1975). This might be interpreted either as a failure to stimulate fusion or as an inhibition of the process of fusion by the bacteria. However, phagosome–lysosome fusion occurs when dead *M. tuberculosis* is phagocytosed (Armstrong and Hart, 1971); the dead organisms undergo, in this respect, the same treatment as most phagocytosed particles. This strongly suggests that the inhibition is an active process. A similar ability to prevent exposure to lysosomal contents is found in some protozoan parasites. There too the organisms must be alive.

At least four substances are known that may, in appropriate conditions, be produced by *M. tuberculosis* and which will inhibit phagosome–lysosome fusion in cultured mouse peritoneal macrophages. It is not clear which, if any, of these is the active material inside the host cell in an infection with *M. tuberculosis*. The inhibitory substances are:

(1) adenosine-3′,5′-cyclic monophosphate (cyclic AMP)
(2) poly(α-L-glutamic acid)
(3) 2,3,6,6′-tetraacyl trehalose 2′-sulphate (sulphatide)
(4) ammonia

Cyclic AMP

Cultures of mouse peritoneal macrophages infected with *M. microti* contain larger amounts of cyclic AMP than uninfected control cultures (Lowrie *et al.*, 1975). This increase did not occur in cultures infected with *M. lepraemurium* (which does not inhibit fusion). It is not clear whether the excess nucleotide was of bacterial or macrophage origin. *Mycobacterium microti* was able to release cyclic AMP into its environment, though the amounts released in the medium used were insufficient to explain the increased levels in the macrophages. *Mycobacterium lepraemurium* isolated from infected animals did not release the nucleotide, but these bacteria are believed to be "leaky" (Dhople and Hanks, 1977) with respect to ATP and might be unable to synthesize cyclic AMP. The capacity of either organism to produce cyclic AMP inside a cell is unknown.

Salmonella typhimurium, like *M. lepraemurium*, did not inhibit fusion and did not increase cyclic AMP levels in infected macrophages (Carrol *et al.*, 1979). The attenuated strain of *M. tuberculosis*, BCG, which inhibits phagosome–lysosome fusion for only a limited time in infected cells, produced a temporary rise in cyclic AMP in the cultures which subsequently declined (Lowrie *et al.*, 1979). Thus the cyclic AMP hypothesis seemed to be corroborated. However, it failed to predict the behaviour of BCG coated with specific antibody. Such coating reversed the inhibition of phagosome–lysosome fusion but had no effect on cyclic AMP production.

Even so, cyclic nucleotides may be important; treatments that increase cyclic AMP in polymorphs have several apparently relevant effects including inhibition of phagocytosis (Ignarro and Cech, 1976), oxidative processes (Spirer *et al.*, 1975), release of lysosomal enzymes (Zurier *et al.*, 1974) and killing of intracellular microorganisms (Bourne *et al.*, 1971). So the appearance of cyclic AMP in the *M. microti*-infected cultures may give important information about the mechanism of inhibition even if it is not itself the direct cause of that process.

Polyglutamic acid

Polyglutamic acid is one of a number of anionic substances which, when added to cultured macrophages, accumulate in secondary lysosomes and inhibit fusion (Hart and Young, 1978). Polyglutamic acid also occurs attached covalently to the cell wall of virulent *M. tuberculosis* (Vilkas and Markovits, 1972) and the attenuated strain BCG (Wietzerbin-Falszpan *et al.*, 1973). Virulent *M. tuberculosis* contains more polyglutamic acid than BCG (Wietzerbin *et al.*, 1975) but there seems to be no correlation between virulence and amounts of polymer in the walls of a series of BCG strains (Phiet *et al.*, 1976). One puzzling fact is that among the pure synthetic polymers only poly(α-D-glutamic acid) inhibits phagosome–lysosome fusion. Poly(α-L-glutamic acid) and poly(γ-D-glutamic acid) (a product of some *Bacillus* spp.) are ineffective (Dr P. d'Arcy Hart, pers. comm.). There is a slight disagreement among the published results about the nature of the mycobacterial polyglutamic acid since Vilkas and Markovits (1972) found some D-glutamic acid residues whereas Lederer and his collaborators considered it to contain only L-glutamic acid. It is clear, however, that the majority of the mycobacterial compound is composed of the L-isomer.

A possible explanation of the failure of synthetic poly(L-glutamic acid) to inhibit fusion is that it is rapidly hydrolysed by peptidases and so does not accumulate; the mycobacterial product is partially amidated (Wietzerbin *et al.*, 1975) and may resist hydrolysis. It is presumably continuously synthesized by the growing bacteria. This, incidentally, might explain why only live mycobacteria inhibit phagosome–lysosome fusion.

A more serious objection to polyglutamic acid as a candidate fusion-inhibiting factor is its site in the host cell. The synthetic polymers accumulate in swollen (secondary) lysosomes. Geisow *et al.* (1980) have shown conclusively that another polyanionic fusion-inhibitor, chlorite-oxidized amylose, is present only in secondary lysosomes and is not transferred to phagosomes unless they fuse with lysosomes. On the other hand it is clear from the French work that mycobacterial polyglutamic acid is covalently attached to the peptidoglycan of the bacterial wall and so is confined to the phagosome unless phagosome–lysosome fusion occurs. Unless fusion is supposed to be a symmetrical process as far as the membranes of the organelles involved are concerned, i.e. inhibitors may act on either of the membranes concerned, mycobacterial polyglutamic acid seems to be in the wrong place to control the process.

Sulphatide

A similar problem of siting arises with sulphatide, another mycobacterial product, though since this is not covalently attached to the bacterium one may suppose that very rapid diffusion after phagocytosis might allow inhibition from inside the lysosome to be postulated. Alternatively, as an amphiphilic substance it might become attached to cell membranes in a suitable site to inhibit fusion. Sulphatide (2,3,6,6′-tretraacyl trehalose 2′-sulphate; Goren, 1970) is, in this context, the major representative of a group of unusual sulphated glycolipids produced by virulent *M. tuberculosis* (Middlebrook *et al.*, 1959). There is a correlation among strains of *M. tuberculosis* between virulence and "strongly acidic lipids", including phospholipids and sulphatides (Goren *et al.*, 1974). (These authors point out that a few strains of low virulence also produce strongly acidic lipids, so that their presence may be a necessary but not a sufficient condition for virulence.)

Applied to cultured mouse peritoneal macrophages as an emulsion sulphatide has striking effects, causing a powerful inhibition of phagosome–lysosome fusion and the formation of swollen lysosomes containing numerous electron-transparent droplets (Goren *et al.*, 1976). The material is also apparently effective when loosely bound to yeast cells, using aluminium ions, reversing the fusion that normally occurs with these organisms. This result goes some way to showing that the sulphatide can act from within the phagosome, with the proviso that the binding of the lipid to the yeast wall (a hydrophilic structure) is likely to be less strong than to the hydrophobic mycobacterial wall, so that release and transfer to lysosomes might have occurred. The authors noted in the experiment involving "coated" yeast that there were a few electron-transparent droplets present in secondary lysosomes, possibly indicating transfer of sulphatide. Quantity is also problematical; it is not clear that the amount of sulphatide present on the mycobacterial surface approaches that added to the macrophages as an emulsion (when uptake amounted to about 1 pg per cell) or even artificially coated on to yeast cells, and it remains to be shown that the "natural" amount is sufficient to inhibit fusion.

Ammonia

The most recent substance, produced by *M. tuberculosis*, found to inhibit phagosome–lysosome fusion is ammonia (Gordon *et al.*, 1980). It is unexpected that this simple molecule should have this rather specific effect on macrophages because other amines tend to enhance fusion (Hart and Young, 1978). Its presence in media in which *M. tuberculosis* has been grown accounts for at least most of the fusion-inhibiting effect of these media. It is thought that the ammonia arises from hydrolysis of asparagine in the medium by asparaginase (Kirchheimer and Whittaker, 1954). Growth on asparagine is unbalanced in that intermediates accumulate (Lyon *et al.*, 1970); presumably ammonia is formed in excess of the amount the bacteria are able to use. It remains to be shown that ammonia can be produced by the bacteria inside cells where presumably nutritional conditions are quite different from those in a medium (and quite unknown). The problem of the site of production being different from the site of action does not arise with such a small and freely diffusible molecule. Moreover, as a weak base it rapidly accumulates in lysosomes (Ohkuma and Poole, 1978).

It must be concluded that the mechanism by which *M. tuberculosis* and its relatives inhibit phagosome–lysosome fusion is not yet known. None of the four fusion-inhibiting substances discussed above is known to fulfil all the requirements, namely:

(1) the substance must be produced by the bacteria in the intracellular environment

(2) the substance must have access to the structure or system controlling fusion

(3) production of the substance must cease, or preformed material must be rapidly degraded, in killed bacteria.

The question may also be asked: whether fusion-inhibition occurs *in vivo*. As discussed in connexion with *M. lepraemurium*, it is often difficult to determine in sections of tissue whether a given bacterium-containing vacuole is a phagosome or a phagolysosome. This means that *quantitative* data needed to confirm fusion inhibition cannot be obtained. Examination of the bone-marrow of mice infected with *M. microti*, exploiting the natural electron-dense label in the macrophage lysosomes, shows that fusion is significantly inhibited by this organism (Mr M. R. Young, pers. comm.).

Cytotoxicity of *Mycobacterium tuberculosis*

The interaction of *M. tuberculosis* and the phagocytic cell does not end with inhibition of fusion, since the bacteria are somewhat cytotoxic and the cell is eventually destroyed (this does not happen with *M. lepraemurium* or, apparently, with *M. leprae*). There is no clear evidence implicating any particular mycobacterial component in this toxicity, but a possible toxic agent is "cord factor". Cord factor (trehalose-6,6′-dimycolate) is produced by *M. tuberculosis* and is, in appropriate dose schedules and with appropriate routes of inoculation, highly toxic to mice (Bloch, 1950). However, *M. lepraemurium* also produces at least some cord factor (Goren *et al.*, 1979) yet is tolerated by cells indefinitely. It would be interesting to compare the amounts of cord factor produced by these two species *in vivo*. The toxicity of cord factor has been attributed to its disruptive effect on mitochondria (Kato, 1968). It should be noted that cord factor, though it has many interesting biological properties, is no longer believed to be responsible for the "cording" characteristic of cultures of virulent *M. tuberculosis* (see Goren, 1975).

Importance of Fusion inhibition

In the experimental system of cultured infected mouse peritoneal macrophages inhibition of phagosome–lysosome fusion confers no special benefit on the mycobacteria. Fusion may be brought about, and the inhibition may be reversed, by coating the bacteria with antibodies (Armstrong and Hart, 1975; Lowrie *et al.*, 1979). The multiplication of the bacteria is unaffected. (This is not the case with some protozoan pathogens that inhibit fusion, where addition of antibody to cause reversal of the inhibition also causes destruction of the parasite (Jones, 1975)). It is, however, increasingly clear that macrophages can vary widely in their physiology, and it may well be that in an intact infected animal the cells may be stimulated or activated in some way such that fusion is lethal to the bacterium. That people and animals can recover from an infection with *M. tuberculosis* indicates that killing mechanisms must exist. It has been shown that recovery from a BCG infection in animals is associated with a great accumulation of lysosomal enzymes (Dannenberg *et al.*, 1972).

Survival in the Macrophage Cytoplasm—*Mycobacterium leprae*

The evidence for the "normal" site of multiplication of *M. leprae* in the infected cell is still incomplete, but the site seems to be the cytoplasm. Very careful timed studies, first with normal mice (Evans and Levy, 1972) and later with thymectomized-irradiated mice (Levy *et al.*, 1975) showed that the appearance of bacteria in this unexpected site coincided with the exponential phase of bacterial growth. In human tissues where rapid multiplication of the organism appears to be occurring (lesions of histoid lepromatous leprosy) and in the tissues of infected nu/nu mice an appreciable proportion of the bacteria seem to be outside vacuoles (P. Draper, unpublished observations). Bacteria have also been seen free in many human cell-types, including axons (Boddingius, 1977) and muscle fibres (Esiri *et al.*, 1972) in biopsies from cases of human lepromatous leprosy, though in these cases no kinetic data about bacterial growth are available. The evidence from the quantitative mouse foot-pad experiments suggests that the route of entry of the bacterium is through a phagocytic vacuole, from which it escapes into the cytoplasm. This route is also employed by some rickettsias (Silverman and Wisseman, 1979; Rikishi and Ito, 1979) and by *Trypanosoma cruzi* (Nogueira, 1974; Kress *et al.*, 1975; Nogueira and Cohn, 1976).

How an organism such as *M. leprae* can escape from a phagosome is not clear. Possible mechanisms include production of an enzyme able to lyse the vacuole or chemical structures on the bacterial surface which allow the organism to fuse with and to pass through the membrane of the vacuole. Neither of these activities has been observed. It should be noted that observations on *M. leprae* are confined to tissues from patients or from experimentally infected animals; no tissue culture system allowing multiplication of the bacteria has been developed.

Once *M. leprae* has escaped it is clearly in a comfortable position since it is remote from all mechanisms for disposing of foreign particles, and short of massive destruction of tissue there is little the host can do to remove the parasite. Extremely slow multiplication and lack of cytotoxicity are presumably adaptations by the organism to its special sort of intracellular existence.

UNSOLVED PROBLEMS

There is much information but little understanding of how the mycobacterial pathogens inhibit intracellular killing. Some questions whose answers would increase understanding may be specified:

(1) How do macrophages kill (or even inhibit multiplication of) mycobacteria?

(2) Is phagosome–lysosome fusion important in the killing mechanism?

(3) How is phagosome–lysosome fusion controlled?

(4) Are the morphological changes that occur in *M. lepraemurium*-infected macrophages caused by a bacterial product? How?

(5) Which if any of the products of *M. tuberculosis* known to affect fusion is active in the infected cell?

(6) Does *M. tuberculosis* inhibit fusion *in vivo*?

(7) How does *M. leprae* escape from the phago(lyso)some?

(8) In which situation does *M. leprae* multiply?

The pathogenic mycobacteria are intriguing biologically and still, unfortunately and despite chemotherapy, important clinically. A proper understanding of their interaction with macrophages seems a worthwhile objective.

SUMMARY

The behaviour of three species of mycobacteria within macrophages is discussed. These organisms occur in phagosomes, in phagolysosomes and in the cytoplasm of the cell, respectively. It is proposed that they form a paradigm for the behaviour of intracellular parasites in general. Knowledge of the ways in which the mycobacteria control the behaviour of the cell is described.

REFERENCES

Armstrong, J. A. and Hart, P. d'Arcy. (1971). Response of cultured macrophages to *Mycobacterium tuberculosis*, with observations on fusion of lysosomes with phagosomes. *Journal of Experimental Medicine* **134**, 713–740.

Armstrong, J. A. and Hart, P. d'Arcy. (1975). Phagosome–lysosome interaction in cultured macrophages infected with virulent tubercle bacilli. Reversal of the usual nonfusion pattern and observations on bacterial survival. *Journal of Experimental Medicine* **142**, 1–16.

Bloch, H. (1950). Studies on the virulence of tubercle bacilli. Isolation and biological properties of a constituent of virulent organisms. *Journal of Experimental Medicine* **91**, 197–217.

Boddingius, J. (1977). Ultrastructural changes in blood vessels of peripheral nerves in leprosy neuropathy. II. Borderline, borderline-lepromatous and lepromatous leprosy patients. *Acta neuropathologica (Berlin)* **40**, 21–39.

Bourne, H. R., Lehrer, R. I., Cline, M. J. and Melmon, K. L. (1971). Cyclic 3′,5′-adenosine monophosphate in the human leukocyte: synthesis, degradation, and effects on neutrophil candidacidal activity. *Journal of Clinical Investigation* **50**, 920–929.

Brown, C. A. and Draper, P. (1970). An electron-microscope study of rat fibroblasts infected with *Mycobacterium lepraemurium*. *Journal of Pathology* **102**, 21–26.

Brown, I. N. and Draper, P. (1976). Growth of *Mycobacterium lepraemurium* in the mouse bone marrow: an ultrastructural study. *Infection and Immunity* **13**, 1199–1204.

Brown, I. N. and Krenzien, H.-N. (1976). Systemic *Mycobacterium lepraemurium* infection in mice: differences in doubling time in liver, spleen, and bone marrow, and a method for measuring the proportion of viable organisms in an inoculum. *Infection and Immunity* **13**, 480–486.

Carrol, M. E. W., Jackett, P. S., Aber, V. R. and Lowrie, D. B. (1979). Phagolysosome formation, cyclic adenosine 3′:5′-monophosphate and the fate of *Salmonella typhimurium* within mouse peritoneal macrophages. *Journal of General Microbiology* **110**, 421–429.

Closs, O. (1975). Experimental murine leprosy: induction of immunity and immune paralysis to *Mycobacterium lepraemurium* in C57BL mice. *Infection and Immunity* **12**, 706–713.

Dannenberg, A. M., Jr, Ando, M. and Shima, K. (1972). Macrophage accumulation, division, maturation, and digestive and microbicidal capacities in tuberculous lesions. III. The turnover of macrophages and its relation to their activation and antimicrobial immunity in primary BCG lesions and those of reinfection. *Journal of Immunology* **109**, 1109–1121.

Dhople, A. M. and Hanks, J. H. (1977). In vitro growth of *Mycobacterium lepraemurium*, an obligate intracellular microbe. *Science* **197**, 379–381.

Draper, P. (1974). The mycoside capsule of *Mycobacterium avium* 357. *Journal of General Microbiology* **83**, 431–433.

Draper, P. and Rees, R. J. W. (1970). Electron-transparent zone of mycobacteria may be a defence mechanism. *Nature* **228**, 860–861.

Draper, P. and Rees, R. J. W. (1973). The nature of the electron-transparent zone that surrounds *Mycobacterium lepraemurium* inside host cells. *Journal of General Microbiology* **77**, 79–87.

Esiri, M. M., Weddell, A. G. M. and Rees, R. J. W. (1972). Infection of murine striated muscle with *Mycobacterium leprae*: a study by light and electron microscopy. *Journal of Pathology* **106**, 73–80.

Evans, M. J. and Levy, L. (1972). Ultrastructural changes in cells of the mouse foot-pad infected with *Mycobacterium leprae. Infection and Immunity* **5**, 238–247.

van Furth, R. (Ed.) (1980). "Mononuclear Phagocytes. Functional aspect." Part II. Nijhoff, The Hague.

Geisow, M. J., Beaven, G. H., Hart, P. d'Arcy and Young, M. R. (1978). Site of action of a polyanion inhibitor of phagosome-lysosome fusion in cultured macrophages. *Experimental Cell Research* **126**, 159–165.

Gordon, A. H., Hart, P. d'Arcy and Young, M. R. (1980). Ammonia inhibits phagosome–lysosome fusion in macrophages. *Nature* **286**, 79–80.

Goren, M. B. (1970). Sulfolipid I of *Mycobacterium tuberculosis*, strain H37Rv. II. Structural studies. *Biochimica et Biophysica Acta* **210**, 127–138.

Goren, M. B. (1975). Cord factor revisited: a tribute to the late Dr Hubert Bloch. *Tubercle* **56**, 65–71.

Goren, M. B., Brokl, O. and Roller, P. (1979). Cord factor (trehalose-6,6′-dimycolate) of in vivo-derived *Mycobacterium lepraemurium. Biochimica et Biophysica Acta* **574**, 70–78.

Goren, M. B., Brokl, O. and Schaefer, W. B. (1974). Lipids of putative relevance to virulence in *Mycobacterium tuberculosis*: correlation of virulence with elaboration of sulfatides and strongly acidic lipids. *Infection and Immunity* **9**, 142–149.

Goren, M. B., Hart, P. d'Arcy, Young, M. R. and Armstrong, J. A. (1976). Prevention of phagosome–lysosome fusion in cultured macrophages by sulfatides of *Mycobacterium tuberculosis. Proceedings of the National Academy of Sciences, U.S.A.* **73**, 2510–2514.

Hart, P. d'Arcy, Armstrong, J. A., Brown, C. A. and Draper, P. (1972). Ultrastructural study of the behaviour of macrophages toward parasitic mycobacteria. *Infection and Immunity* **5**, 803–807.

Hart, P. d'Arcy and Young, M. R. (1978). Manipulations of the phagosome–lysosome fusion response in cultured macrophages. Enhancement of fusion by chloroquine and other amines. *Experimental Cell Research* **114**, 486–490.

Ignarro, L. J. and Cech, S. Y. (1976). Bidirectional regulation of lysosomal enzyme secretion and phagocytosis in human neutrophils by guanosine 3′-5′-monophosphate and adenoisine 3′-5′-monophosphate. *Proceedings of the Society for Experimental Biology and Medicine* **151**, 448–452.

Ignarro, L. J. and George, W. J. (1974). Hormonal control of lysosomal enzyme release from human neutrophils: elevation of cyclic nucleotide levels by autonomic neurohormones. *Proceedings of the National Academy of Sciences, U.S.A.* **71**, 2027–2031.

Jackett, P. S., Aber, V. R. and Lowrie, D. B. (1978a). Virulence and resistance to superoxide, low pH and hydrogen peroxide among strains of *Mycobacterium tuberculosis. Journal of General Microbiology* **104**, 37–45.

Jackett, P. S., Aber, V. R. and Lowrie, D. B. (1978b). Virulence of *Mycobacterium tuberculosis* and susceptibility to peroxidative killing systems. *Journal of General Microbiology* **107**, 273–278.

Jackett, P. S., Aber, V. R. and Lowrie, D. B. (1980). The susceptibility of strains of *Mycobacterium tuberculosis* to catalase-mediated peroxidative killing. *Journal of General Microbiology*, **121**, 381–386.

Jones, T. C. (1975). Phagosome–lysosome interaction with *Toxoplasma. In* "Mononuclear Phagocytes in Immunity, Infection and Pathology". (Ed. R. van Furth), pp. 595–607. Blackwell Scientific, Oxford.

Jones, T. C. and Hirsch, J. G. (1972). The interaction between *Toxoplasma gondii* and mammalian cells. II. The absence of lysosomal fusion with phagocytic vacuoles containing living parasites. *Journal of Experimental Medicine* **136**, 1173–1194.

Kato, M. (1968). Studies of a biochemical lesion in experimental tuberculosis in mice. VIII. Effect of derivatives and chemical analogues of cord factor on structure and function of mouse liver mitochondria. *American Review of Respiratory Disease* **98**, 668–676.

Kim, K.-S., Salton, M. R. J. and Barksdale, L. (1976). Ultrastructure of superficial mycosidic integuments of *Mycobacterium* sp. *Journal of Bacteriology* **125**, 739–743.

Kirchheimer, W. F. and Whittaker, C. K. (1954). Asparaginase of mycobacteria. *American Review of Tuberculosis* **70**, 920–921.

Klebanoff, S. J. (1969). Antimicrobial activity of catalase at acid pH. *Proceedings of the Society for Experimental Biology and Medicine* **132**, 571–574.

Kress, Y., Bloom, B. R., Wittner, M., Rowen, A. and Tanowitz, H. (1975). Resistance of *Trypanosoma cruzi* to killing by macrophages. *Nature* **254**, 394–396.

Lefford, M. J. and Mackaness, G. B. (1977). Suppression of immunity to *Mycobacterium lepraemurium* infection. *Infection and Immunity* **18**, 363–369.

Levy, L., Ng, H., Evans, M. J. and Krahenbuhl, J. L. (1975). Susceptibility of thymectomized and irradiated mice to challenge with several organisms and the effect of dapsone on infection with *Mycobacterium leprae. Infection and Immunity* **11**, 1122–1132.

Lowrie, D. B., Aber, V. R. and Jackett, P. S. (1979). Phagosome–lysosome fusion and cyclic adenosine 3′:5′-monophosphate in macrophages infected with *Mycobacterium microti, Mycobacterium bovis* BCG and *Mycobacterium lepraemurium. Journal of General Microbiology* **110**, 431–441.

Lowrie, D. B., Jackett, P. S. and Ratcliffe, N. A. (1975). *Mycobacterium microti* may protect itself from intracellular destruction by releasing cyclic AMP into phagosomes. *Nature* **254**, 600–602.

Lyon, R. H., Hall, W. H. and Costas-Martinez, C. (1970). Utilization of amino acids during growth of *Mycobacterium tuberculosis* in rotary cultures. *Infection and Immunity* **1**, 513–520.

Middlebrook, G., Coleman, C. M. and Schaefer, W. B. (1959). Sulfolipid from virulent tubercle bacilli. *Proceedings of the National Academy of Sciences, U.S.A.* **45**, 1801–1804.

Murray, H. W. and Cohn, Z. A. (1979). Macrophage oxygen-dependent antimicrobial activity. I. Susceptibility of *Toxoplasma gondii* to oxygen intermediates. *Journal of Experimental Medicine* **150**, 938–949.

Murray, H. W., Juangbhanich, C. W., Nathan, C. F. and Cohn, Z. A. (1979). Macrophage oxygen-dependent antimicrobial activity. II. The role of oxygen intermediates. *Journal of Experimental Medicine* **150**, 950–964.

Nishiura, M., Izumi, S., Mori, T., Takeo, K. and Nonaka, T. (1977). Freeze-etching study of human and murine leprosy bacilli. *International Journal of Leprosy* **45**, 248–254.

Nishiura, M., Uehira, K., Hasegawa, T. and Takeuchi, M. (1972). The morphological difference between human and murine leprosy bacilli as revealed by the freeze-etching technic. *International Journal of Leprosy* **40**, 89–90.

Nogueira, N. (1974). The escape of *T. cruzi* from the vacuolar system of macrophages. *Journal of Cell Biology* **63**, 246a.

Nogueira, N. and Cohn, Z. (1976). *Trypanosoma cruzi*: mechanism of entry and intracellular fate in mammalian cells. *Journal of Experimental Medicine* **143**, 1402–1420.

Ohkuma, S. and Poole, B. (1978). Fluorescence probe measurement of the intralysosomal pH in living cells and the perturbation of pH by various agents. *Proceedings of the National Academy of Sciences, U.S.A.* **75**, 3327–3331.

Phiet, P. H., Wietzerbin, J., Zissman, E., Petit, J. F. and Lederer, E. (1976). Analysis of the cell wall of five strains of *Mycobacterium tuberculosis* BCG and of an attenuated human strain, W115. *Infection and Immunity* **13**, 677–681.

Rikisha, Y. and Ito, S. (1979). Intracellular localization of *Rickettsia tsutsugamushi* in polymorphonuclear leukocytes. *Journal of Experimental Medicine* **150**, 703–708.

Sbarra, A. J., Selvaraj, R. J., Paul, B. B., Mitchell, G. W., Jr and Louis, F. J. (1979). Myeloperoxidase and leukocyte function. *In* "Lysosomes in Applied Biology and Therapeutics" (Eds J. T. Dingle, P. J. Jacques and I. H. Shaw), Vol. 6, pp. 267–274. North-Holland, Amsterdam.

Silverman, D. J. and Wisseman, C. L., Jr. (1979). In vitro studies of rickettsia-host cell interactions: ultrastructural changes induced by *Rickettsia rickettsii* infection in chicken embryo fibroblasts. *Infection and Immunity* **26**, 714–727.

Spirer, Z., Zakuth, V., Golander, A. and Bogair, N. (1975). The influence of cyclic nucleotides (c-AMP and c-GMP) on the nitrous blue tetrazolium reduction by human polymorphonuclear leukocytes. *Experientia* **31**, 118–120.

Vilkas, E. and Markovits, J. (1972). Sur la présence d'un acide polyglutamique dans les parois de *Mycobacterium tuberculosis* souche Peurois. *Comptes rendus hebdomadaires des séances de l'Académie des sciences* **275C**, 913–915.

Wietzerbin, J., Lederer, E. and Petit, J.-F. (1975). Structural study of the poly-L-glutamic acid of the cell wall of *Mycobacterium tuberculosis* var. hominis, strain Brévannes. *Biochemical and Biophysical Research Communications* 62, 246–252.

Wietzerbin-Falszpan, J., Das, B. C., Gros, C., Petit, J.-F. and Lederer, E. (1973). The amino acids of the cell wall of *Mycobacterium tuberculosis* var. bovis, strain BCG. Presence of poly(L-glutamic acid). *European Journal of Biochemistry* 32, 525–532.

Zurier, R. B., Weissman, G., Hoffstein, S., Kammermann, S. and Tai, H. H. (1974). Mechanism of lysosomal enzyme release from human leukocytes. II. Effects of cAMP and cGMP, autonomic agonists, and agents which affect microtubule function. *Journal of Clinical Investigation* 53, 297–309.

DISCUSSION

Smith Dr Draper has talked only about the intracellular survival and growth of mycobacteria, but in fact observations on mycobacteria have been the fountain of similar work with other microbes. Just to take a few: *Toxoplasma gondii* survives and grows within macrophages by inhibiting granule fusion like tubercle bacilli. *Leishmania donovani*, like *Mycobacterium leprae*, escapes into the cytoplasm to grow. In the bacterial field *Salmonella typhimurium* like *M. leprae* is resistant to granule fusion and prevention of granule fusion may occur in infections with *Legionella*. Hence, although Dr Draper has talked only about mycobacteria he has illustrated much similar work throughout microbiology.

Braude Are you talking, Dr Draper, about activated macrophages as well, or just about "virgin" macrophages, so to speak? The reason I ask is that there seems to be striking evidence that macrophages can kill tubercle bacilli after the individual develops tuberculin hypersensitivity. I wonder—if that is the case—whether the processes that you describe are inhibited? For example, is phagosome–lysosome fusion inhibited in the activated macrophage?

Draper I do not think anyone knows. This is the mouse peritoneal macrophage system and people are beginning to distinguish between various kinds of activated macrophage. Activation seems a rather specific process and yet one can bring about not dissimilar changes by rather nonspecific mechanisms. For example, macrophages grown in medium with 50% serum certainly develop a tremendous level of lysosomal enzymes which is sometimes regarded as one of the characteristics of activated macrophages. If you are talking about activation by immunological mechanisms, then they are not activated. The fact that even in the days before chemotherapy patients got better from tuberculosis must surely indicate that macrophages can kill tubercle bacilli, so the mechanism is there if one can find it.

Valdimarsson Can I comment on the question of activation? It is mainly

Zanvil Cohn's group who have been looking into this recently and they, I think, draw a distinction between macrophages which are simply elicited from the peritoneal cavity by various chemicals and macrophages taken from animals which have been infected and then re-infected. Chemically induced macrophages are to some extent activated, but they do not produce H_2O_2 and other oxygen reduction products so well *in vitro* as those from animals re-infected shortly before the macrophages are harvested. These are the activated ones which seem able to produce hydrogen peroxide and other oxygen reduction products. It looks from their work as if activated macrophages, that is to say immunologically activated macrophages, are able at least in some systems to kill by hydrogen peroxide and perhaps also by singlet oxygen and hydroxy radicals. I think, therefore, that the question of activation is extremely important in the context of this discussion.

Mogensen In relation to what Dr Valdimarsson said, I can add that chemically elicited macrophages are generally less restrictive to the replication of viruses than are normal resident macrophages, whereas specifically activated macrophages are more restrictive. So it is true that there are differences between elicited and activated macrophages in relation to microorganisms.

Mims I would like to say how unfortunate this word "activation" is. It is so complex; there are so many parameters to be measured; cells of very different properties all enjoying the same word "activation". To get an idea of what is going on look at the issue before last of the *Journal of the Reticulo-endothelial Society*, where the macrophage properties that you can measure—enzymes, functional properties, surface markers—have been delineated in terms of whether the macrophages are resident, thioglycolate-induced, BCG-induced, or whatever. It is a very complicated matter. Can I comment on this exciting suggestion of Dr Draper, so relevant to our theme, that the mycobacteria for their own purposes produce epitheloid cells as a better place in which they can multiply? Does anyone know whether in tuberculous lesions there are many mycobacteria present in and multiplying in epitheloid cells?

Draper I was talking about *M. lepraemurium* and I do not know the answer for *M. tuberculosis.* Could I make another comment about activation? In an infection, the chances are that the first encounter that the bacterium has with a cell is not going to be with an activated macrophage unless the person has been vaccinated. So by and large one is interested, at least to begin with, in what happens in the unactivated macrophage.

Easmon Please correct me if I am wrong, but I thought that in the presence of antibody directed against *M. tuberculosis*, phagolysozyme fusion did in fact occur but the organism survived. So even if you overcome the inhibition of fusion, the organism still survives.

Draper Yes, that is certainly true in the mouse peritoneal macrophage system, but one can then turn this on its head and say that these are not activated macrophages. It is clear that macrophages can under some circumstances kill mycobacteria: that is a clinical observation because people recover. It is also pretty clear that cultivated peritoneal macrophages can kill hardly anything, not even *M. smegmatis* that never caused a disease in its life. It may well be that the killing mechanism simply does not exist there, which is why one cannot be certain that phagosome–lysosome fusion has anything to do with killing. On the other hand, the inhibition is a very clearly defined phenomenon and my guess is that it is important to the bacterium in a cell that could otherwise kill it.

Mims Since one of the aims of our meeting is to make bridges between viruses and the other infectious agents, I want to comment on the inhibitors of lysosomal fusion. From a virus's point of view, once it gets into a vacuole and is exposed to lysosomal enzymes, that may well be the end of it. It must make haste to adsorb to the surface membrane of the vacuole and release its messengers and get going in the cell. After talking to Philip d'Arcy Hart, we thought if we could inhibit lysosomal fusion we might make it easier for a virus to infect the cell. So we added poly-D-glutamic acid to our cell system, then added our virus (mouse cytomegalovirus) and sure enough we increased the infectivity of the virus—as measured by plaque-forming units—by ten- to a hundred-fold. We were very excited. But then it occurred to us, and it was soon apparent from reading the literature, that poly-D-glutamic acid does many things beside inhibit lysosomal fusion, including exerting important membrane effects, and there were a variety of ways in which the poly-D-glutamic acid could have been acting. Just because we were interested in lysosomal fusion, that does not mean to say that was the way it was acting.

Draper One of the theories that I have always held is that *M. lepraemurium* actually thrives on being in the phagosome–lysosome because it is surrounded by small peptides and other agreeable things, so if it could be prevented from getting into its phagosome–lysosome it should not do so well. That goes back to the days when Celia Fildes was at the National Institute for Medical Research and we looked at her infected fibroblasts and found that in cells which do not have many lysosomes the bacteria do not multiply nearly so well. However, in whole animals Philip d'Arcy Hart showed that injections of polyglutamic acid actually made *M. lepraemurium* infection much worse. I am really saying just the same as you: in any system these things can have many effects.

Mims There is at least one virus that is said not to initiate infection unless it is exposed to lysosomal enzymes. That is reovirus, which needs to be uncoated by lysosomal enzymes before it can initiate infection.

Arbuthnott In talking about polyglutamic acid and sulphatide you said that you thought these could be produced, but you found it difficult to envisage how they gained access to the lysosome or how they influenced the fusion process. I was just wondering whether it is possible that small amounts of these compounds could become associated with the host cell membrane in some way and then have an indirect effect on fusion. Is there any evidence that sulphatide or polyglutamic acid become bound to macrophage membranes?

Draper No; I do not think anyone knows where the sulphatide is in the bacterial cell. It has been a question of extract a kilogram of tubercle bacilli with the appropriate solvent and you can isolate some sulphatide. I do not think anyone has the faintest idea whether it is in the wall or the cytoplasm or where. The polyglutamic acid is certainly part of the peptidoglycan, because it was originally picked up in purified peptidoglycan preparations. That might mean that it is deeply buried in the bacterial wall.

Smith There was one thing about Goren's experiments that I found intriguing: why did he put the sulphatide on yeast? Why did he not try to put the sulphatide back on a nonpathogenic *Mycobacterium*.

Draper A simple technical reason. With yeast you can do the work by light microscopy; with mycobacteria you need tedious electron microscopy.

Peters Just to return to this question of activated macrophages and the point that Dr Draper made about the macrophages being in an inactive stage when they first meet the tubercle bacillus, is there any information on the relative susceptibility of macrophages in various states of elicitation or activation? Of course, macrophages could quite easily be activated by other stimuli which make them more or less susceptible and this may have some bearing in clinical practice on susceptibility to infection.

Draper The whole classic studies centre around the people at the Trudeau Institute who showed that guinea-pigs infected with a variety of organisms including, *Listeria* and corynebacteria, develop infections from which they recover. The suggestion—at least the one that I have always accepted as being reasonable—is that this is because these bacteria nonspecifically activated the macrophages.

Peters I take that point, but that does not relate to the question of initial infection: that relates to the capacity of activated macrophages perhaps to kill the organism. If one thinks of it in various phases, presumably there is a stage of uptake of organism and then a stage of killing. I wondered, in relation to the question we are considering, whether there is any knowledge of the relative roles of these phenomena. It may be, for example, that the more that can be taken up the more can be effectively killed.

van Furth I wonder whether we are really speaking about the right part of the cell biology. We all think about fusion of phagosomes and lysosomes, but since the work of Tulkens and Steinman and his group at the Rockefeller University we know there is also another phenomenon: namely the membrane shuttle. In this, part of the outer membrane goes inside the cell, fuses with the phagosome and then returns to the outer membrane. That is a very quick process, which most probably takes one way in and one way out in the order of 10 or 20 minutes. What might be possible is that when you are looking for fusion and nonfusion with mycobacteria this membrane shuttle is inhibited. We know that on the outer membrane of phagocytes enzymes can be activated which will start metabolic events. As Segal has shown, by the shuttle these membrane enzymes move to the phagosome and it might well be that this is inhibited after ingestion of mycobacteria. When you have activated macrophages it could well be that the shuttle is much faster (more membrane goes in) or the metabolism might be higher and the cells kill more efficiently.

Wilton In relation to that—and Dr Draper would know better than I —I seem to remember experiments where mycobacteria were coated with specific antibody or, more accurately, opsonized with serum and although phagosome–lysosome fusion occurred they resisted any antibacterial effects of the lysosome contents. That is the first point. The second point, which is a rather roundabout way of looking at it, is this: when the phagosome is formed it is essentially the outer cell membrane and presumably has the same receptor array as the outer part of the membrane—for instance, the C3b receptor or the Fc receptor. There are pointers in the literature suggesting that IgG and complement are necessary for killing intracellularly as well as for particle binding and internalization. One therefore thinks in terms—as just mentioned by Professor van Furth—of the metabolic stimulation which follows events such as binding to Fc and C3b receptors, remembering that this will also be going on within the phagosome.

Draper The cultured mouse peritoneal macrophage is not an ideal system because it seems to be pretty defective in the ability to kill mycobacteria, but I do not think that this affects the usefulness of the system as indicating inhibition of fusion. You are absolutely right about the antibody. If you coat mycobacteria with antibody before putting them into mouse peritoneal macrophages, fusion is no longer inhibited. In fact, if you coat them with normal serum and are rather careless about washing it off, inhibition is reversed. But once again, the naïve recipient of a first infection would not have antituberculosis antibodies around, so this tells you how BCG works but it does not tell you about the initial stages of tuberculosis in a nonimmune person.

Wilton Except that I think you said that these bacteria were opsonized with serum. There was, as I remember, no evidence that there was any specific antibody.

Draper There were two parts to that experiment. Specific antibody was sufficiently strongly bound to the bacteria for one to be able to wash them afterwards and still have fusion inhibition reversed. But if you used normal globulin, apparently without antitubercular specificity (although mycobacteria are so ubiquitous that it is possible there was a little there) providing you did not wash the bacteria carefully it looked as though almost any globulin would serve to reverse the inhibition.

Valdimarsson In relation to intracellular killing by mononuclear phagocytes, the role of complement should be investigated. Very little is known about that. There is a possibility that complement may participate directly in killing by macrophages, as it seems to do in the case of neutrophils. When we are discussing compartmentalization of organisms within the macrophage, one question that comes to mind is this. To what extent could this be due to effects by the microorganism on complement outside and inside the phagocytic vacuole? For instance, do these organisms release something which breaks down C3b on the surface of the organisms? Has anyone looked into that relation of mycobacteria?

Quie I wonder about the proteases of mycobacteria. Perhaps these proteases activate C3 and this provides opsonic activity or cell membrane perturbation.

Valdimarsson I am thinking more in terms of the organism being coated with C3b because if the organism destroys that C3b it may thereby prevent fusion since there is some evidence that the presence of C3b facilitates various metabolic events, possibly including fusion.

Quie Professor van Furth's laboratory has evidence that C3b does indeed influence intracellular killing of *Staph. aureus* by macrophages and peripheral monocytes but I do not believe that there is similar evidence with granulocytes.

van Furth Indeed, you need stimulation of the Fc and C3b receptor on the monocyte membrane to obtain optimal killing of bacteria. We have done the same experiments with the granulocytes and found that you need to trigger the Fc receptor and the complement (C3b) receptor to get maximum killing. However, with granulocytes the situation is a little different, because without any serum in the environment about 70% of the bacteria are killed; when you add the above-mentioned serum components you get a killing of about 95%. So serum has an additional effect. The basic background level for killing in the granulocyte is much higher than in the monocyte. Monocytes do not kill any bacteria in the absence of serum.

Valdimarsson Certainly neutrophils need *Candida albicans* to be coated with C3b before they can kill. In the absence of C3b, candidas which are ingested by neutrophils are not killed in our system.

van Furth Can you kill mycobacteria *in vitro* with hydrogen peroxide or oxygen radicals?

Draper Douglas Lowry has measured this. Lack of susceptibility to hydrogen peroxide is one of the virulence factors and although there are many such factors, there is certainly a relation between susceptibility to hydrogen peroxide and virulence.

van Furth Is that in concentrations which you expect to occur intracellularly? All these studies have been done *in vitro* and it is difficult to say that there is any biological significance. I do not know the answer but it is important that we should know how macrophages kill microorganisms.

Smith This is an old chestnut. For many years both for tubercle bacilli and for brucellae there has been an association between catalase activity and virulence. Virulent strains tend to have more catalase activity although the correlation is not absolute. More recently, a correlation between virulence and presence of superoxide dismutase in strains has been suggested. However, I do not think anyone knows whether these enzymes have a real function intracellularly in neutralizing some of the killing mechanisms of phagocytes.

Mims With regard to relevance, it is important to remember that although we can wash out mouse peritoneal macrophages so well, and so many beautiful studies have been done with them, it is not necessarily the relevant thing to do. I say this because Brian Rodgers in my laboratory has recently shown that if you try to infect mouse peritoneal macrophages with influenza virus nothing happens, but if you take alveolar macrophages there is a totally different picture. We know that the metabolism and appearance of alveolar macrophages is quite different and it is wrong to suppose that macrophages from anywhere in the body will respond to infection in the same way, even if they all have the same IGa or Fc receptors.

Peters With regard to the role of complement, it may be worth noting that patients with complement deficiency, including C3 deficiency, do not seem to have any special problem with tuberculosis.

Valdimarsson Have they been exposed?

Peters That is hard to answer but I think that one of the C3 deficiency patients in Boston had.

Quie There are so few patients with C3 deficiency, I would judge that those who have been so described have been in locations where exposure to tuberculosis is not so great.

Peters One family with C3 deficiency, in whom the major manifestation is nephritis, are Palestinian refugees living in Kuwait.

van Furth What would you do in the case of a patient with C3 deficiency? I would hesitate to give any live vaccine to these patients until we know a little more about it.

Peters What may be important is the extent to which they have intracellular complement in macrophages, but you are talking about complement coated by serum.

Valdimarsson We also have to consider the possibility that the macrophages can actually deliver C3 directly into the phagosome.

Peters That is the point I was making.

Valdimarsson I should like to make a comment relating to the susceptibility of patients with C3 deficiency. We know that phagocytes from patients with myeloperoxidase deficiency are completely incapable of killing *C. albicans in vitro*. In spite of that, only one of the 10 or so patients reported with this abnormality has had candidiasis which coincided with the onset of diabetes. This is in spite of the fact that *C. albicans* is everywhere. Even if we know that a certain component of the defence system is important for the protection against an organism, that does not necessarily mean that an individual lacking this component is susceptible to infections with that organism, because there are many other host factors which may compensate. However, if the defence system is further perturbed by an intercurrent illness, the underlying defect may give rise to specific problems, as in the myeloperoxidase deficient patient who developed diabetes.

Peters You have to put a weighting on the relative importance of the mechanism.

Braude There are two things that distinguish *M. tuberculosis* from the other mycobacteria. They are its ability to throw a lot of niacin into the medium and its possession of di-mycolyl-trehalose. I wondered whether either of these had been examined for its ability to inhibit fusion.

Draper The cord factor (di-mycolyl-trehalose) is not unique to *M. tuberculosis*. It has recently been shown to be in *M. lepraemurium.*

Braude I am talking about the human pathogenic mycobacteria. Is it present in any of the others?

Draper I think cord factors are present in many mycobacteria. There is a little in *M. leprae.*

Viral Interaction with Phagocyte Functions

SØREN C. MOGENSEN

Institute of Medical Microbiology,
University of Aarhus,
Denmark.

INTRODUCTION

Virus infections often predispose to secondary bacterial invasion, especially in the respiratory tract. Influenza complicated by bacterial pneumonia is the prototype of a viral infection that enhances the susceptibility of the host to bacterial disease, a fact that has been well documented both for the natural infection in humans (Stuart-Harris, 1965) and for experimental infections in laboratory animals (for references, see Jakab, 1977). Earlier concepts of the mechanisms by which viruses render the lungs more susceptible to bacterial infection have focused on the importance of viral-induced damage to the mucociliary transport mechanisms of the bronchopulmonary tree (Harford *et al.*, 1946) and on the effects of oedema of the lung (Harford and Hara, 1950). However, during the last 15 years or so, attention has been directed towards functional lesions induced by virus infections in the host phagocytic cells.

PHAGOCYTIC CELL SYSTEMS

Cells of two major systems are able to respond to local invasion and multiplication of microorganisms by accumulating in infectious foci and ingesting and inactivating the invading microorganisms, namely cells of the mononuclear phagocyte system (the reticuloendothelial system) and polymorphonuclear leukocytes. Indeed, it was these cell systems that were analysed by Metchnikoff (1892) by the end of the last century and attributed by him an important role in the resistance to bacterial infection through engulfment and digestion of invading microorganisms. Since most of the studies on the deleterious action of virus infections on host phagocytic functions have dealt with the interaction of viruses with macrophages, a brief survey of current concepts of the mononuclear phagocyte system will be given.

Metchnikoff (1892) classified phagocytic cells as *macrophages* and *microphages* (polymorphonuclear leukocytes) on morphological and functional grounds. Mononuclear phagocytes residing in various organs and tissues were, according to Metchnikoff, closely related and belonged to a "macrophage system". This system was further elaborated by Aschoff (1924), who grouped reticular cells of the spleen and lymph nodes and reticuloendothelial cells of the lymph and blood sinuses as well as histiocytes, splenocytes and blood monocytes in a unifying cell system called the "reticuloendothelial system", a term which has since been widely accepted and used. However, our current knowledge of phagocytic mononuclear cells has prompted re-evaluation of the classification of these cells. On the basis of morphology, function, and kinetics of development all highly phagocytic mononuclear cells and their precursors fit into one cell lineage called the "mononuclear phagocyte system" (van Furth *et al.*, 1972). Mononuclear phagocytes originate from precursor cells of the bone marrow. Following maturation of these cells into promonocytes and monocytes, the monocytes are transported via the blood to organs and tissues, where they finally develop into macrophages. These are histiocytes of the connective tissue, Kupffer cells of the liver, alveolar macrophages of the lung, free and fixed macrophages of the spleen, lymph nodes and bone marrow, and macrophages monitoring serous spaces such as the pleural and peritoneal cavities. Osteoclasts of bone tissue and microglial cells of the nervous system have been included more tentatively in the system.

From an anatomical point of view, cells of the mononuclear phagocyte system are well suited to function as a barrier against microbial invasion and dissemination. They are long-lived and strategically placed at the portal of entry of many infections (e.g. the respiratory tract) and are widely distributed in close contact with the circulating blood in most organs of the body, thus encountering the microorganism early in the infection. From a functional point of view, the ability of the mononuclear phagocyte system to provide an influx of new cells from the bone marrow and blood monocyte compartment into foci of infection and the ability of the cells to take up and digest microorganisms may be decisive in determining the outcome of the infection. Polymorphonuclear leukocytes, on the other hand, are very short-lived and do not constitute a fixed barrier system in the body, although they are able to react to chemotactic stimuli and to ingest and degrade microorganisms to an even greater extent than macrophages.

VIRUS REPLICATION IN PHAGOCYTES

The ability of phagocytic cells to support virus growth has been dealt with in several reviews (Allison, 1974; Gresser and Lang, 1966; Mims, 1964; Mogensen, 1979; Morahan and Morse, 1979; Silverstein, 1970). Generally, most authors have been interested in this virus–phagocyte interaction as a means of explaining the outcome of the virus infection in question. However, many of the data obtained from these studies may provide valuable clues as to how virus infections may interfere with phagocyte functions and thereby predispose to secondary infection.

Macrophages are either intrinsically resistant (nonpermissive) or susceptible (permissive) to virus replication. The nonpermissive virus–macrophage interaction results in an abortive infection. The internalized virus is either eclipsed without subsequent efficient replication or it is destroyed in the phagolysosome. In the permissive situation, the virus replicates productively in the macrophage. This may cause cytopathic effects or death of the macrophage, or the cell may become persistently infected without obvious cytopathic changes (Mogensen, 1979; Morahan and Morse, 1979). Almost no studies have been made of the ability of polymorphonuclear leukocytes to support virus replication, probably because these cells are very short-lived and do not survive for long in culture. Mims (1964) concluded that, given the opportunity, polymorphonuclear leukocytes take up virus particles quite readily, but that there is no evidence that they can support virus replication.

When attempting to analyse the numerous and often conflicting data on virus–macrophage interactions, it is important to realize that a number of variables may influence the outcome of this interaction both *in vivo* and *in vitro*. Examples of such variables are given in the following.

The Strain and Type of the Virus

Closely related viruses, different serotypes, and even different strains of the same virus may vary in their ability to induce productive infection of macrophages. This has been shown for influenza, Newcastle disease, ectromelia, vaccinia, lymphocytic choriomeningitis, mouse hepatitis, and herpes simplex viruses (reviewed by Mogensen, 1979). Both naturally occurring variants and variants obtained by adaptation to a particular host have been used. Of these, the naturally occurring strains or types may be more suited to the analysis of interactions of pathogenetic importance, since adaptation or attenuation procedures may result in mere artefacts with little bearing on the natural situation. An example of the difference between naturally occurring types of the same virus is the interaction of mouse peritoneal macrophages with herpes simplex virus type 1 and type 2. Although mouse macrophages are rather restrictive in the replication of both virus types, the restriction of the type 1 virus is far more pronounced than that of type 2 (Mogensen, 1977a). The adaptation by Lindenmann *et al.* (1978) of an influenza virus to growth in high titres with gross cytopathic changes in macrophage cultures, although in its native form it did not replicate in macrophages, may be quoted as an example of an artificially induced difference in virus–macrophage interaction.

The Species and Strain of Animal

The interaction of viruses with macrophages from different animal species may vary widely. This is not surprising in view of the marked species specificity of many virus infections. However, differences in the effect of viruses on macrophages from members of the same species are also known. Most of these studies have been done in mice, because of the availability of different inbred and congenic strains. Genetically determined variation in virus–macrophage interactions has been shown for infections with flavi-, mouse hepatitis, herpes simplex, murine cytomegalo-, and influenza viruses (reviewed by Mogensen, 1979). In most instances resistance or susceptibility of macrophages has been found to be inherited as monogenic, autosomal dominant traits, but Mogensen (1977b) found that resistance of macrophages to herpes simplex virus type 2 is governed by an X-linked dominant gene, thereby stressing the possible importance of the sex of the animal when analysing virus-macrophage interactions. Another important implication of these studies is that the outcome of virus–macrophage interactions requires individual assessment with each virus–host system; for instance, macrophages that resist flaviviruses are susceptible to mouse hepatitis virus and *vice versa*.

The Age of the Animal

The ability of macrophages to restrict virus replication has been shown to be age-dependent in that macrophages from mature animals are much more restrictive than macrophages from suckling or weanling animals (reviewed by Mogensen, 1979). The basic nature of this maturation process has not been disclosed, but at least for herpes simplex virus type 1 the infection has been shown to be aborted in adult macrophages. All major components of the virus are synthesized, but errors seem to occur in the assembly of the virus particles (Stevens and Cook, 1971). Also herpes simplex virus type 2 has been shown to replicate more efficiently in macrophages from weanling mice than in macrophages from adult mice (Mogensen, 1978).

Induction and Cultivation of Macrophages

During induction, harvest and cultivation, macrophages may lose their native properties, or new ones may be gained. For instance, the widely used induction of peritoneal exudates by inflammatory agents such as mineral oil, thioglycolate or proteose–peptone to increase macrophage yields is not only affecting the macrophage population quantitatively, but also qualitatively. No comparative studies have been performed thus far to compare the influence of various inducing agents on virus–macrophage interactions, but recent studies have shown that they may actually increase the permissiveness of macrophages to virus infection (Lopez and Dudas, 1979). On the other hand, macrophages from mice inoculated with various immunomodulators such as pyran and *Corynebacterium parvum* (Morahan and Morse, 1979) or resident macrophages from nude mice (Mogensen and Andersen, 1978) show increased restriction of virus growth. Culture conditions, for instance the type and concentration of serum used (Lavelle and Bang, 1971) and the length of incubation before viral inoculation (Lopez and Dudas, 1979) have also been found to influence the outcome of the virus–macrophage interaction.

VIRAL INTERFERENCE WITH PHAGOCYTIC ANTIBACTERIAL ACTIVITY *IN SITU*

Almost all *in situ* studies of the mechanisms by which a virus infection may predispose to secondary bacterial invasion have focused on acute respiratory infections, especially those caused by influenza and Sendai virus. As mentioned in the introduction, earlier studies have stressed the importance of the pathological lesions induced by the virus infection in the lung. Desquamation of the bronchial epithelium was thought to impair the mucociliary transport mechanisms of the lungs responsible for the physical translocation of inhaled bacteria (Harford *et al.*, 1946). It was proposed, moreover, that pulmonary oedema might promote bacterial multiplication by providing an excellent growth medium and indirectly impair phagocytosis by diluting the inflammatory exudate (Harford and Hara, 1950). However, using radiolabelled bacteria, Green and Kass (1964) showed that viable bacteria in the lungs after aerosol challenge of normal mice disappeared almost completely after a few hours, whereas radioactivity was only marginally reduced during the same period. By the immunofluorescent method, the inhaled bacteria were found to be localized mainly within alveolar macrophages. They concluded that the phagocytic activity of alveolar macrophages constitutes the main clearance mechanism of the lung, and that mechanical mucociliary transport only comprises a small fraction of the clearing process.

Since these discoveries, studies of the influence of virus infections on the *in situ* bactericidal activity of the lungs have focused on the effect of viruses on the phagocytic clearance mechanisms. A number of studies have shown that infection of mice with respiratory pathogens like influenza and Sendai viruses causes a marked decrease in the phagocytic clearance of inhaled bacteria followed by multiplication of the organisms (Jakab and Green, 1972, 1974; Jakab *et al.*, 1979; Klein *et al.*, 1969; Warshauer *et al.*, 1977), or the appearance of endogenous pathogens (Jakab, 1974). The impairment of the bactericidal activity is maximal at a time when the pathological lesions caused by the virus are most severe, that is approximately a week after infection with a sublethal dose of virus. However, even under these circumstances the physical translocation of bacteria by the mucociliary apparatus was not found to be notably impaired (Jakab and Green, 1972, 1974; Warshauer *et al.*, 1977). The minor importance of damage to the physical transport mechanisms of the lungs was also stressed by Klein *et al.* (1969) and Goldstein *et al.* (1972) in experiments with reovirus and encephalomyocarditis virus, respectively. These viruses induced only minimal pathological changes in the lungs of infected mice, but impaired nevertheless the pulmonary antibacterial mechanisms. However, the suppression of host antibacterial defences during influenza virus infection in mice was localized to the lungs with no alteration of microbicidal activity of the liver and spleen (Jakab *et al.*, 1979).

The hypothesis that viral infections of the respiratory tract promote secondary bacterial infection through the development of edema within the lung was tested by Jakab and Green (1974). They examined quantitatively the bactericidal activity of consolidated and nonconsolidated areas of the same lung one week after a sublethal infection of mice with Sendai virus. Their data demonstrated that the intrapulmonary bactericidal activity was depressed in nonconsolidated as well as in consolidated areas, whereas bacterial multiplication above the value of initial deposition was limited to the consolidated areas.

Studies at the cellular level of the reduced phagocytic bactericidal activity *in situ* following viral infection have not provided unequivocal results. Jakab and Green (1976) and Silverberg *et al.* (1979), using infection of mice with Sendai virus and *Staphylococcus aureus*, found that the ingestion of bacteria by alveolar macrophages, as measured by the intra- and extracellular location of staphylococci in histological sections of lungs and in lung lavage fluid immediately after bacterial challenge, was unaffected by the preceding virus infection, whereas Warshauer *et al* (1977), using influenza virus and *Staphylococcus albus*, found that the ingestive process was decreased in virus-infected animals. However, it was found in all of these studies that the intracellular digestion of bacteria failed in virus-infected mice with subsequent multiplication of the staphylococci in the macrophages as a result. The basis of this impairment of intracellular digestion may be the reduced lysosomal enzyme content (Warr *et al.*, 1979) or the phagosome–lysosome fusion defect (Silverberg *et al.*, 1979) of macrophages from Sendai virus infected mice.

VIRAL INTERFERENCE WITH PHAGOCYTOSIS *IN VITRO*

Several studies have tried to identify the virus-induced defects in the function of phagocytic cells by examining the phagocytosis process *in vitro*. The advantage of *in vitro* experiments over *in situ* analysis is that it is possible to examine the interaction between phagocytes and microorganisms directly without any interference of other defence mechanisms mediated by factors such as antibody, complement or lymphocytes present in the intact animal. However, in analysing the results, due attention should be paid to the possible alteration of phagocyte functions during the *in vitro* cultivation required for the establishment and infection of the cultures to be used in the phagocytosis assay.

Two main approaches have been made in these studies. Phagocytic cells are either harvested from virus-infected animals at various times after the infection and examined in phagocytosis assays *in vitro*, or they are collected from normal animals, exposed to the virus *in vitro* and then examined for defects in phagocytosis. Although the results of such studies vary considerably depending on the cell type and assay conditions, it has been possible to define some of the steps involved in impairment of the phagocytosis process.

Virus Infection *In Vivo*

This "semi-*in vitro*" approach allows the virus–phagocyte interaction to take place in the intact animal, thereby avoiding the artefact of *in vitro* cultivation and infection of the phagocytic cells before the phagocytosis assay. On the other hand, an observed alteration of the phagocytic potential of the cells cannot be unequivocally ascribed to a direct effect of the virus on the cell, since it might as well be caused by intermediate helper or suppressor factors generated by the virus in the animal. Nevertheless, this approach seems to reveal most accurately the influence of the virus–host interaction on phagocyte functions.

Again, most studies have been done with influenza and Sendai virus infections of the respiratory tract of mice. The overall picture of these studies is that alveolar macrophages obtained by lung lavage at various times after a pulmonary virus infection may show defects in binding (Warr and Jakab, 1979), ingestion (Degré, 1970; Jakab *et al.*, 1980; Sawyer, 1969; Warr and Jakab, 1979) and intracellular killing (Taylor *et al.*, 1974; Warr and Jakab, 1979) of various microorganisms at some stage of the infection. Some of the studies have shown one or another of these parameters to be unaffected or even augmented by the virus infection. This is probably due to differences in timing of the experiments, as it has been shown that phagocytic parameters may fluctuate widely during the course of infection (Jakab *et al.*, 1980).

The defect in ingestion of microorganisms may be related to the suppression of Fc receptor-mediated ingestion of erythrocytes by alveolar macrophages from mice infected with Sendai virus as described by Warr *et al.* (1979). The suppression of this activity was maximal 7 days after the virus infection, that is at a time, when the mice are most susceptible to secondary bacterial pneumonia. In contrast, complement receptor-mediated ingestion, which only occurs with activated macrophages, was increased during the same period, indicating that the virus infection is accompanied by macrophage activation in spite of defective phagocytosis.

The reduced intracellular microbicidal activity of pulmonary macrophages from virus-infected animals has also been studied. Jakab *et al.* (1980) have described a defect in the phagosome–lysosome fusion of alveolar macrophages derived from mice infected with Sendai virus. Lysosomes of alveolar macrophages were prelabelled with acridine orange, and after challenge of the cells with *Candida krusei*, the discharge of the dye from lysosomes into yeast-containing phagosomes was determined by fluorescence microscopy. The phagosome–lysome fusion was progressively inhibited during the course of infection, peak inhibition correlating in time with maximal virus-induced suppression of pulmonary bactericidal activity. By electron microscopy, Silverberg *et al.* (1979) have demonstrated a phagosome–lysosome fusion defect as the main alteration in the function of lung macrophages from Sendai virus-infected mice challenged *in vivo* with *Staphylococcus aureus.*

Virus Infection *In Vitro*

Several studies have been aimed at elucidating the question whether the defect in phagocytosis induced by virus infections is a direct effect of the virus on the phagocytic cell. Pertinent to this problem is also the question whether the permissiveness of the phagocyte for virus replication may be related to such a defect.

In contrast to the striking effect of Sendai and influenza virus infections *in vivo* on the phagocytic potential of alveolar macrophages, most studies have failed to detect any reduction of either ingestion or intracellular microbicidal activity of mouse macrophages after infection of the cells with these viruses *in vitro* (Mills, 1979; Nugent and Pesanti, 1979; Taylor *et al.*, 1974; Verini and Lief, 1979). As regards the ingestive capability, no difference was detected in either the number of macrophages ingesting the microorganisms or the average number of organisms per macrophage between virus-infected and control cultures. However, Sawyer (1969) has described a reduction in the number of macrophages containing at least one *Pneumococcus*, and Lemercier *et al.* (1979) has reported that the number of *Candida albicans* cells per macrophage in phagocytosis assays was lower after influenza virus infection of the culture. The phagosome–lysosome fusion defect of macrophages obtained from Sendai virus-infected mice described by Jakab *et al.* (1980) was not found in macrophages infected *in vitro* with influenza virus (Nugent and Pesanti, 1979). It thus seems that a direct effect of viruses on the phagocytosis of macrophages is either absent or at least very difficult to detect. Any possible defect is unrelated to the ability of the virus to replicate productively in macrophages. Macrophages are permissive for Sendai virus replication (although without production of any cytopathic effect: Mills, 1979), whereas influenza virus infection is aborted in macrophages (Nugent and Pesanti, 1979).

Virus infection of polymorphonuclear leukocytes *in vitro* regularly leads to inhibition of their ability to ingest bacteria and yeasts. This is best documented for influenza virus (Fisher and Ginsberg, 1956; Larson *et al.*, 1977; Merchant and Morgan, 1950; Sawyer, 1969), but has also been shown with mumps virus (Merchant and Morgan, 1950) and Coxsackie virus (Kantoch and Dubowska-Inglot, 1960). Viruses do not replicate in polymorphonuclear leukocytes, but heat inactivation was found to destroy the inhibitory action of influenza and mumps viruses, while neutralization with specific immune serum affected the inhibitory activity of mumps virus but not that of influenza virus (Merchant and Morgan, 1950). The inhibition of phagocytosis by influenza virus was related by Fisher and Ginsberg (1956) to a block in glycolysis of virus-treated cells, but this relationship was later questioned by Sawyer (1969).

VIRAL INTERFERENCE WITH CHEMOTAXIS

The ability of phagocytic cells to react to chemotactic stimuli and thereby accumulate at sites of inflammation is generally regarded as an important event in the host defence against infectious diseases. Factors which counteract this function might, therefore, be expected to result in increased susceptibility to infection. If the microorganisms themselves are able to interfere with chemotaxis, this function can be considered a virulence factor of the microorganism with a detrimental effect on the elimination of the infection in question and on the ability of the host to resist secondary invasion by other microorganisms.

Viral interference with chemotaxis has been the subject of several studies in recent years. Again, the interest has focused on influenza virus. It has been well documented that incubation with influenza virus can inhibit the chemotaxis of mononuclear leukocytes from humans (Kleinerman *et al.*, 1974; Pike *et al.*, 1977) and mice (Kleinerman *et al.*, 1976) as well as of polymorphonuclear leukocytes from humans (Larson *et al.*, 1977; Ruutu *et al.*, 1977; Schlesinger *et al.*, 1976) and rats (Ruutu, 1977). Human mononuclear chemotaxis was also inhibited by herpes simplex virus but not by vaccinia, polio or reovirus (Kleinerman *et al.*, 1974), whereas polymorphonuclear leukocyte chemotaxis was inhibited by measles, respiratory syncytial, mumps, varicella-zoster and cytomegalovirus (Park *et al.*, 1977).

The importance of these observations was stressed by the finding of reduced chemotaxis of mononuclear phagocytes during natural infection with influenza virus (Kleinerman *et al.*, 1975) and of polymorphonuclear leukocytes after immunization with this virus (Baum and Douglas, 1979). Also patients with measles (Anderson *et al.*, 1974) and recurrent herpes simplex virus infections (Rabson *et al.*, 1977) have shown defective chemotaxis of polymorphonuclear leukocytes. The subnormal chemotactic response of cells from patients with influenza (Pike *et al.*, 1977) and herpes simplex virus infections (Rabson *et al.*, 1977) was normalized if the patients were treated with the immunostimulant levamisole or if the leukocytes were treated *in vitro* with the drug.

In experimental animals the accumulation and exudation of mononuclear (Kleinerman *et al.*, 1976) and polymorphonuclear (Ruutu, 1977) leukocytes into the peritoneal cavity after inoculation of a chemical irritant was found to be reduced after influenza virus infection. It is interesting that this effect could be achieved after intranasal inoculation of the virus (Kleinerman *et al.*, 1976).

The mechanisms by which viruses can interfere with chemotaxis is not well understood. Apparently, the effect is caused by a direct interaction of the virus with leukocytes, but it is not dependent on replication in the cells and is not caused by virus induced cell death (Kleinerman *et al.*, 1974). UV-inactivated influenza virus still caused some depression of monocyte (Kleinerman *et al.*, 1976) and polymorphonuclear (Park *et al.*, 1977) chemotaxis, although not to the same degree as live virus, whereas the effect of herpes simplex virus on monocytes was abolished by UV inactivation (Kleinerman *et al.*, 1974). The inhibitory effect of influenza virus on polymorphonuclear leukocytes was not affected by inactivation of virus infectivity with Tween 80 and ether (Ruutu *et al.*, 1977). On the other hand, treatment with specific antiserum (Larson *et al.*, 1977; Ruutu *et al.*, 1977) or gentle heating sufficient to inactivate virus infectivity and the neuraminidase, but not the haemagglutinin (Larson *et al.*, 1977), abolished the effect. However, bacterial neuraminidase was not found to inhibit polymorphonuclear motility (Ruutu *et al.*, 1977). Pretreatment of polymorphonuclear leukocytes with amantadine hydrochloride, which inhibits the penetration (but not adsorption) and uncoating of influenza A virus has been claimed by Schlessinger *et al.* (1976) to partially protect the cells against the effect of influenza virus, although in the experiments by Ruutu *et al.* (1977) the inhibition of polymorphonuclear chemotaxis by influenza virus was not affected by amantadine.

It is difficult to reach any conclusion as to which properties of the virus may be responsible for the inhibition of leukocyte chemotaxis. However, most data indicate that the effect is not dependent on infectivity but rather related to some surface property of the virus (not necessarily the haemaglutinin or the neuraminidase) interacting with the cell surface.

CONCLUDING REMARKS

The experimental studies reviewed herein have clearly shown that virus infections can adversely affect the function of mononuclear and polymorphonuclear leukocytes. This may lead to defects in the antimicrobial defence provided by these cells and should therefore be considered a potential mechanism by which viruses may counteract host defences and predispose to secondary infections. The approach of the review has been purely mechanistic with special emphasis on the effect of virus infections on the phagocytic clearance mechanisms *in situ* and on various aspects of phagocytosis and chemotaxis. No attempt has been made to elucidate viral interference with the immune response, although macrophages are known to play an important role in the inductive phase of immunity.

This work was supported by the Danish Medical Research Council grant No. 512–20475 and the Aarhus University Research Foundation grant No. 7131–01–2.

REFERENCES

Allison, A. C. (1974). Interactions of antibodies, complement components and various cell types in immunity against viruses and pyogenic bacteria. *Transplantation Reviews* 19, 3–55.

Anderson, R., Sher, R., Rabson, A. R. and Koornhof, H. J. (1974). Defective chemotaxis in measles patients. *South African Medical Journal* **48**, 1819–1820.

Aschoff, L. (1924). Das reticulo-endotheliale System. *Ergebnisse der Inneren Medicin und Kinderheilkunde* **26**, 1–118.

Baum, J. and Douglas, R. G. (1979). The effect of immunization on polymorphonuclear leukocyte chemotaxis in influenza. *Acta Virologia* **23**, 433–436.

Degré, M. (1970). Synergistic effect in viral–bacterial infection. II. Influence of viral infection on the phagocytic ability of alveolar macrophages. *Acta Pathologica et Microbiologica Scandinavica, B* **78**, 41–50.

Fisher, T. N. and Ginsberg, H. S. (1956). The reaction of influenza viruses with guinea pig polymorphonuclear leucocytes. III. Studies on the mechanism by which influenza viruses inhibit phagocytosis. *Virology* **2**, 656–664.

van Furth, R., Cohn, Z. A., Hirsch, J. G., Humphrey, J. H., Spector, W. G. and Langevoort, H. L. (1972). The mononuclear phagocyte system: a new classification of macrophages, monocytes, and their precursor cells. *Bulletin of the World Health Organization* **46**, 845–852.

Goldstein, E., Buhles, W. C., Akers, T. G. and Vedros, N. (1972). Murine resistance to inhaled *Neisseria meningitidis* after infection with an encephalo-myocarditis virus. *Infection and Immunity* **6**, 398–402.

Green, G. M. and Kass, E. H. (1964). The role of the alveolar macrophage in the clearance of bacteria from the lung. *Journal of Experimental Medicine* **119**, 167–176.

Gresser, I. and Lang, D. J. (1966). Relationships between viruses and leucocytes. *Progress in Medical Virology* **8**, 62–130.

Harford, C. G. and Hara, M. (1950). Pulmonary edema in influenzal pneumonia of the mouse and the relation of fluid in the lung to the inception of pneumococcal pneumonia. *Journal of Experimental Medicine* **91**, 245–259.

Harford, C. G., Smith, M. R. and Wood, W. B. (1946). Sulfonamide chemotherapy of combined infection with influenza virus and bacteria. *Journal of Experimental Medicine* **83**, 505–518.

Jakab, G. J. (1974). Effect of sequential inoculations of Sendai virus and *Pasteurella pneumotropica* in mice. *Journal of the American Veterinary Medical Association* **164**, 723–728.

Jakab, G. J. (1977). Pulmonary defense mechanisms and the interaction between viruses and bacteria in acute respiratory infections. *Bulletin Europeen de Physiopathologie Respiratoire* **13**, 119–135.

Jakab, G. J. and Green, G. M. (1972). The effect of Sendai virus infection on bactericidal and transport mechanisms of the murine lung. *Journal of Clinical Investigation* **51**, 1989–1998.

Jakab, G. J. and Green, G. M. (1974). Pulmonary defense mechanisms in consolidated and nonconsolidated regions of lungs infected with Sendai virus. *Journal of Infectious Diseases* **129**, 263–270.

Jakab, G. J. and Green, G. M. (1976). Defect in intracellular killing of *Staphylococcus aureus* within alveolar macrophages in Sendai virus-infected murine lungs. *Journal of Clinical Investigation* **57**, 1533–1539.

Jakab, G. J., Warr, G. A. and Knight, M. E. (1979). Pulmonary and systemic defenses against challenge with *Staphylococcus aureus* in mice with pneumonia due to influenza

A virus. *Journal of Infectious Diseases* 140, 105–108.

Jakab, G. J., Warr, G. A. and Sannes, P. L. (1980). Alveolar macrophage ingestion and phagosome–lysosome fusion defect associated with virus pneumonia. *Infection and Immunity* 27, 960–968.

Kańtoch, M. and Dubowska-Inglot, A. (1960). Inhibition of phagocytic activity of leukocytes by Coxsackie viruses. I. The influence of viral concentration and temperature on the inhibition of phagocytosis. *Pathologia et Microbiologia* 23, 83–94.

Klein, J. O., Green, G. M., Tilles, J. G., Kass, E. H. and Finland, M. (1969). Effect of intranasal reovirus infection on antibacterial activity of mouse lung. *Journal of Infectious Diseases* 119, 43–50.

Kleinerman, E. S., Daniels, C. A., Polisson, R. P. and Snyderman, R. (1976). Effect of virus infection on the inflammatory response. Depression of macrophage accumulation in influenza-infected mice. *American Journal of Pathology* 85, 373–382.

Kleinerman, E. S., Snyderman, R. and Daniels, C. A. (1974). Depression of human monocyte chemotaxis by herpes simplex and influenza viruses. *Journal of Immunology* 113, 1562–1567.

Kleinerman, E. S., Snyderman, R. and Daniels, C. A. (1975). Depressed monocyte chemotaxis during acute influenza infection. *Lancet* ii, 1063–1066.

Larson, H. E., Parry, R. P., Gilchrist, C., Luquetti, A. and Tyrrell, D. A. J. (1977). Influenza viruses and staphylococci *in vitro*: some interactions with polymorphonuclear leucocytes and epithelial cells. *British Journal of Experimental Pathology* 58, 281–288.

Lavelle, G. C. and Bang, F. B. (1971). Influence of type and concentration of sera *in vitro* on susceptibility of genetically resistant cells to mouse hepatitis virus. *Journal of General Virology* 12, 233–238.

Lemercier, G., Mavet, S., Burckhart, M. F. and Fontanges, R. (1979). Interactions entre le virus grippal et le macrophage alvéolaire de souris: étude *in vitro*. *Annals de Microbiologie (Institut Pasteur)* 130A, 119–132.

Lindenmann, J., Deuel, E., Fanconi, S. and Haller, O. (1978). Inborn resistance of mice to myxoviruses: macrophages express phenotype *in vitro*. *Journal of Experimental Medicine* 147, 531–540.

Lopez, C. and Dudas, G. (1979). Replication of herpes simplex virus type 1 in macrophages from resistant and susceptible mice. *Infection and Immunity* 23, 432–437.

Merchant, D. J. and Morgan, H. R. (1950). Inhibition of the phagocytic action of leucocytes by mumps and influenza viruses. *Proceedings of the Society for Experimental Biology and Medicine* 74, 651–653.

Metchnikoff, E. (1892). "Leçons sur la pathologie comparée de l'inflammation". Masson, Paris.

Mills, J. (1979). Effects of Sendai virus infection on function of cultured mouse alveolar macrophages. *American Review of Respiratory Disease* 120, 1239–1244.

Mims, C. A. (1964). Aspects of the pathogenesis of virus diseases. *Bacteriological Reviews* 28, 30–71.

Mogensen, S. C. (1977a). Role of macrophages in hepatitis induced by herpes simplex virus types 1 and 2 in mice. *Infection and Immunity* 15, 686–691.

Mogensen, S. C. (1977b). Genetics of macrophage-controlled resistance to hepatitis induced by herpes simplex virus type 2 in mice. *Infection and Immunity* **17**, 268–273.

Mogensen, S. C. (1978). Macrophages and age-dependent resistance to hepatitis induced by herpes simplex virus type 2 in mice. *Infection and Immunity* **19**, 46–50.

Mogensen, S. C. (1979). Role of macrophages in natural resistance to virus infections. *Microbiological Reviews* **43**, 1–26.

Mogensen, S. C. and Andersen, H. K. (1978). Role of activated macrophages in resistance of congenitally athymic nude mice to hepatitis induced by herpes simplex virus type 2. *Infection and Immunity* **19**, 792–798.

Morahan, P. S. and Morse, S. S. (1979). Macrophage-virus interactions. *In* "Virus–Lymphocyte Interactions: Implications for Disease", pp. 17–35. Elsevier/North-Holland, Oxford.

Nugent, K. M. and Pesanti, E. L. (1979). Effect of influenza infection on the phagocytic and bactericidal activities of pulmonary macrophages. *Infection and Immunity* **26**, 651–657.

Park, B. H., Chiba, Y., Ramirez, R. I. and Ogra, P. L. (1977). Viral suppression of neutrophil chemotaxis in man. *Federation Proceedings* **36**, 1189.

Pike, M. C., Daniels, C. A. and Snyderman, R. (1977). Influenza-induced depression of monocyte chemotaxis: reversal by levamisole. *Cellular Immunology* **32**, 234–238.

Rabson, A. R., Whiting, D. A., Anderson, R., Glover, A. and Koornhof, H. J. (1977). Depressed neutrophil motility in patients with recurrent herpes simplex virus infections: In vitro restoration with levamisole. *Journal of Infectious Diseases* **135**, 113–116.

Ruutu, P. (1977). Depression of rat neutrophil exudation and motility by influenza virus. *Scandinavian Journal of Immunology* **6**, 1113–1120.

Ruutu, P., Vaheri, A. and Kosunen, T. U. (1977). Depression of human neutrophil motility by influenza virus in vitro. *Scandinavian Journal of Immunology* **6**, 897–906.

Sawyer, W. D. (1969). Interaction of influenza virus with leukocytes and its effect on phagocytosis. *Journal of Infectious Diseases* **119**, 541–556.

Schlesinger, J. J., Ernst, C. and Weinstein, L. (1976). Inhibition of human neutrophil chemotaxis by influenza virus. *Lancet* **i**, 650–651.

Silverberg, B. A., Jakab, G. J., Thomson, R. G., Warr, G. A. and Boo, K. S. (1979). Ultrastructural alterations in phagocytic functions of alveolar macrophages after parainfluenza virus infection. *Journal of the Reticuloendothelial Society* **25**, 405–416.

Silverstein, S. (1970). Macrophages and viral immunity. *Seminars in Hematology* **7**, 185–214.

Stevens, J. G. and Cook, M. L. (1971). Restriction of herpes simplex virus by macrophages. An analysis of the cell–virus interaction. *Journal of Experimental Medicine* **133**, 19–38.

Stuart-Harris, C. H. (1965). "Influenza and other virus infections of the respiratory tract", pp. 28–46. Edward Arnold, London.

Taylor, R. N., Dietz, T. M., Maxwell, K. W. and Marcus, S. (1974). Effect of influenza virus infection on phagocytic and cytopeptic capasities of guinea pig macrophages. *Immunological Communications* **3**, 439–455.

Verini, M. A. and Lief, F. S. (1979). Interaction between 6/94 virus, a parainfluenza type 1 strain, and mouse macrophages. *Infection and Immunity* **24**, 720–728.

Warr, G. A. and Jakab, G. J. (1979). Alterations in lung macrophage antimicrobial activity associated with viral pneumonia. *Infection and Immunity* **26**, 492–497.

Warr, G. A., Jakab, G. J., Chan, T. W. and Tsan, M. F. (1979). Effects of viral pneumonia on lung macrophage lysosomal enzymes. *Infection and Immunity* **24**, 577–579.

Warr, G. A., Jakab, G. J. and Hearst, J. E. (1979). Alterations in lung macrophage immune receptor(s) activity associated with viral pneumonia. *Journal of the Reticuloendothelial Society* **26**, 357–366.

Warshauer, D., Goldstein, E., Akers, T., Lippert, W. and Kim, M. (1977). Effect of influenza viral infection on the ingestion and killing of bacteria by alveolar macrophages. *American Review of Respiratory Disease* **115**, 269–277.

DISCUSSION

Anderson I would like to ask one question about the data on inhibition of chemotaxis. You were suggesting that this was a surface adherence phenomenon between the virus and the cells. I wonder how that could be true since it occurred with Tween 80 and ether inactivated virus which would presumably have been stripped of its envelope and cell receptors.

Mogensen One only study has shown that ether and Tween inactivated viruses still reduce chemotaxis, but maybe stripped envelope components are still active in reducing chemotaxis.

Mims I used to believe that macrophages did everything and were responsible for everything, but now I have developed considerable scepticism. With nearly all the virus infections that we know about, virus does not replicate in macrophages. In other virus infections the macrophage is often a very restrictive cell type in which infection is aborted. You get antigens produced without much infectious virus, or a low infectious virus yield, and the macrophage is not a very susceptible cell. We have been studying mouse cytomegalovirus and here the avirulent strain grows very well in macrophages whereas the virulent strain hardly grows at all in them. This inverts our normal ideas about the macrophage as a determinant of virulence. I am not sure that the effects on phagocytosis and chemotaxis which we are talking about today have anything to do with virus replication in the cell. Dr Anderson has referred indirectly to possible neuraminidase surface effects and someone said that *in vivo* the effects are on polymorphs as well as on macrophages.

There is one infection to which macrophages are susceptible: that caused by lactic dehydrogenase virus. I inject a mouse this afternoon and tomorrow morning it has 10^{10} virus infectious doses per ml of plasma and the only susceptible cell in the body is the macrophage. The macrophage is almost unaffected by it except that it is unable to clear certain endogenous enzymes which build up in the blood and give the only signs that the mouse has been infected.

I feel that the macrophage story in relation to virulence has become less clear over the years, although we have to concentrate on it as it is still often important.

Mogensen Yes, I agree that macrophage replication of viruses as related to virulence is not a simple black and white picture, but it might be that in some virus infections macrophage activity has nothing to do with the overall outcome of the infection—for instance, death from encephalitis—whereas it has something to do with what happens in the visceral organs.

Stuart-Harris I want to discuss a little bit more this question of macrophages in relation to different races of mice. You mentioned that a number of viruses may behave differently in their rate of multiplication in different breeds of mice and that this is correlated with the extent to which they replicate in macrophages. You mentioned influenza virus amongst these. Were you talking about the A2G breed of mice in that connection, and has it been shown that the macrophage does not support the growth of influenza virus in that race compared with the ordinary Swiss mice?

Mogensen Yes, it was the A2G mouse. I was referring to the work of Haller and Lindenmann. They have shown that there is a correlation between the ability of macrophages to support replication of the virus and resistance of the mice; but I must admit that recent findings indicate that it is the interferon sensitivity of the cells that determines the outcome of the infection.

Stuart-Harris There is another comment that I should like to make, if I may, in relation to parainfluenza viruses. The production of fusion factor, which I believe is one of the surface antigens of parainfluenza virus, may be one way of interfering with the host's defences, because it has some relationship to the integrity of the host cell. It has now been shown that the fusion factor is a vital antigen in relation to infection and antibody against it is requisite for protection.

Mims If I can just comment on those results you referred from the work of Dr Haller and his colleagues. I feel we must regard them as somewhat irrelevant for infectious disease processes with influenza virus because the strain of influenza used, as you will recall, was one highly adapted to mouse peritoneal macrophages: an irrelevant cell type for natural influenzal infection.

Mogensen I agree. Differences between the virulence of certain types or strains of the same virus may tell us more about the real situation if they are naturally occurring variants—for instance, herpes simpex virus type 1 and type 2—rather than laboratory adapted variants.

Sweet Could I ask a question about impairment of phagocyte function in respiratory infections? I think the evidence is quite clear that uptake of bacteria and yeast by phagocytes is impaired in influenza-infected animals, but is there any evidence that these cells are impaired with regard to their phagocytosis of the virus itself?

Mogensen I have seen no such studies.

Sweet It seems to me that if we are interested in the effects of virus on host defence mechanisms we should also consider what advantage this is to the virus as well as to the superinfecting bacteria.

Wilton Sir Charles, were you suggesting that fusion factor might inhibit function because it formed polykaryons?

Stuart-Harris I do not know how it actually works in the host, but it is obviously one of the mechanisms whereby the virus attacks the host cells. Whether or not it promotes the multiplication of itself by that process I do not know. Many of us thought until quite recently that it was a relatively irrelevant property, but it is quite clear that if one is trying to immunize against parainfluenza virus it is essential that vaccine preparations should contain enough of the fusion factor as well as the haemagglutinin.

Wilton I am not a virologist, so I cannot speak about virulence factors or the virulence mechanism as far as that is concerned, but certainly polykaryons of macrophages are phagocytic.

Sweet If I can just add to that, we have done some work with polymorphs produced in the upper respiratory tract of ferrets during influenza infection. These phagocytes are just as capable of phagocytosing virus as are peritoneal exudate cells from uninfected animals. So these infected nasal inflammatory phagocytes seem unimpaired with respect to their phagocytosis of virus.

Smith We have heard that influenza or Sendai virus infection exacerbates bacterial infection. Are there any mixed infection experiments with viruses? For example, if a mouse is given Sendai virus would a subsequent herpesvirus infection go more quickly in view of the fact that Sendai virus inactivates the phagocytes? Have experiments of this type been done?

Mims There have been double infection experiments. If they interfere with each other, it may be because they are growing competitively in the same cell system in the body, or perhaps because of macrophage activation or interferon induction.

Lambert Can I ask more about the quantitative side of the experiments in the first part of the paper? With influenza and Sendai viruses what sort of infecting dose do you need to produce these effects on bacterial clearance and phagocytosis? Are they quantitatively situations which could be matched in real life?

Mogensen First of all, I must say these are not my own studies; the data were mainly from the work of Jakab and Warr and others. As far as I remember, the mice were infected with fairly high doses of virus intranasally and developed an acute infection with maximum virus titres in the lungs after two or three days.

Draper This is probably a silly question, but how actually do viruses get into cells? What I am thinking is that if viruses do not multiply in macrophages, then it is not in their interest to get into a macrophage, so it may resist uptake by macrophages. Is it possible that viruses actually stimulate uptake by the cells they are really after as, for example, *Toxoplasma* stimulates phagocytosis by all sorts of cells that are not normally phagocytic?

Smith *Chlamydia* do this.

Quie The membrane of granulocytes is perturbed by C5a, the major serum chemotactic factor, which activates the oxidative metabolism of granulocytes. This action may be stimulatory in one instance, but also might be toxic in another. Workers in Umea, Sweden, have shown that a mixture of microbes and antiserum with phagocytic cells produces in the latter an immediate chemiluminescence response which occurs within seconds, followed by a somewhat diminished chemiluminescence response at 11 min. This chemiluminescence may be caused by humoral component or antigen–antibody complex, which stimulates a metabolic response and I wonder if something like this has taken place when polymorph responses are abnormal *in vitro*.

As far as inhibition of chemotaxis is concerned, one possibility is that exocytosis of specific granules may result in loss of an necessary protease. Neutrophils produce fibronectin which participates in adherence and therefore chemokinesis and chemotaxis. Some of the observations that you presented would be consistent with that possibility. Granulocytes appear to have a local membrane response, rather than a one-hit total cell response. After certain kinds of perturbation these cells may be left with less than complete metabolic or locomotory responsiveness.

Valdimarsson I had two questions and Dr Quie has dealt with one of them. In relation to the disparity between the *in vivo* and *in vitro* Sendai mouse system, I wanted to ask what serum concentration was used *in vitro*, because it is possible that the disparity could be explained on the basis of depletion of complement factors in the lung mucosa, whilst if a high serum concentration was used *in vitro* nonlimiting amounts of complement may have been present.

Mogensen I do not recall the serum concentration used in these experiments.

Williams Will interferon interfere with phagocytosis?

Quie Interferon stimulates metabolism which results in chemiluminescence and increased locomotion.

van Furth And activates macrophages to become more cytotoxic for tumour cells and probably also for bacteria as shown by Michael Rabinowitz and others in Paris.

Williams It seems very strange, in that case, that we have macrophages full of virus and therefore producing a lot of interferon, which are not able to function properly.

van Furth I am not an interferon expert, but I wonder whether immune interferon would be better than leukocyte interferon.

Anderson It may be that a macrophage infected with virus produces interferon, but the effect is exerted not on it but on the next macrophage down the line.

Williams But we are told that interferon stimulates and the macrophages are not stimulated, they are retarded.

Anderson The infected ones are retarded, but the interferon-treated ones are stimulated. What I am postulating is that they are two quite different populations of macrophages.

Peters One other theoretical possibility in virus or, indeed, other types of infections is the presumably nonspecific effect of an acute load of immune complexes on the function of various cells. Using tests of splenic function and the clearance of antibody-coated erythrocytes, for example, there is clinical evidence, in a variety of circumstances where there is a load of circulating immune complexes, of depression of mononuclear phagocytic function. So this is yet another mechanism which might be involved in perturbation of phagocytic cells.

Smith Professor Mims, surely you do not really believe that macrophage–virus interactions are not important in virus infection?

Mims I do not think they are as important as I used to!

Smith That is different.

Mims One thing that is not relevant to what has been said—and perhaps I will deal with this tomorrow—is that you can coat a virus with antibody and, because of the Fc receptors on mononuclear cells, you can in some instances enhance the infectivity of that virus for mononuclear cells. This has been clearly shown for dengue and for other arthropod-borne viruses.

Braude I want to ask Professor Mims a question about his diminished enthusiasm towards macrophages and viruses. As I remember your studies with pox virus in mice, you made the remarkable observation that after the virus multiplied in the skin it went to the liver and then nothing happened for a while, and then it came back again to the skin. I guess it went from the respiratory tract to the liver, then to the skin and then produced mouse pox. The thing that struck me was that something happened to the phagocytic cells in the liver so they were no longer able to restrain and keep the virus there. I wonder if this is not a remarkable example of what we have been talking about, namely that the virus in the Kupffer cells interfered with their ability to hang on to the virus and allowed it to escape again.

Mims In that particular infection I do believe macrophages are important. But even there they have a dual role. First, the Kupffer cells act as barriers between the sinusoidal lumen and the hepatic cell in the case of ectromelia virus. Second, my colleague, Bob Blanden, showed that although cytotoxic T cells protected against the same virus in the mouse liver this was not enough by itself. T cells must act in cooperation with a circulating mononuclear cell or macrophage which seemed to become activated, helping with the cleaning up of the infectious focus in quite a different way. So I think that, as always, things get more complicated the more you look at them.

Anderson To go back to what was said quite early on about the correlation between susceptibility of macrophages to herpes simplex virus, according to the genotype of mouse involved, have you compared the natural killer cell activity, which also varies with genotype in those different strains of mouse?

Mogensen I have not, but I know that Carlos Lopez at the Sloan Kettering in New York has found a correlation between resistance and high NK cell activity in strains of mice resistant or susceptible to herpes simplex virus type 1. But he is not looking at the liver infection with herpes simplex virus type 1 but at the central nervous system infection, because his marker for resistance or susceptibility is death of the animal from encephalitis. Therefore, I think that in one organ one cell type may be responsible for resistance while in another organ it may be another cell type.

Bacterial Interference with the Immune Response

GIUSEPPE FALCONE and MARIO CAMPA

Institute of Microbiology,
University of Pisa,
Pisa, Italy.

The result of the host–parasite encounter will depend on interactions between the host defence mechanisms and the ability of the parasite to make these mechanisms ineffective.

Though specific, acquired immunity is of primary importance for host survival, natural immunity determines events that may or may not result in infection, besides allowing the infected host to survive long enough to mount an adequate specific immune response.

Genetic factors may play a major role in natural resistance to many infectious agents. In mice, for instance, resistance to *Rickettsia tsutsugamushi* and *Listeria monocytogenes* is unigenic and autosomal; to type 2 herpes simplex virus, unigenic and X-linked; to *Toxoplasma gondii*, polygenic and autosomal; to *Salmonella typhimurium*, polygenic, both autosomal and X-linked. However, in all cases of autosomal resistance known so far, the genes are not *H-2* linked, and therefore do not seem to control specific immune responsiveness, but rather the expression of nonspecific immune mechanisms. In the case of resistance to *Salmonella typhimurium* this consists of an effective parasite killing in the spleen and liver by bone marrow-derived macrophages. It seems that a single gene may be responsible for the resistance to a group of microorganisms (Rosenstreich *et al.*, 1980). In man, research is more difficult and we do not have such clear-cut data regarding natural resistance. However, it is hoped that we will gain more information in this area by future studies with *in vitro* systems.

A microorganism that succeeds in overcoming the various and complex mechanisms of the host's natural immunity by more or less sophisticated strategies will be able to invade and grow in the host, thereby causing infection and eventually disease. This aspect of the host–parasite relationship will be discussed by others. Here we deal with the possible mechanisms by which a parasite may affect the specific immune response once the infection has been established.

Usually the infection is terminated by the development of effective protective immunity; however, when the host is unable to mount and maintain an adequate immune response, the microorganisms can survive and continue to multiply within the host tissues. This may be influenced by environmental factors such as nutritional state (Chandra, 1974) and intercurrent diseases (Wheelock *et al.*, 1971; Bryceson, 1974), or by genetic defects (O'Brien *et al.*, 1979). It has been shown, for instance, that CBA/N mice are poor producers of antibodies to certain T-independent antigens, as they are markedly deficient in a B lymphocyte subpopulation (O'Brien *et al.*, 1979); furthermore, patients with lepromatous leprosy seem unable to control the infection, due possibly to a defective macrophage function or, more likely, to a T lymphocyte-associated defect (Godal, 1978; Bullock, 1978). Apart from these or similar situations, the host should be able to control the infection; but where this does not take place, the parasite itself may have contrived a way to avoid the powerful mechanisms of the host immune response. This seems plausible if one considers that microorganisms have undergone a slow evolutionary process with their hosts. The close and prolonged association which has resulted may, therefore, be the consequence of the parasite's ability to adapt itself to the ever-changing conditions in the host tissues, and also its capacity to influence the host physiological systems, including the immune system (Schwab, 1975). In this context, the ability of bacterial constituents such as lipopolysaccharide (LPS) to induce phenotypic and functional maturation of both B and T lymphocytes, should be considered. A great deal of work has shown that bone marrow B lymphocyte precursors undergo stepwise differentiation to antigen-reactive B cells, after LPS stimulation. The various steps of this maturation process are characterized by the appearance of different markers on the cell membrane which are expressed with the following temporal sequence: immunoglobulin M (IgM), the antigen associated with the immune response genes (Ia), the receptor for the third complement component (C3) and immunoglobulin D (IgD) (Ryser and Vassalli, 1974; Hämmerling *et al.*, 1976; Watson, 1977;

Sitia *et al.*, 1979; Hoffmann *et al.*, 1979). LPS is also able to stimulate T lymphocyte precursors to differentiate and express TL and Thy 1.2 antigens (Scheid *et al.*, 1973; Scheid *et al.*, 1975; Hämmerling *et al.*, 1976; Watson, 1977).

Parasite interaction with the host immune system is not limited to its effect on lymphoid tissue maturation but also includes quantitative (potentiation or suppression) and qualitative (affinity, restricted heterogeneity, and predominant class of antibodies produced) modulation of the immune response. This has been reviewed by Schwab (1977).

To escape the host's antimicrobial activity, parasites contrive sophisticated mechanisms capable of interfering either with natural immunity factors, the regulatory system of the immune response, or with its effector mechanisms. In normal animals, immunocompetence is maintained by a delicate balance between stimulatory cells and suppressor cells. Therefore, any depression of the immune response that may occur during infection could be correlated with a strong stimulation of suppressor cells by the parasite, rather than with a deficit of stimulatory cells.

LPS may represent a paradigmatic example for understanding all mechanisms that are known so far to have been devised by microorganisms to modulate the host immune response. It also constitutes the best example of a chemically well characterized bacterial constituent able to affect host immune response by inhibiting both cell-mediated immunity (CM: Lagrange *et al.*, 1975; Gill and Liew, 1979; Vallera *et al.*, 1980) and antibody production to T-dependent (Johnson *et al.*, 1967; Franzl and McMaster, 1968; McMaster and Franzl, 1968; Nakano *et al.*, 1976; Persson, 1977; Walker and Weigle, 1978) and T-independent antigens (Scott and Diener, 1976; Braley-Mullen *et al.*, 1977), both *in vitro* (Scott and Diener, 1976; Walker and Weigle, 1978; Vallera *et al.*, 1980) and *in vivo* (Johnson *et al.*, 1967; Franzl and McMaster, 1968; McMaster and Franzl, 1968; Lagrange *et al.*, 1975; Nakano *et al.*, 1976; Braley-Mullen *et al.*, 1977; Persson, 1977; Gill and Liew, 1979).

Since the results of Johnson *et al.* (1967), Franzl and McMaster (1968), and McMaster and Franzl (1968), it has been quite clear that LPS in mice may either potentiate or depress the immune response to a given antigen, depending on the dose, route and time interval between LPS and antigen administration. In fact, if LPS is given together with or immediately before the antigen, potentiation of the immune response occurs, whereas LPS given 1 or 2 days before antigen causes a marked depression. In addition, LPS has been shown to induce selective depletion of the T-dependent areas in the spleen and lymph nodes (Johnson *et al.*, 1967; McMaster and Franzl, 1968); the histological alterations observed were similar to those brought about by LPS in the thymus (Rowlands *et al.*, 1965).

All these data seemed to indicate that the LPS immunosuppressive capacity was either due to the direct cytotoxic effect on T-lymphocytes of its toxic moiety, the lipid A, or could be ascribed to LPS-induced release of adrenal hormones, which are known to be toxic mainly for T lymphocytes (Rowlands *et al.*, 1965). This hypothesis, however, turned out to be in conflict with the finding that lipid A is mitogenic for B lymphocytes (Peavy *et al.*, 1973), and that LPS can make a T-dependent antibody response, T-independent (Möller *et al.*, 1972; Sjöberg *et al.*, 1972). In mice, besides the variable regions of immunoglobulins, another recognition structure may exist on B lymphocytes, namely the receptor for B mitogens such as LPS, lipoprotein (LP) (Melchers *et al.*, 1975) and *Nocardia* water-soluble mitogen (NWSM) (Bona, 1979). The interaction of LPS or LP with the corresponding receptor has been shown to lead to differentiation of resting B cells into mature cells which produce immunoglobulins with the same specificity as those on their cell membrane. In other words, these mitogens circumvent the H-2 restriction and the need for antigen-specific T helper cells or factors for B cells to grow (polyclonal activation). This aspect has been reviewed by Melchers (1980). The potentiating effect of LPS on antibody formation (adjuvant effect) seems to be due to its mitogenic activity on B lymphocytes and to its capacity to stimulate macrophages (Hoffman *et al.*, 1977; Hoffman *et al.*, 1979), or T helper cells (Armerding and Katz, 1974; Norcross and Smith, 1977), or, more likely, both (McGhee *et al.*, 1979).

Specific antibodies for an antigen have been shown to suppress the immune response to the same antigen, probably by binding to the antigen and thus preventing it from reaching the antigen-reactive cells (Uhr and Möller, 1968) or, in the form of antigen–antibody complexes, by blocking the activity of the specific effector T cells (Mackaness *et al.*, 1974). More recently, it has also been suggested that antibodies can suppress the immune response by directly affecting B lymphocytes (Sinclair, 1978). However, the adjuvant effect of LPS does not seem to be responsible for its suppressive activity. Although a marked increase in immunoglobulin levels, as a result of LPS-induced polyclonal B cell activation, has been observed in animals injected with LPS 2–3 days before antigen administration, the specific antibody titre to the antigen used was found to be the same, if not lower, than that of controls (Persson, 1977). In addition, LPS-induced suppression was found not to be transferable by serum (Gill and Liew, 1979). Several studies have clearly shown that LPS immunosuppression is due to the activation of suppressor cells. Uchiyama and Jacobs (1978), and McGhee *et al.* (1980a, b), have demonstrated that these cells are T lymphocytes. Goodman and Weigle (1979) have suggested that LPS activates T cells that may also suppress the LPS polyclonal activation of B cells. However, it should be pointed out that the activation mechanism of suppressor T cells by LPS is still largely unknown. Several reports indicate that LPS also activates suppressor B lymphocytes. Persson (1977) has shown that in mice given high doses of *E. coli* LPS intraperitoneally 2–3 days before intravenous administration of sheep red blood cells (SRBC), both IgM and IgG responses to the antigen were inhibited. Furthermore, spleen cells, taken from mice which had been inoculated with LPS alone 2–3 days previously, were unable to mount a normal primary response to SRBC *in vitro*. Since this suppression was not removed when spleen cell suspensions were depleted of either T cells or macrophages, it was concluded that LPS activated suppressor B cells. Koenig and Hoffman (1979), have also shown that LPS activates suppressor cells capable of inhibiting the *in vitro* primary response to SRBC, even when added *in vitro* to murine spleen cell cultures before or together with the antigen. These suppressor cells have been characterized phenotypically as Ig^+, Ia^+, CR^+, Ly-B-2^+ and PC 1^-. In addition, these authors reported that LPS does not induce suppressor macrophages or suppressor T cells, nor are macrophages or T cells required for the generation of suppressor B cells by LPS.

Several reports have demonstrated that LPS may also affect cell mediated immunity. Lagrange *et al.* (1975) have observed that LPS depresses delayed-type hypersensitivity reaction (DTH) to SRBC in mice, when given 2–3 days before the antigen, and has a potentiating effect when administered 2 days after the antigen (Lagrange and Mackaness, 1975). In these experiments, the total haemagglutinin titre was maximum when the greatest depression of DTH to the same antigen occurred. Using the same experimental model, Gill and Liew (1979) showed the same reverse relationship, this time between the specific antibody titre to SRBC and DTH; the depression of DTH to SRBC was not transferable by serum but was due to the activation of specific suppressor B cells. Very recently, Vallera *et al.* (1980) have shown that LPS prevents the development of cytotoxic T cells when added *in vitro* at the beginning to a mixed lymphocyte culture (MLC), in which spleen cells of BALB/c mice were used as "responders" to X-rayed spleen cells of C57BL/6 mice. The depression was due neither to T cells nor to macrophages acting directly or through the release of prostaglandins although macrophages are known to produce prostaglandins when treated with LPS (Kurland and Bockman, 1978), and increased prostaglandin levels are known to inhibit lymphocyte proliferative responses (Goodwin *et al.*, 1977). The direct activation of suppressor B cells by LPS was, therefore, responsible for the depression. LPS (Colizzi and Bozzi, 1979), or *Pseudomonas aeruginosa* (Campa *et al.*, 1976; Campa *et al.*, 1980a), possibly through its LPS, may also inhibit contact sensitivity to oxazolone by activating specific suppressor B cells.

Jacobs and Morrison (1975) and Poe and Michael (1976) have shown that it is possible to dissociate the adjuvant activity of LPS from its mitogenic effect on B lymphocytes. Furthermore, a detoxified, polysaccharide-rich fraction from *Serratia marcescens* LPS, though nonmitogenic for B cells, has been shown to potentiate, in mice, both the *in vivo* (Behling and Nowotny, 1977) and *in vitro* (Frank *et al.*, 1977) antibody responses to SRBC, when given together with or after the antigen. Similar dissociation between adjuvant effect and mitogenic activity for B lymphocytes has also been reported for *Staphylococcus aureus* peptidoglycan (Dziarski, 1979).

Although Behling and Nowotny (1977) have reported that the non-mitogenic polysaccharide-rich fraction from *Serratia marcescens* LPS was not only able to enhance but also to inhibit the *in vivo* antibody production to SRBC, it now seems quite clear that the mitogenicity for B lymphocytes of LPS is a necessary prerequisite for its immunosuppressive activity, i.e. it requires the integrity of lipid A (Nakano *et al.*, 1976; Braley-Mullen *et al.*, 1977; Walker and Weigle, 1978) Koenig and Hoffmann, 1979; Vallera *et al* 1980). Similar correlation between mitogenicity and suppressive activity has been reported by Dziarski (1979) for *Staphylococcus aureus* peptidoglycan.

Therefore, even though the mechanism by which LPS in conjunction with an antigen activates specific suppressor B cells has not yet been fully investigated, all these findings allow us to postulate that LPS induces nonspecific expansion of B cell clones, including the suppressor B cell precursors, and that the antigen brings about a further proliferation of the corresponding suppressor B cells. On the other hand, if one considers that approximately 50% of the antibody-forming cells, polyclonally activated by LPS, produce autoantibodies (Dresser, 1978; Izui *et al.*, 1979), and that an antigen-reactive cell can be inhibited by an antibody against its surface immunoglobulins, the hypothesis may be expressed as follows: anti-idiotypic antibodies, produced after LPS polyclonal activation of B cells, may selectively block the corresponding antigen-reactive cells by binding to their surface immunoglobulins. In other words, LPS-induced suppressor B cells are anti-idiotypic antibody-producing B cells. In agreement with Jerne's theory (1974) that an antigenic determinant might induce antibody-producing B cells and corresponding suppressor B cells, we could postulate that LPS might likewise induce antibody-producing B cells and corresponding suppressor B cells in a polyclonal manner. The finding that normal mouse serum inhibits in mice the activity of LPS-induced suppressor B cells but not their induction (Koenig and Hoffmann, 1979), supports this hypothesis, in that antibodies produced by these suppressor cells could bind to serum immunoglobulins rather than to those on the surface of antigen-reactive cells.

The hypothesis that suppressor B cells are anti-idiotypic antibody-producing cells implies that they do not need cell–cell interaction in order to inhibit other cell activity. However, Gill and Liew (1979) have reported that suppressor B cells do not produce soluble factors, while Persson (1977) has suggested that suppressor B cells, possibly through antibody production, may activate suppressor T lymphocytes through the mechanism proposed by Gershon *et al.* (1974). Kempf and Rubin (1979), on the contrary, have reported that normal mouse spleen cells polyclonally stimulated by LPS, release a factor that is capable of suppressing the primary anti-SRBC response of murine spleen cells *in vitro.* It was found that B cells were essential for production of this suppressive factor. Similar results were obtained by Vallera *et al.* (1980) who showed that LPS induces the release of a factor from activated B cells with a marked modulatory effect on the T cell subpopulation involved in the generation of cell-mediated cytotoxicity in the murine mixed lymphocyte culture. Although it is not yet known whether this factor is an immunoglobulin, the importance of these results is that LPS may induce reduction in T cell reactivity. Suppression of DTH and hypergammaglobulinaemia due to polyclonal stimulation of B lymphocytes could be, in fact, two linked phenomena (Hudson *et al.*, 1976; Poels and Van Niekerk, 1977). One might, therefore, postulate that parasite-derived B cell mitogens may modulate the immune response *in vivo* in favour of the infecting microorganism. We could now consider the following findings in the light of this hypothesis: (1) *S. aureus* induces specific suppressor B cells capable of inhibiting DTH to the same microorganism (Easmon and Glynn, 1979); (2) *P. aeruginosa* inhibits contact sensitivity to oxazolone by activating specific suppressor B cells (Campa *et al.*, 1975, 1976, 1980a); (3) an acidic polysaccharide from *Serratia piscatorum* affects antibody response to SRBC in the same way (Matsumoto *et al.*, 1977). On the other hand, it is known that *S. aureus* peptidoglycan (Dziarski, 1979) and protein A (Forsgren *et al.*, 1976; Romagnani *et al.*, 1980), three outer membrane proteins (Chen *et al.*, 1980) as well as the whole cells of *P. aeruginosa* (Garzelli *et al.*, 1979a), and the acidic polysaccharide from *Serratia piscatorum* (Matsumoto *et al.*, 1977) are B mitogens.

Indeed, microorganisms can activate other suppressor cell types: examples include macrophages and T cells by *Mycobacterium lepraemurium* (Bullock *et al.*, 1978), macrophages by *Mycobacterium tuberculosis* (Katz *et al.*, 1979), T cells by BCG, *Mycobacterium habana* and *Mycobacterium simiae* (Watson and Collins, 1980), T cells by *Streptococcus mutans* (Lamb *et al.*, 1979) and T lymphocytes by group A streptococcal pyrogenic exotoxin (Cunningham and Watson, 1978).

It would be interesting to test the possibility that parasite-derived B cell mitogens may modulate CMI *in vivo* in favour of the infecting microorganism, especially in those infections caused by microorganisms with mitogenic properties for B lymphocytes in which CMI, though playing an important role in controlling the infection, is depressed. It is known, however, that almost all microorganisms have such mitogenic properties, as do peptidoglycans from various Gram positive and Gram negative bacteria (Damais *et al.*, 1975), purified protein derivative (Sultzer and Nilsson, 1972), type III pneumococcal polysaccharide (Coutinho and Möller, 1973) endotoxin protein (Sultzer and Goodman, 1976), in addition to those already mentioned.

It has been reported that in mice at least one in three B cells reacts with LPS

(Andersson *et al.*, 1972) and the LPS-reactive B cells differ from those B cells which are stimulated by LP (Melchers *et al.*, 1975), peptidoglycan (Damais *et al.*, 1975), or *Nocardia* (Bona, 1979). Although a single B cell may have receptors for different B mitogens (Andersson *et al.*, 1979), it appears that a large part, if not all, of B lymphocytes can have receptors for B cell mitogens. Since LPS reverses tolerance to immunity even in the presence of suppressor T cells (Louis *et al.*, 1973), it would seem that B lymphocytes could be easily activated by such mitogens, and autoimmune diseases could be the consequence. Cunningham (1974) has observed that LPS induces a dramatic rise in antibody production against isologous erythrocytes in mice. Furthermore, it has been shown that experimental infection by *P. aeruginosa*, a B cell mitogen (Garzelli *et al.*, 1979a), induces in mice increased numbers of splenic plaque-forming cells against SRBC and trinitrophenyl-SRBC, as well as against isologous, bromelain-treated erythrocytes (Garzelli *et al.*, in preparation). This circumvention of tolerance, which may have important clinical implications, can be viewed as a further illustration of the influence of bacteria on immune regulation.

Some reports, however, have suggested that LPS-induced suppression is not due to suppressor cells (Nakano *et al.*, 1976; Diamanstein *et al.*, 1976; Braley-Mullen *et al.*, 1977; Walker and Weigle, 1978), but rather to the fact that high doses of LPS, administered some time before an antigen, strongly stimulate B cells to proliferate which, as a result, temperarily lose their capacity to respond to any antigen. This temporary exhaustion of antibody-forming cell precursors only lasts for a few days. A similar mechanism has been suggested to explain the capacity of *P. aeruginosa* to inhibit the antibody response to SRBC in mice, since this suppressive state was not transferable by lymphoid cells from *P. aeruginosa*-treated mice to syngeneic recipients, and since this microorganism is at least as mitogenic for B lymphocytes, as is *E. coli* LPS (Garzelli *et al.*, 1979a). It has also been reported that *P. aeruginosa* inhibits contact sensitivity to oxazolone by activating suppressor B cells which interfere with the inductive phase of the immune reaction (Campa *et al.*, 1976, 1980a; Garzelli *et al.*, 1979b). *P. aeruginosa*, therefore, represents a good example of how a bacterial constituent with mitogenic properties for B lymphocytes can depress the host immune response, either through activation of suppressor cells or because of its capacity to function as a polyclonal activator of B lymphocytes.

Another mechanism by which LPS may alter the host immune response is by interfering with lymphocyte circulation (Freitas and de Sousa, 1976). Lymphocyte trapping, which may limit the expression of the specific subset of T cells at the periphery, has been reported in mice after injection of *Corynebacterium parvum* (Frost and Lance, 1978) or *Bordetella pertussis* extracts (Taub *et al.*, 1972), in rats with active infection with *Mycobacterium lepraemurium* (Bulloch,

1976), and in mice infected with *P. aeruginosa* (Campa *et al.*, 1979). In this last case, the disturbance of lymphocyte circulation seems to be due to the suppressor B cells activated by the microorganism. It has, therefore, been suggested that lymphocyte trapping may represent another mechanism by which suppressor cells can regulate the immune response (Campa *et al.*, 1980b). However, it must be noted that attempts to restore the immune response by eliminating the trapping mechanism have been unsuccessful (Lefford and Mackaness, 1977).

Metha *et al.* (1973) found a proteolytic enzyme in colonic fluid which, unlike other proteases, hydrolyses human serum IgA immunoglobulins to yield Fabα and intact Fcα fragments. This enzyme is elaborated by normal microbial flora of the human gastrointestinal tract. The enzyme is a metal-dependent, neutral endopeptidase inactive on human IgG, IgM and IgE, but highly specific for IgA1, in which it cleaves a peptide bond in the hinge region of the heavy chains (Kilian *et al.*, 1980). IgA2 is resistant to this enzyme owing to the deletion of 13 amino acids in the region that contains the enzyme-susceptible peptide bond (Plaut *et al.*, 1974).

The fact that in man IgA2 immunoglobulins represent approximately 50% of the total IgA in colostrum, while only 10% in the serum, suggests that their relatively high concentration in the secretions could confer a selective advantage at the level of mucous membranes populated by masses of microorganisms, since they are resistant, unlike IgA1, to IgA protease. The evolution of IgA2 may have been influenced by IgA protease in that evolutionary pressures may have determined the development of epithelial cell membrane transport pathways which favour the passage into secretions of IgA2 as opposed to IgA1 (Plaut *et al.*, 1974). On the other hand, it is also possible to speculate that microorganisms, in response to secretory IgA, underwent mutation manifested by IgA protease production (Plaut *et al.*, 1975).

The high specificity of IgA protease is of great relevance if one considers the central role that this class of immunoglobulins exerts in the functional organization of the secretory immune system and especially at the sites normally populated by microorganisms able to produce IgA protease. In the mouth IgA antibodies against *Streptococcus mutans*, for instance, may inhibit colonization of the teeth by this cariogenic microorganism. This suggests that salivary IgA may exert a fundamental influence on the bacterial colonization of mucous membranes. Since such colonization plays an important part in the full expression of the virulence of bacterial pathogens responsible for such diseases as streptococcal pharyngitis, bacterial diarrhoeas, dental caries and peridontitis, local conditions that modify the effects of secretory IgA antibodies could influence adherence and colonization and thus the onset and progress of mucosal and dental diseases. It is, therefore, reasonable to postulate that IgA protease released by *Streptococcus sanguis*, an ubiquitous microorganism in the gastrointestinal tract may, through the cleavage of secretory IgA, reduce the ability of these immunoglobulins to prevent colonization of the gastrointestinal tract by transient microorganisms, some of which may be pathogenic (Genco *et al.*, 1975). Localized or systemic infections by *Streptococcus pneumoniae*, *Haemophilus influenzae* (Kilian *et al.*. 1979; Male, 1979; Mulks *et al.*, 1980), or *Neisseria meningitidis* (Plaut *et al.*, 1975), all of which produce IgA protease, are also preceded by nasopharyngeal colonization; even in these cases the complex host and bacterial factors involved in establishing and maintaining the carrier state and in the transition from this condition to tissue invasion are not well known. However, since host, local or systemic, humoral or cellular responses may affect this transition, it seems possible that IgA protease, by interfering with the early interactions between invading microorganisms and secretory IgA, may influence the colonization process and eventually the onset of disease.

Furthermore, IgA protease could play a major role in the case of *Neisseria gonorrhoeae* infections (Plaut *et al.*, 1975; Plaut *et al.*, 1977; Blake *et al.*, 1979). A marked and rapid cleavage of IgA by IgA protease, in fact, may account for the reinfection of patients with high specific antibody levels (Blake *et al.*, 1979).

The possibility exists that microorganisms may also elaborate nonspecific antibody proteases as suggested by the finding that *Tetrahymena pyriformis* produces a protease similar to papain able to cleave immunoglobulins in to monovalent Fab fragments, which, by binding to the antigenic determinants of the parasite, protect it from circulating antibodies. Moreover, since these fragments do not activate complement, a further reduction in the effectiveness of the immune response occurs (Eisen and Tallare, 1977).

By inactivating the antibody defence mechanisms, the production of specific IgA or nonspecific antibody proteases, may allow microorganisms to escape immunologic attack.

REFERENCES

Andersson, J., Coutinho, A. and Melchers, F. (1979). Mitogen-activated B-cell blasts reactive to more than one mitogen. *Journal of Experimental Medicine* **149**, 553–564.

Andersson, J., Sjöberg, O. and Möller, G. (1972). Induction of immunoglobulin and antibody synthesis *in vitro* by lipopolysaccharides. *European Journal of Immunology* **2**, 349–353.

Armerding, D. and Katz, D. H. (1974). Activation of T and B lymphocytes *in vitro*. II. Biological and biochemical properties of an allogeneic effect factor (AEF) active in triggering specific B lymphocytes. *Journal of Experimental Medicine* **140**, 19–37.

Behling, U. H. and Nowotny, A. (1977). Immune adjuvancy of lipopolysaccharide and a non toxic hydrolytic product demonstrating oscillating effects with time. *Journal of Immunology* **118**, 1905–1907.

Blake, M., Holmes, K. K. and Swanson, J. (1979). Studies on gonococcus infection XVII. IgA1-cleaving protease in vaginal washings from women with gonorrhea. *Journal of Infectious Diseases* **139**, 89–92.
Bona, C. (1979). Modulation of immune responses by Nocardia immunostimulants. *Progress in Allergy* **26**, 97–136.
Braley-Mullen, H., Hayes, N. and Sanders, M. (1977). Suppression of IgM responses to type III pneumococcal polysaccharide by lipopolysaccharide (LPS). *Cellular Immunology* **30**, 300–309.
Bryceson, A. (1974). "Progress in Immunology II" Vol. 3, pp. 161–170. Elsevier/North-Holland, Amsterdam.
Bullock, W. E. Jr. (1976). Perturbation of lymphocyte circulation in experimental murine leprosy. II. Nature of the defect. *Journal of Immunology* **117**, 1171–1178.
Bullock, W. E. (1978). Leprosy: a model of immunological perturbation in chronic infection. *Journal of Infection Diseases* **137**, 341–354.
Bullock, W. E., Carlson E. M. and Gershon, R. K. (1978). The evolution of immunosuppressive cell populations in experimental mycobacterial infection. *Journal of Immunology* **120**, 1709–1716.
Campa, M., Garzelli, C. and Falcone, G. (1975). Depression of contact sensitivity and enhancement of antibody response in *Pseudomonas aeruginosa*-infected mice. *Infection and Immunity* **12**, 1252–1257.
Campa, M., Garzelli, C., Ferrannini, E. and Falcone, G. (1976). Evidence for suppressor cell activity associated with depression of contact sensitivity in *Pseudomonas aeruginosa* infected mice. *Clinical and Experimental Immunology* **26**, 355–362.
Campa, M., Ferrannini, E., Garzelli, C., Colizzi, V. and Falcone, G. (1979). Disturbance of lymphocyte circulation by *Pseudomonas aeruginosa* infection in oxazolone-sensitized mice. *Current Microbiology* **2**, 283–286.
Campa, M., Colizzi, V., Garzelli, C., Toca, L. and Falcone, G. (1980a). *Pseudomonas aeruginosa* infection: activation of B suppressor cells which affect cell cooperation in the induction phase of contact sensitivity to oxazolone in mice. *Current Microbiology*, **4**, 173–175.
Campa, M., Toca, L., Garzelli, C., Colizzi, V. and Falcone, G. (1980b). Reversal of *Pseudomonas aeruginosa*-induced disturbance of lymphocyte circulation in oxazolone-sensitized mice by cyclophosphamide. *Immunology Letters*, **2**, 123–131.
Chandra, R. K. (1974). Rosette-forming T lymphocytes and cell-mediated immunity in malnutrition. *British Medical Journal* **iii**, 608–609.
Chen, Y. U., Hancock, E. W. and Mishell, R. I. (1980). Mitogenic effects of purified outer membrane proteins from *Pseudomonas aeruginosa*. *Infection and Immunity* **28**, 178–184.
Colizzi, V. and Bozzi, L. (1979). A mechanism for the depression of contact sensitivity with B-cell mitogens. *Annales d'Immunologie (Institut Pasteur)* **130c**, 659–673.
Coutinho, A. and Möller, G. (1973). Mitogenic properties of the thymus-independent antigen pneumococcal polysaccharide SIII. *European Journal of Immunology* **3**, 608–613.
Cunningham, A. J. (1974). Large numbers of cells in normal mice produce antibody components of isologous erythrocytes. *Nature* **252**, 749–751.
Cunningham, C. M. and Watson, D. W. (1978). Suppression of antibody response

by Group A streptococcal pyrogenic exo-toxin and characterization of the cells involved. *Infection and Immunity* 19, 470–476.

Damais, C., Bona, C., Chedid, L., Fleck, Y., Nauciel, C. and Martin Y. P. (1975). Mitogenic effect of bacterial peptidoglycans possessing adjuvant activity. *Journal of Immunology* 115, 268–271.

Diamantstein, T., Keppler, W., Blitstein-Willinger, E. and Ben-Efraim, C. (1976). Suppression of the primary immune response *in vivo* to sheep red blood cells by B-cell mitogens. *Immunology* 30, 401–407.

Dresser, D. W. (1978). Most IgM-producing cells in the mouse secrete auto-antibodies (rheumatoid factor). *Nature* 274, 480–483.

Dziarski, R. (1979). Relationships between adjuvant, immunosuppressive, and mitogenic activities of staphylococcal peptidoglycan. *Infection and Immunity* 26, 508–514.

Easmon, C. S. F. and Glynn, A. A. (1979). The cellular control of delayed hypersensitivity to *Staphylococcus aureus* in mice. *Immunology* 38, 103–108.

Eisen, H. and Tallan, I. (1977). *Tetrahymena pyriformis* recovers from antibody immobilization by producing univalent antibody fragments. *Nature* 270, 514–515.

Forsgren, A., Svedjelund, A. and Wigzell, H. (1976). Lymphocyte stimulation by protein A of *Staphylococcus aureus*. *European Journal of Immunology* 6, 207–213.

Frank, S., Specter, S., Nowotny, A. and Friedman, H. (1977). Immunocyte stimulation *in vitro* by nontoxic bacterial lipopolysaccharide derivatives. *Journal of Immunology* 119, 855–860.

Franzl, R. E. and McMaster, P. D. (1968). The primary immune response in mice. I. The enhancement and suppression of hemolysin production by a bacterial endotoxin. *Journal of Experimental Medicine* 127, 1087–1107.

Freitas, A. A. and de Sousa, M. (1976). Control mechanisms of lymphocyte traffic. Altered distribution of ^{51}Cr-labeled mouse lymph node cells pretreated *in vitro* with lipopolysaccharide. *European Journal of Immunology* 6, 269–273.

Frost, P. and Lance, E. M. (1978). On the mechanism of action of adjuvants. *Immunology* 35, 63–68.

Garzelli, C., Colizzi, V., Campa, M., Bozzi, L. and Falcone, G. (1979a). Depression of the antibody response in *Pseudomonas aeruginosa*-injected mice. *Infection and Immunity* 24, 32–38.

Garzelli, C., Colizzi, V., Campa, M., Bozzi, L and Falcone, G. (1979b). Depression of contact sensitivity by *Pseudomonas aeruginosa*-induced suppressor cells which affect the induction phase of immune response. *Infection and Immunity* 26, 4–11.

Genco, R. J., Plaut, A. G. and Moellering, R. C., Jr. (1975). Evaluation of human oral organisms and pathogenic *Streptococcus* for production of IgA protease. *Journal of Infectious Diseases* 131S, 17–21.

Gershon, R. K., Mokyr, M. B. and Mitchell, M. S. (1974). Activation of suppressor T cells by tumour and specific antibody. *Nature* 250, 594–596.

Gill, H. K. and Liew, F. Y. (1979). Regulation of delayed-type hypersensitivity. IV. Antigen-specific suppressor cells for delayed-type hypersensitivity induced by lipopolysaccharide and sheep erythrocytes in mice. *European Journal of Immunology* 9, 101–106.

Godal, T. (1978). Immunological aspects of leprosy—Present status. *Progress in Allergy* 25, 211–242.

Goodwin, J. S., Bankhurst, A. D. and Messner, R. P. (1977). Suppression of human T-cell mitogenesis by prostaglandin: existence of a prostaglandin producing suppressor celi. *Journal of Experimental Medicine* 146, 1719–1734.

Goodman, M. G. and Weigle, W. O. (1979). T Cell regulation of polycolonal B cell responsiveness. I. Helper effects of T cells. *Journal of Immunology* 122, 2548–2553.

Hämmerling, U., Chin, A. F. and Abbott, J. (1976). Ontogeny of murine B lymphocytes: sequence of B-cell differentiation of surface-immunoglobulin-negative precursors to plasma cells (Induction of surface markers). *Proceedings of National Academy of Sciences,* U.S.A. 73, 2008–2012.

Hoffmann, M. K., Galanos, C., Koenig, S. and Oettgen, H. F. (1977). B-cell activation by lipopolysaccharide. Distinct pathways for induction of mitosis and antibody production. *Journal of Experimental Medicine* 146, 1640–1647.

Hoffmann, M. K., Koenig, S., Mittler, R. S., Oettgen, H. F., Ralph, P., Galanos, C. and Hammerling, U. (1979). Macrophage factor controlling differentiation of B cells. *Journal of Immunology* 122, 497–502.

Hudson, K. M., Byner, C., Freeman, J. and Terry, R. J. (1976). Immunodepression, high IgM levels and evasion of the immune response in murine trypanosomiasis. *Nature* 264, 256–258.

Izui, S., Kobayakawa, T., Louis, J. and Lambert, P. H. (1979). Induction of thymocytotoxic autoantibodies after injection of bacterial lipopolysaccharides in mice. *European Journal of Immunology* 9, 338–341.

Jacobs, D. M. and Morrison, D. C. (1975). Dissociation between mitogenicity and immunogenicity of TNP-lipopolysaccharide, a T-dependent antigen. *Journal of Experimental Medicine* 141, 1453–1458.

Jerne, N. K. (1974). Towards a network theory of the immune system. *Annales d'Immunologie (Institut Pasteur)* 125C, 373–389.

Johnson, A. G., Jacobs, A., Abrams, G. and Merrit, K. (1967). "Germinal centers in immune response", pp. 214–220. Springer-Verlag, New York.

Katz, P., Goldstein, R. A. and Fauci, A. S. (1979). Immunoregulation in infection caused by *Mycobacterium tuberculosis*: the presence of suppressor monocytes and the alteration of subpopulation of T lymphocytes. *Journal of Infectious Diseases* 140, 12–21.

Kempf, K. E. and Rubin, A. S. (1979). Generation by lipopolysaccharide of a late-acting soluble suppressor of antibody synthesis. *Cellular Immunology* 43, 30–40.

Kilian, M., Mestecki, J., Kulhavy, R., Tomana, M. and Butler, W. T. (1980). IgA1 protease from *Haemophilus influenzae, Streptococcus pneumoniae, Neisseria meningitidis*, and *Streptococcus sanguis*: comparative immunochemical studies. *Journal of Immunology* 124, 2596–2600.

Kilian, M., Mestecky, J. and Schrohenloher, R. E. (1979). Pathogenic species of the genus *Haemophilus* and *Streptococcus pneumoniae* produce immunoglobulin A1 protease. *Infection and Immunity* 26, 143–149.

Koenig, S. and Hoffmann, M. K. (1979). Bacterial lipopolysaccharide activates suppressor B lymphocytes (regulation of humoral immunity). *Proceedings of the National Academy of Sciences, U.S.A.* **76**, 4608–4612.

Kurland, J. I. and Bockman, R. (1978). Prostaglandin E production by human blood monocytes and mouse peritoneal macrophages. *Journal of Experimental Medicine* **147**, 952–957.

Lagrange, P. H. and Mackaness, G. B. (1975). Effects of bacterial lipopolysaccharide on the induction and expression of cell-mediated immunity. II. Stimulation of the efferent arc. *Journal of Immunology* **114**, 447–451.

Lagrange, P. H., Mackaness, G. B., Miller, T. E. and Pardon, P. (1975). Effects of bacterial lipopolysaccharide on the induction and expression of cell-mediated immunity. I. Depression of the afferent arc. *Journal of Immunology* **114**, 442–446.

Lamb, J. R., Kontiainen, S. and Lehner, T. (1979). Generation of specific T-cell suppressor function induced by *Streptococcus mutans* in monkeys and mice. *Infection and Immunity* **26**, 903–909.

Lefford, M. J. and Mackaness, G. B. (1977). Suppression of immunity to *Mycobacterium lepraemurium* infection. *Infection and Immunity* **18**, 363–369.

Louis, J. A., Chiller, J. M. and Weigle, W. O. (1973). The ability of bacterial lipopolysaccharide to modulate the induction of unresponsiveness to a state of immunity. *Journal of Experimental Medicine* **138**, 1481–1495.

Mackaness, G. B., Lagrange, P. H., Miller, T. E. and Ishibashi, T. (1974). Feed-back inhibition of specifically sensitized lymphocytes. *Journal of Experimental Medicine* **139**, 543–599.

Male, C. J. (1979). Immunoglobulin A1 protease production by *Haemphilus influenzae and Streptococcus pneumoniae. Infection and Immunity* **26**, 254–261.

Matsumoto, T., Monoyama, N., Ootsu, K. and Hokan, T. (1977). Effect of an acid polysaccharide produced by *Serratia piscatorum* on immune response in mice. II. Stimulatory effects in normal and immunologically impaired animals. *Immunology* **32**, 121–129.

McGhee, J. R., Farrar, J. J., Michalek, S. M., Mergenhagen, S. E. and Rosenstreich, D. L. (1979). Cellular requirements for lipopolysaccharide adjuvanticity. A role for both T lymphocytes and macrophages for *in vitro* responses to particulate antigens. *Journal of Experimental Medicine* **149**, 793–807.

McGhee, J. R., Kiyono, H., Michalek, S. M., Babb, J. L., Rosenstreich, D. L. and Mergenhagen, S. E. (1980a). Lipopolysaccharide (LPS) regulation of the immune response: T lymphocytes from normal mice suppress mitogenic and immunogenic responses to LPS. *Journal of Immunology* **124**, 1603–1611.

McGhee, J. R., Michalek, S. M., Babb, J. L., Kiyono, H., Rosenstreich, D. L. and Mergenhagen, S. E. (1980b). "Microbiology—1980", pp. 49–60. American Society for Microbiology, Washington, DC.

McMaster, P. D. and Franzl, R. E. (1968). The primary immune response in mice. II. Cellular responses of lymphoid tissue accompanying the enhancement or complete suppression of antibody formation by a bacterial endotoxin. *Journal of Experimental Medicine* **127**, 1109–1126.

Mehta, S. K., Plaut, A. G., Calvanico, N. J. and Tomas, T. B. Jr. (1973). Human immunoglobulin A: production of an Fc fragment by an enteric microbial proteolytic enzyme. *Journal of Immunology* **111**, 1274–1276.

Melchers, F. (1980). "The Molecular Basis of Microbial Pathogenicity", pp. 285–306. Weinheim: Verlag Chemie.

Melchers, F., Braun, V. and Galanos, C. (1975). The lipoprotein of the outer membrane of *Escherichia coli*: a B-cell mitogen. *Journal of Experimental Medicine* **142**, 473–482.

Möller, G., Andersson, J. and Sjöberg, O. (1972). Lipopolysaccharides can convert heterologous red cells into thymus-independent antigen. *Cellular Immunology* **4**, 416–424.

Mulks, M. H., Kornfeld, S. J. and Plaut, A. G. (1980). Specific proteolysis of human IgA by *Streptococcus pneumoniae* and *Haemophilus influenzae*. *Journal of Infectious Diseases* **141**, 450–456.

Nakano, M., Tanabe, M. J., Saito, T. and Shimizu, T. (1976). Immunosuppressive effect of bacterial lipopolysaccharide on antibody response. *Japanese Journal of Microbiology* **20**, 53–58.

Norcross, M. A. and Smith, R. T. (1977). Regulation of B-cell proliferative responses to lipopolysaccharide by a subclass of thymic T cells. *Journal of Experimental Medicine* **145**, 1299–1315.

O'Brien, A. D., Scher, I., Campbell, G. H., Mac Dermott, R. P. and Formal, S. B. (1979). Susceptibility of CBA/N mice to infection with *Salmonella typhimurium*: influence of the X-linked gene controlling B lymphocyte function. *Journal of Immunology* **123**, 720–724.

Peavy, D. L., Shands, J. W., Adler, W. H. and Smith, R. T. (1973). Mitogenicity of bacterial endotoxins: characterization of the mitogenic principle. *Journal of Immunology* **111**, 352–357.

Persson, U. (1977). Lipopolysaccharide-induced suppression of the primary immune response to a thymus-dependent antigen. *Journal of Immunology* **118**, 789–796.

Plaut, A. G., Gilbert, J. V., Artenstein, M. S. and Capra, J. D. (1975). *Neisseria gonorrhoeae* and *Neisseria meningitidis*: extracellular enzyme cleaves human immunoglobulin A. *Science* **190**, 1103–1105.

Plaut, A. G., Gilbert, J. V. and Wistar, R. Jr. (1977). Loss of antibody activity in human immunoglobulin A exposed to extracellular immunoglobulin A proteases of *Neisseria gonorrhoeae* and *Streptococcus sanguis*. *Infection and Immunity* **17**, 130–135.

Plaut, A. G., Wistar, R. Jr and Capra, J. D. (1974). Differential susceptibility of human IgA immunoglobulins to streptococcal IgA protease. *Journal of Clinical Investigation* **54**, 1295–1300.

Poe, W. J. and Michael, J. G. (1976). Separation of the mitogenic and antigenic responses to bacterial lipopolysaccharide. *Immunology* **30**, 241–248.

Poels, L. G. and Van Niekerk, C. C. (1977). *Plasmodium berghei*: immunosuppression and hypergammaglobulinemia. *Experimental Parasitology* **42**, 235–247.

Romagnani, S., Giudizi, G. M., Almerigogna, F., Nicoletti, P. L. and Ricci, M. (1980). Protein A of *Staphylococcus aureus* is mitogenic for IgG-bearing, but also for a subpopulation of IgM-and/or IgD-bearing human lymphocytes. *Immunology* **39**, 417–425.

Rosenstreich, D. L., O'Brien, A. D., Groves, M. G. and Taylor, B. A. (1980). "The Molecular Basis of Microbial Pathogenicity", pp. 101–114. Weinheim: Verlag Chemie.

Rowlands, D. T. Jr., Claman, H. N. and Kind, P. D. (1965). The effect of endotoxin on the thymus of young mice. *American Journal of Pathology* **46**, 165–176.

Ryser, J. E. and Vassalli, P. (1974). Mouse bone marrow lymphocytes and their differentiation. *Journal of Immunology* **113**, 719–728.

agents. The determined state of the precursor cell. *Journal of Experimental Medicine* **138**, 1027–1032.

Scheid, M. P., Hoffmann, M. K., Komuro, K., Hämmerling, U., Abbott, J., Boyse, E. A., Cohen, G. H., Hooper, J. A., Schulof, R. S. and Goldstein, A. L. (1973). Differentiation of T cells induced by preparations from thymus and by nonthymic

Scheid, M. P., Goldstein, G. and Boyse, E. A. (1975). Differentiation of T cells in nude mice. *Science* **190**, 1211–1213.

Schwab, J. H. (1975). Suppression of the immune response by microorganisms. *Bacteriological Reviews* **39**, 121–143.

Schwab, J. H. (1977). "Microbiology—1977", pp. 366–373. American Society for Microbiology, Washington DC.

Scott, D. W. and Diener, E. (1976). Effect of lypopolysaccharide on the induction of tolerance to polymerized flagellin. *Journal of Immunology* **116**, 1220–1223.

Sinclair, N. R. St C. (1978). Immunoregulation by antibody and antigen–antibody complexes. *Transplantation Proceedings* **10**, 349–353.

Sitia, R., Abbott, J. and Hämmerling, U. (1979). The ontogeny of B lymphocytes. V. Lipopolysaccharide-induced changes of IgD expression on murine B lymphocytes. *European Journal of Immunology* **9**, 859–864.

Sjöberg, O., Andersson, J. and Möller, G. (1972). LPS can substitute for helper cells in the antibody response *in vitro*. *European Journal of Immunology* **2**, 326–331.

Sultzer, B. M. and Goodman, G. W. (1976). Endotoxin protein: a B-cell mitogen and polyclonal activator of C_3H/HeJ lymphocytes. *Journal of Experimental Medicine* **144**, 821–827.

Sultzer, B. M. and Nilsson, B. S. (1972). PPD tuberculin. A B-cell mitogen. *Nature New Biology* **240**, 198–200.

Taub, R. H., Rosett, W., Adler, A. and Morse, S. I. (1972). Distribution of labeled lymph node cells in mice during the lymphocytosis induced by *Bordetella pertussis*. *Journal of Experimental Medicine* **136**, 1581–1593.

Uchiyama, T. and Jacobs, D. M. (1978). Modulation of immune response by bacterial lypopolysaccharide (LPS): cellular basis of stimulatory and inhibitory effects of LPS on the *in vitro* IgM antibody response to a T-dependent antigen. *Journal of Immunology* **121**, 2347–2351.

Uhr, J. W. and Möller, G. (1968). Regulatory effect of antibody on the immune response. *Advances in Immunology* **8**, 81–84.

Vallera, D. A., Gamble, C. E. and Schmidtke, J. R. (1980). Lypopolysaccharide-induced immunomodulation of the generation cell-mediated cytotoxicity. II. Evidence for the involvement of a regulatory B lymphocyte. *Journal of Immunology* **124**, 641–649.

Walker, S. M. and Weigle, W. O. (1978). Effect of bacterial lypopolysaccharide on the *in vitro* secondary antibody response in mice. I. Description of the suppressive capacity of lypopolysaccharide. *Cellular Immunology* **36**, 170–179.

Watson, J. (1977). Differentiation of B lymphocytes in C_3H/HeJ mice: the induction

of Ia antigens by lypopolysaccharide. *Journal of Immunology* **118**, 1103–1108.
Watson, S. R. and Collins, F. M. (1980). Development of suppressor T cells in mice heavily infected with mycobacteria. *Immunology* **39**, 367–373.
Wheelock, E. F., Toy, S. T. and Stjernholm, R. L. (1971). Interaction of viruses with human lymphocytes. *Progress in Immunology* 1, 787–801.

DISCUSSION

Braude Has anyone shown that LPS is a mitogen for human B cells?

Campa Yes, LPS is also active on human B lymphocytes.

Wilton Lida Ivanyi, who was with our group until a couple of years ago, showed that it was a mitogen for human B cells, but not anything like as powerful a mitogen as it is for the mouse B cell. In the mouse there was a dissociation of mitogenicity and antigenicity, which was difficult to investigate in the human for obvious reasons.

Smith Why in some cases do you get stimulation of suppressor cells and in other cases stimulation of T or B cells to give high antibody or cell mediated immunity? There is no answer to that one as far as I can see at the moment.

Valdimarsson Has anyone convincingly demonstrated that LPS stimulation induces suppressor B cells? Is this something that has been demonstrated *in vivo* with cell transfer experiments or is it a theory? I am not quite clear.

Campa Yes, it has been clearly demonstrated. There are several reports both *in vivo* and *in vitro* showing that LPS can directly activate B suppressor cells.

Braude Do you think that the bi-adjuvant activity of LPS represents an important modulation of the immune response? Let me explain what I mean by bi-adjuvant activity. When you give LPS shortly before another antigen you get an enhanced immune response from the second antigen. Do you think that has significance when Gram negative organisms are present in mixed infections in helping to enhance the immunity to the other organism?

Campa It could be possible, but I also think that LPS by polyclonally stimulating B cell precursers may leave the host temporarily without defence. This could enhance infection by a second microorganism.

Williams Is there any evidence that the lymphocyte has any role to play in the early stages of infection: firstly, during the period of initiation of infection when the organisms are lodged and getting their foothold and, secondly, in the acute phase of the established illness?

Anderson I can only speak for viral infections because my knowledge of bacterial infections is vanishingly small. Certainly in several systems it has been shown that if you suppress lymphocyte function by such drugs as cyclophosphamide and prevent any sort of lymphocyte reaction, those infections which are normally tolerated and cleared are converted to fatal pneumonic disease. For example, if you inoculate a mouse intranasally with a relatively small amount of Sendai virus the mouse will normally clear the virus from its lungs within about seven days. If, just prior to inoculation, the mouse is given cyclophosphamide (admittedly in large doses) there is no lymphocyte response, as demonstrated histologically at the site of infection or by measuring any of the various parameters of lymphocyte activity and a fulminating viral pneumonia develops which kills the mouse.

Potter May I add that the same thing is true of influenza. When cyclophosphamide is used to limit lymphocyte activity in influenza virus infected mice the result is a very protracted illness compared to untreated animals. My concern is that one cannot assume that the effect of cyclophosphamide is specifically related to lymphocytes; cyclophosphamide probably has a large number of effects, any one of which could be the mediator of this protracted illness.

Valdimarsson There are relatively few clean experiments of nature which tell us about the importance of specific immunity in primary infection. Probably the best example is the fatal measles virus infection in children who lack T cells or those with T cell deficiency who tend to develop systemic vaccinia after smallpox vaccination. There are a number of other examples but I think, on the whole, that specific lymphocyte reactivity does not significantly interfere with the initial stages of primary infections, but it certainly helps to eradicate primary infections in many instances.

Stuart-Harris I hesitate to speak about a bacterial subject, but I have been waiting patiently for a day and a half to hear somebody mention it. Now discussion on the lymphocyte has given me the opportunity, as no one else has raised it. Pertussis is a bacterial infection which is characterized by a rather striking lymphocytosis, which I believe has been shown to be due to the production of a lymphocyte-promoting factor. Can anyone explain why we have all these excellent lymphocytes in whooping cough which seem to be quite impotent to restrain infection?

Valdimarsson At least in experimental systems lymphocytosis in whooping cough appears to be due mainly to mobilization of lymphocytes from lymphoid organs into the circulation by some unknown properties of the organism. It is a shift of relatively small lymphocytes into the circulation.

Smith Before we go on I should like to emphasise one point. Professor Williams referred to the initiation of the infection. He asked whether lymphocytes are important in the initiation of infection; we all know they are important in recovery.

Valdimarsson I tried to cover that. They probably do not have any significant effect in the initial phases of the primary infection by most organisms, but they are certainly important in the eradication of infection in many instances.

Mims I wonder whether in any of these infections with LPS-producing microorganisms there is demonstrable disturbance of the immune response to other antigens?

Campa Yes. In our laboratory we have shown that *Ps. aeruginosa* is able to depress contact sensitivity by activating B suppressor cells, possibly through its LPS.

Mogensen What is the outcome of bacterial infections in LPS-insensitive C_3H/HeJ mice compared with other substrains of C_3H mice?

Braude One outcome is that disseminated gonococcal infections in LPS-resistant mice are less lethal.

Mogensen C_3H/HeJ mice are also more resistant to at least some virus infections.

Draper I am worried by this lipopolysaccharide story. The human race has been living with Gram negative bacteria producing LPS in its gut for as long as its history. How is it that it has these very dramatic effects? One would have thought that some mechanism would by now have developed to enable us to cope with it. To pick up what was said in another connection this morning, is it true that there is lipopolysaccharide and lipopolysaccharide?

van Furth We live with LPS but only in the gastrointestinal tract and the portal vein. LPS is cleared by Kupffer cells in the liver. Only when the infection is in another place do you have problems, because you then have LPS in the circulation. This also occurs in liver cirrhosis, when there is a shunt between the portal vein and the large circulation.

Peters I would like to make a general point. As I see it, just because a LPS-producing organism is lethal that does not bear upon the question of whether it has immunosuppressive properties. There are obviously other mechanisms which are more important. Certainly, in clinical practice whereas viral infections are commonly complicated by secondary infections, it is unusual under ordinary circumstances of bacterial infection to see clinical evidence of interference with the immune response. It is not nearly such an important factor.

Smith It has not been studied as much in the bacterial as in the viral field.

Wilton David Morrison has twice recently reviewed the LPS literature from two different points of view. The first striking thing is that its effects are mutually antagonistic. LPS can do anything. It can turn on, turn off, switch on, switch off. I would make two points about the turning on and about the suppressor B cell. LPS is the only adjuvant that you can administer in advance. It does not have to be given, like the bacterial adjuvant or the oil-based adjuvant, simultaneously with the antigen. If you pre-inject them you get the immune deviation that was described by Geoffrey Asherson.

The second thing is that it was not appreciated that the LPS preparations used by many people until a few years ago contained protein. The isolated protein has different effects from the parent LPS. It has to be said that a lot of interpretations put on LPS mechanisms may have to be re-thought when people work with LPS protein or LPS in a purified, defined form.

Campa Yes, I agree with you. You need to inject LPS two or three days before the antigen in order to get suppression, but LPS-induced suppression is not always mediated by suppressor cells. There could be another explanation: LPS-induced polyclonal stimulation of B-precursor cells may lead to a temporary exhaustion of precursor cells, so that when you inject the antigen it does not encounter the right cells, and you get suppression.

Wilton There are two further points. One is the evidence of Allison and Davies that the adjuvanticity of LPS is apparently T-cell mediated. The second point is that LPS-activated macrophages produce very large amounts of prostaglandins which are inhibitory to lymphocyte mitogenesis. That may be the basis of the suppression.

Campa I can answer your second point. It has been shown that LPS-induced suppression is not due to prostaglandin released by macrophages after stimulation by LPS but rather to direct activation of B suppressor cells.

van Furth Are you saying, Dr Wilton, that most probably suppression is the work of the macrophages producing prostaglandins?

Wilton No, what I am saying is that it can be shown, at least *in vivo*, that if you take lymphocyte cultures which would normally be driven by antigen or mitogen and increase the number of macrophages above about 10 or 15% you start getting suppressive effects. Those effects are prostaglandin-mediated suppression and can be inhibited by indomethacin. I am not disagreeing that there is a B cell suppressor mechanism. There are other LPS induced suppressor mechanisms which should also be considered.

Jeljaszewicz Two things trouble me a little. The first is that probably the majority of findings with LPS are more or less laboratory experiments and there seems to be not too much clinical evidence about the role of LPS during natural infection. The second thing is that in most Gram negative infections specific antibody does not seem to play a very significant role in protection. I would be interested to hear the views of people more experienced with Gram negative organisms on the antigen which is claimed to be commonly present in most normal healthy humans. What is the relation of this antigen to interference with the immune response?

Braude I think that LPS contributes considerably to human infection syndromes. There is no question but that LPS is important in acute bacteraemia. In our hospital, for example, the occurrence of shock in septicaemia is about five times as common in bacteraemia due to Gram negative organisms, which contains LPS, as in that due to Gram positive bacteria, which do not contain LPS. There is no other way to account for the striking difference in the incidence of shock than the presence of LPS. Furthermore, the shock that is produced during the course of Gram negative bacteraemia is identical to the shock that is produced in patients when they are given LPS intravenously for one reason or another.

One of the first studies along this line was done at the National Cancer Institute in the late 1940s. The object was to see whether or not the tumour necrotic effect occurring in experimental animals treated with LPS could be reproduced in human beings. It was found that the injection of Shear's polysaccharide (Serratia LPS) did not have any effect on tumours but it did reproduce a syndrome that was identical to human Gram negative bacteraemia.

Another thing that made us appreciate the role of LPS in human beings was the transfusion reactions seen in the early 1950s from blood contaminated with cold growing Gram negative organisms. These Gram negative bacteria are completely avirulent. They can grow in the blood bank but they are unable to grow at body temperature, so they are unable to produce a progressive infection in human beings. Yet transfusions contaminated with cold growing Gram negative organisms (usually species of pseudomonads) produce a horrible type of transfusion reaction, almost always fatal, that has clinical manifestations identical to the syndrome of Gram negative shock that we see now.

I am aware of the fact that there are some people—particularly Joe Shands—who question the role of LPS in Gram negative infections, but he has dealt exclusively not with acute bacteraemias but with slowly progressive Gram negative infections such as *Salmonella* infections of animals, where the element of sudden invasion of the bloodstream by Gram negative bacteria is not a factor. I think his arguments are irrelevant to the question whether or not LPS is important in overwhelming Gram negative bacteraemia.

When you asked about a common antigen I think you were perhaps referring to the Kunin antigen. I do not think this is very important. I think it is a fragmentary antigen of the core glycolipid. We have been interested instead in the core glycolipid antigen on the theory that since this is uniformly present in all Gram negative organisms we might prepare an antiserum against it in an attempt to neutralise LPS toxin in the treatment of Gram negative bacteraemia. In experimental animals, our studies leave no doubt that antibody to core glycolipid is very effective in treatment as well as prophylaxis against a variety of Gram negative organisms, regardless of species.

So, in answer to your two questions, yes, I believe that LPS is a very important factor in acute bacteraemias and that the common antigen, if you mean the core glycolipid, is also important.

Williams I do not think Dr Braude has really answered Professor Jeljaszewicz's question. We agree that lipopolysaccharide is a toxic substance and when injected into man it has a very marked effect on all tissues, including the blood vessels and lymphocytic system. It is not surprising that one can show that lymphocytes *in vitro* are affected by LPS, but possibly not more than any of the other cells in the body: the liver cells or the brain or the lining of the gastrointestinal tract are also affected by LPS. It is interesting for the immunologist to show how LPS affects the lymphocytes, but it has not necessarily got anything to do with infection. The question is whether lymphocytes which have been damaged by LPS lose their ability to produce specific antibody or whether they return to normal function.

Braude May I say just one further word? I do not know whether or not LPS during infection does have any effect on the lymphocytes along the lines that you question. I simply wanted to answer the question whether or not LPS is operative during infections and I do not think there is any doubt about the fact that it is with respect to its circulatory effects, although we have not been dealing much with that because it is not an immune function necessarily. The collapse of the circulation is one of the most important, striking and uniform effects of both LPS and Gram negative bacteraemia.

Easmon Could I change the subject from LPS to bacterial polysaccharides, particulary capsular polysaccharides, and perhaps try and make a case for a more direct interference with immune response? With capsulated strains of pneumococci and with *Haemophilus influenzae* type B, it is certain that opsonic antibody is important in the course of the disease. With *H. influenzae* type B in particular there seems to be a problem in infants with their capacity to respond to the capsular polysaccharide as an immunogen. There has certainly been a lot of work on pneumococcal polysaccharide and more recently on *H. influenzae* type B capsular polysaccharide which suggests that early on in life something on the surface of these organisms may trigger off the activity of suppressor cells as opposed to antibody-producing cells. This may not only impair the capacity of the individual to produce a suitable antibody response during the course of the acute infection, but attempts to immunize with capsular material might have the danger of producing tolerance if these immunogens are given early in life.

The other point is that in *H. influenzae* type B or pneumococcal infections the presence of persistent antigenaemia is very often associated with a poor prognosis. I wonder if anyone would like to develop the point that the antigenaemia, particularly with the polysaccharide capsular antigen, may have fairly disastrous effects on the immunocompetence of the patient's mononuclear phagocyte system during the acute phase of the infection which are reflected in the poor clinical response to infection.

Quie A small number of very young children have been immunized with the pneumococcal polysaccharides but there is no evidence that tolerance has developed. There is minimal antibody response in the very young, but when they are re-immunized at 18 months or older the antibody response is very similar to those infants that had not been exposed to polysaccharide in early life. Tolerance, described in experimental animals, has never been demonstrated in humans, as far as I know.

Easmon There have also been studies using purified *H. influenzae* type B immunogen in which it has signally failed to produce an antibody response in children under the age of two years. Given to older children, the polysaccharide stimulated a satisfactory humoral response.

Quie An interesting report from Boston recently has suggested that IgG subclass 2 may be missing in patients who do not respond to the polysaccharide vaccines. Hodgkin's disease patients have low levels of IgG subclass 2. Another experiment of nature, if you will, is the Wiscott-Aldrich syndrome. These patients are incapable of responding to polysaccharide antigens but respond quite normally to protein antigens.

Mims One fascinating thing that I believe came out of those pneumococcal vaccine studies was that when you give children of various ages this 14 valent antigen the younger ones respond very poorly to the pneumococcal types that most commonly cause trouble in children of that age. That suggests to me, although it is only a possibility, that they have a genetically determined defect and make a poor antibody response to those pneumococcal types. Hence their susceptibility. It is very similar to the results with childhood meningococcal meningitis obtained by Dr Whittle and his colleagues from West Africa; poor antibody responses to the relevant meningococcal type was associated with meningococcal meningitis and there were indications that this was genetically determined.

I wonder if I could refer to the cleavage of IgA, which I think is very interesting. I understand that his has now been extended to *H. influenzae* and *Pneumococcus*. I should like to suggest that it may turn out to be irrelevant because of the very interesting finding reported a year or two ago with *Tetrahymena pyriformis*. This is a free-living microorganism, known to produce a protease which cleaves IgA. In fact in this report the process was called "fabulation". If a free-living animal like that can do it, you could argue that it is a useful protease and maybe was developed for other purposes. Perhaps it was turned to use against host defences by the gonococci, but it could be a protease still produced for other purposes. I thought it was an interesting finding.

Campa I agree. In addition I would like to say that in abscesses polymorphs can produce proteases. So we do not know the real importance of these enzymes in relation to infection.

Wilton I think that Robbins would go even further; he has suggested that the IgA protease of gonococci might even be a virulence determinant because it allows the organism to attach to epithelial cells.

Smith I wonder if I might just change the tack a little, I think there is an area here where the bacteriologists are much behind the virologists and certainly behind the parasitologists. This is in avoidance of the immune response by antigenic shift and drift. There has been the marvellous work of Cross and others showing how the trypanosomes avoid the immune response to produce chronic infection. We all also know, of course, the work with the influenza virus. Amongst bacteria antigenic shift and drift occurs with *Borrelia recurrentis* and *Campylobacter fetus*. It has also been suggested for some of the dental organisms that remain in the mouth for long periods.

Mims Although antigenic variation is so important in trypanosomiasis and the molecular biological basis of this has been worked out in terms of shifts in gene expression during development of the trypanosome, influenza is not comparable because you do not get antigenic shift during the infection of a given individual. There are two virus infections where it has been suggested that this occurs. One is visna disease of sheep and the other is equine infectious anaemia. So, although it is not unknown in viruses, the influenza example is rather different.

Smith I think the people at the Forsythe Institute in Boston made the suggestion that antigenic shift occurred in oral organisms. I do not know whether Dr Wilton would like to comment on that?

Wilton I do not know whether they have taken it very much further than the initial observation that there seemed to be what they called antigenic drift amongst oral streptococci. *Streptococcus sanguis* was the one that was chosen. But the mention this morning of Derek Elwood's work with the chemostat is interesting because I often wonder whether bacteria growing as you have suggested in tissues under growth-limiting and rate-limiting conditions, might not express antigens of which we have no knowledge at all. Therefore, when we talk about antigenic modulation for bacteria we are even further in the dark because they may be producing antigens *in vivo* one knows nothing about and we are studying the wrong ones because they are the ones identifiable in the test tubes. It is going to be doubly difficult to talk about protective antigens.

Smith Does anyone else wish to talk about antigenic drift?

Valdimarsson Could we drift away from infection altogether for a while? I want to refer to a comment which was made in the introduction and that is the possibility of autoimmune phenomena caused by LPS. Does anybody know whether measurements of autoantibodies have been made on patients who have survived endotoxin shock or whether they tend to develop autoimmune phenomena after such shock?

Campa Cunningham has shown that there is a dramatic increase in antibodies against erythrocytes in mice.

Peters Am I not right in thinking that that occurred in strains already susceptible to develop autoimmune haemolytic anaemia?

Campa No, it was in resistant strains.

Peters Could I come back to the title: the evidence that bacterial infection perturbs the immune response in a biologically important way. We have heard evidence that lipoplysaccharide can do so. We have heard other evidence that lipopolysaccharide in its own right, probably through nonclassical immunological mechanisms, such as the production of hypotension and disseminated intravascular coagulation can cause death, which is clinically very relevant but not really to the point of this discussion. Is there any hard evidence that important immunosuppressive events occur after bacterial infections in the way, as I said earlier, that they occur after measles or various other virus infections?

Mims I think there are examples. One of them is lepromatous leprosy where we know that in the infected individual there is a suppressor population which reduces immune responses to a lot of unrelated antigens. I feel that there are not too many examples from bacteriology and that where they exist they are more likely to be bacteria that grow in cells and invade lymphoreticular tissues.

Peters By destruction of lymphocytes, you mean?

Mims As I will show tomorrow, it can be achieved by more subtle ways than destruction.

Braude Thyroiditis is probably an auto-immune disease and there is considerable evidence now that thyroiditis in human beings is usually due to mumps virus. I think therefore that mumps virus infection of the thyroid can induce autoimmunity.

Peters That was not my point. I am sure that there are circumstances where viral infection can produce autoimmunities. The question is "do bacteria produce a direct influence on immune responses?".

Quie Examples may be poststreptococcal glomerular nephritis and rheumatic fever. In rheumatic fever there seems to be an association between elevated circulating antibodies to some of the streptococcal products and damage to the heart. The immune system has been perturbed somehow and there is some pretty good evidence now that T cells in these patients respond differently to some of the streptococcal antigens than T cells from nonrheumatic subjects.

Peters There are a number of examples of chronic bacterial infection producing immune complex disease which might be considered eventually to have repercussions on the immune system; and there are conditions like *Mycoplasma* pneumonia with which autoimmunity is associated. But I was not thinking of examples of that kind where other explanations are possible.

Valdimarsson Perhaps I could tell one story relevant to your point. In the superficial fungal infection, chronic mucocutaneous candidiasis, some patients develop generalized anergy but sometimes the anergy is restricted to *Candida*. Quite often this anergy is associated with a serum factor which blocks cellular immunity *in vitro*, as judged by various techniques. It has been demonstrated now quite convincingly that his inhibitory factor is probably mannan released from *Candida* into the circulation of these patients. It is notable that these patients are only superficially infected.

In the patients in whom suppression is not selective for *Candida*, it also affects the reponse of lymphocytes to PHA. I think that is a reasonably good example of perturbation of the immune system by fungi.

Mims If by a perturbation we mean alterations, I think Professor Peters is right in saying that most of the examples given are not strictly to the point. If we mention mumps thyroiditis we should also mention ankylosing spondylitis and *Klebsiella* infections, where the connection is fairly well tied even to certain *Klebsiella* subtypes.

Peters In *Klebsiella* infections there are no perturbations of the immune response that have been identified. There is a specific disease that is associated, but evidence of perturbation of the immune response is lacking. It is a consequence of that particular infection in that genetically prone individual and as I see it not within the remit of our title.

Viral Interference with the Immune Response

C. A. MIMS

Guy's Hospital Medical School,
London, UK.

INTRODUCTION

Immune defences against virus infections are for the most part the same as those against bacterial, rickettsial, protozoal and other infections. But there are differences of emphasis. These arise first because viruses, unlike most bacteria, must enter cells to replicate. Viruses are best kept out of susceptible cells, whereas the host attempts to enclose invading bacteria within phagocytic cells. This generally leads to destruction of the infectious agent, but some viruses replicate in phagocytes, and a virus opsonin can then enhance and encourage infection. A second reason for a difference of immunological emphasis in virus infections is because infected cells generally bear virus-specified antigens on their surfaces. This is true even for many viruses such as pox viruses or adenoviruses that do not mature from the cell membrane by budding. Virus-infected cells therefore become targets for immune destruction, and this is a major determinant both for host defences and for immunopathology.

Viruses, like all infectious agents, must come to terms with host defences. In a fascinating variety of ways successful viruses have learnt to evade or subvert host defences and thus promote their survival in the host and their continued existence as infectious agents. I shall classify the ways in which viruses interfere with host immune responses. When a particular phenomenon reduces the effectiveness of host defences I shall refer to it as if it were a virus strategy. Even if this is seldom justified, it is nevertheless an interesting way of looking at virus–host interactions. The interplay between virus and host has been a constant feature of evolutionary history, and it can be assumed that any mechanism of interference that is possible and would give advantage to an infected virus will have been "discovered" and utilized. In some cases the type of interference is well established, while in others we still await the discovery of good examples.

INTERFERENCE WITH THE ACTION OF ANTIBODIES

Antibodies protect against virus infections in several ways. First by combining with the surface of the virus and preventing attachment to susceptible cells, they act as neutralizing antibodies. Second, by combining with virus antigen on the surface of infected cells they render them susceptible to complement-mediated or perhaps more importantly to cell-mediated cytolysis. Third, by combining with viral antigens either free or in virus particles or cell debris, they initiate inflammatory events just like any other antigen–antibody complex. The inflammatory events bring serum components and circulating leukocytes to the site of the interaction, and this results in antiviral effects whose exact mode of action and role is still poorly defined.

There are many examples of virus interference with the action of antibodies (Table I). For instance, large quantities of viral antigens or non-infectious virus particles are sometimes liberated during the infection and these tend to mop up antibody which might otherwise usefully combine with virus particles or with infected cells. The immune complexes thus formed are common in systemic virus infections, but it is not known whether the diversion of antibodies has significant effect on the course of the infection.

Another method of interference is when viruses fail to produce antigens on the surface of infected cells. This takes place in persistent virus infections caused by herpesviruses, leukaemia viruses, or papovaviruses. In the case of EB virus in leukocytes, herpes simplex in dorsal root ganglion cells, or polyoma virus in tubular epithelial cells in the kidney, the virus remains in the cell in a latent form without expressing antigens on the cell surface. This renders it insusceptible to immune attack. The infected cell may also be less susceptible to immune attack if there is a low density of virus antigens expressed on the cell surface. This has been shown to occur for instance in simian foamy virus infections (Hooks *et al.*, 1976).

Many viruses, including picornaviruses, influenza, spread from cell to cell after liberation of virus particles into extracellular fluid where they are susceptible to any neutralizing antibodies that may be present. However, when a virus spreads directly from cell to cell without entering extracellular fluids, so that its spread is not restricted by neutralizing antibodies, it can be said to have evaded the action of these antibodies. This is characteristic of herpes simplex, cytomegalovirus, mumps or foamy virus infections (Hooks *et al.*, 1976). In a cell monolayer neutralizing antibodies will prevent extracellular virus infecting the first set of cells, but if this has already occurred the antibodies fail to inhibit the subsequent spread of the infection and the development of plaques. This is more likely to be important if the infected cells are less susceptible to immune destruction, either because there is a low density of virus antigen on the cell surface, or because of a local shortage of complement as appears to be the case in the central nervous system (Albrecht, 1978).

TABLE I.
Virus interference with the action of antibodies.

Type of interference	Mechanism	Examples	Status[a]
(1) Virus infection induces non-neutralizing or poorly neutralizing antibodies	Antibodies of poor affinity or directed against irrelevant virus antigens	LDH[b] virus in mice ADV[c] in mink EIA[d] virus in horses LCM[e] virus in mice	++
(2) Virus spreads directly from cell to cell	Neutralizing anti bodies less effective in preventing virus spread	Herpes simplex CMV[f] Foamy virus Vaccinia	++
(3) Virus antigens not produced on infected cell surface[g]	Infected cell is not susceptible to immune lysis	Papovaviruses, Herpes simplex, EB virus } latent state Leukemia virus in mouse cells	++
(4) Virus infection induces low levels of protective antibody	Virus and infected cells less susceptible to immune elimination	CMV (mice) Thymic necrosis virus (mice)	+

TABLE I *cont.*

Type of interference	Mechanism	Examples	Status[a]
(5) Antibody-mediated loss of virus antigen from infected cell surface	Antibody "caps" with virus antigen; complex is then lost by shedding or cytosis	Measles	+(SSPE)
(6) Virus induces Fc receptors on surface of infected cell	Infected cell binds IgG antibodies non-specifically and is protected from immune destruction	Herpes simplex Varicella-zoster CMV	+
(7) Virus infection induces a slowly evolving protective antibody response	Virus replication proceeds further before being halted	CMV (mice)	±
(8) Neutralizing antibody acts as enhancing antibody	Antibody assists virus entry into susceptible phagocyte (bearing Fc receptors)	Dengue and certain other arboviruses	±
(9) Free virus antigens combine with antibody	Antibody is "mopped up" and unavailable for antiviral action elsewhere	Many virus infections, e.g. measles, yellow fever	—
(10) Virus antigens produced on the membranes of intracellular vacuoles rather than on cell surface	Infected cell less susceptible to immune lysis	Alphaviruses, cornaviruses	—

[a] Status of phenomenon as a method of interference.
[b] Lactic dehydrogenase.
[c] Aleutian disease virus.
[d] Equine infectious anaemia.
[e] Lymphocytic choriomeningitis.
[f] Cytomegalovirus.
[g] Or virus antigens produced in a very low density on cell surface, so that infected cell is less susceptible to immune lysis.

A few enveloped viruses produce antigens on the membranes of intracellular vacuoles and are released from the cell after budding into these vacuoles. Flaviviruses and coronaviruses mature in this fashion and also visna virus in macrophages (O. Narayan, pers. comm.). There have been few investigations of virus antigens on the outer cell membrane, but if they are absent or present only in low density a degree of insusceptibility to immune defences might be predicted.

Another useful "device" is to make use of antibodies to get rid of viral antigens on the cell surface. This depends on the phenomenon called capping, in which substances are induced to move in the fluid matrix comprising the cell membrane after binding with antibody. Virus antigens on the cell surface combine with specific antibody and then move to one pole of the cell where they are either shed to the exterior as immune complexes, or taken into the cell by cytosis. The antibodies that should have prepared the infected cell for immune destruction are diverted from this purpose and used to rid the cell of virus-specific surface antigens, making it less susceptible to immune cytolysis. This phenomenon has been beautifully documented for measles virus (Lampert *et al.*, 1975) and in persistent measles (SSPE) it probably promotes persistence of the infection in the central nervous system in spite of the presence of large amounts of antibody. Capping presumably occurs during primary acute measles virus infection but it is not known whether it is an important mechanism of interference with immune defences under these circumstances. It might be expected to occur in many other virus infections and would then tend to make infected cells resistant to immune cytolysis but few if any studies have been made. In any case it is difficult to assess the importance of capping unless it could be prevented in the infected host, and this could not be done without causing serious interference with cell function.

Certain viruses escape the action of antibodies in a very indirect and interesting way. Neutralizing antibodies combine with virus particles and generally prevent them attaching to susceptible cells. The virus antibody complex is then likely to attach to phagocytic cells (e.g. macrophages) because they bear Fc receptors on their surface. This leads to phagocytosis, and usually the virus is degraded and inactivated even though it might otherwise have been able to initiate infection in the phagocyte. Because it entered the cell coated with antibody it is noninfectious. Sometimes, however, the antibody-coated virus successfully infects the phagocyte, and in this case the antibody can be said to have taken the virus into the susceptible cell. Instead of neutralizing infectivity it has actually enhanced it. There are good examples of this from dengue virus, which both *in vitro* and *in vivo* (Halstead, 1979) shows antibody-mediated infection of mononuclear phagocytes bearing Fc receptors, and also for other arboviruses such as West Nile virus (Peiris and Porterfield, 1979).

An interference with antibody action that looks very much like a virus strategy is seen in certain herpesvirus infections. Cells infected with herpes simplex, varicella-zoster or cytomegalovirus develop Fc receptors on their surface (Westmoreland and Atkins, 1974; Furukawa *et al.*, 1975). The Fc receptors react with IgG antibodies and appear to be virus-coded, sometimes appearing quite early in the infection cycle (Adler *et al.*, 1978; Ogata and Shigeta, 1979). Their function is not established, but they are likely to be important because they bind aggregated IgG antibodies, which are not capped but act as blocking antibodies and prevent immune recognition of the infected cell. The infected cell thus enjoys considerable protection against antibody (or cell-mediated) immune lysis (Adler *et al.*, 1978). Fc receptors are also present on the surface of the virus particle (Baucke and Spear, 1979).

It can be said that viruses sometimes interfere with the effectiveness of antibody responses by inducing low levels of protective antibody. Many viruses that persist in the body for long periods never induce very high titres of neutralizing antibodies. For instance, mice infected as infants with mouse thymic virus undergo a lifelong infection and never form detectable antibodies (Ross *et al.*, 1979) and in mice persistently infected with cytomegalovirus neutralizing antibodies are present only in low titres. This would theoretically favour persistance although there is no direct evidence that this is a significant factor, and indeed it is difficult to think of an experiment which would provide convincing evidence. Perhaps more importantly, the antibody response evolves sluggishly in certain virus infections, such as CMV in mice or in man. In the latter infection, neutralizing antibodies are not detectable in the serum until 5 weeks after the onset of the illness. The outcome of any infection depends on a race between virus replication and the speed with which host defences can be brought into play. If a key antibody is produced a day or two later it may give a decisive advantage to the infecting virus, enabling it to spread through the body and replicate in a way that would not otherwise have been possible. This is a theoretically important phenomena but few studies have been made of the kinetics of production of protective antibodies in relation to the extent of infection.

Finally, viruses may induce antibodies which combine with the virus particle or with the infected cell without neutralizing or eliminating them, and indeed sometimes protecting them from the action of good quality antibodies or from the attentions of immune cells (see below). There are many examples, mostly in persistent virus infections. Mice persistently infected with LDH virus for instance have very high titres (10^5) of serum antibodies that react with virus antigens in fluorescent antibody tests. Antibodies combine with circulating virus particles but fail to neutralize them, as demonstrated by a substantial reduction in virus titre after reacting the virus–antibody complexes with antiglobulins (Notkins *et al.*, 1968). The ineffectual antibodies may be of low affinity, or could theoretically be directed against irrelevant virus antigens on the infected cell surface or on the virus particle. This last possibility is not too difficult to imagine for a reovirus for instance, where neutralizing antibodies must be directed against a strategically important but minor virus component representing only 1% of viral polypeptides and less than 2% of the outer virus surface (Weiner and Fields, 1977).

It is suggested above that the infecting virus is responsible when antibodies are produced in small amounts or are of poor quality. A positive role for the virus has been proposed (Mims, 1978), in which it was pointed out that viruses invading the lymphoreticular tissues where immune responses are generated have the opportunity to interfere with these responses. Infection of lymphoreticular tissue is a feature of nearly all persistent virus infections, and it is also seen in certain other virus infections where there is systemic spread during a longish incubation period (e.g. mumps, rubella, and measles). This matter is discussed more fully for cell-mediated immunity (see below), and there are various theoretical mechanisms by which antibody responses could be rendered less effective. But invasion of lymphoreticular tissue is obviously not the only cause of ineffective antibody responses. For instance, both the magnitude of antibody responses and their avidity are under genetic control (Katz and Steward, 1975). Also, molecular mimicry could be mentioned, antigens of the infectious agent resembling those of host tissues and thus inducing tolerance rather than protective immune responses. So far there is not evidence that this ever occurs in virus infections.

INTERFERENCE WITH THE ACTION OF CELL-MEDIATED IMMUNITY

The antiviral action of cell mediated immunity is expressed in the following ways:

(1) Infected cells bearing viral antigens on their surface are lysed by cytotoxic T cells.

(2) T cells of another kind (helper and delayed hypersensitivity T cells) after interacting with viral antigen in tissues, differentiate and locally liberate lymphokines. They also liberate the important antiviral substance interferon (type II). Lymphokines cause circulating leukocytes to leave blood vessels and then monocytes are attracted to the tissue site, arrested, and activated. Activated monocytes (macrophages) show increased phagocytic activity and increased ability to inactivate virus particles and infected cell debris.

(3) Interferon causes increased production of natural killer cells, which are capable of lysing a variety of cells including those infected with certain viruses.

This may turn out to be an important antiviral defence although it is immunologically nonspecific, because it appears within a day or two of infection, before there has been time for the generation of regular immune responses.

This picture of cell-mediated immunity defences is a greatly simplified one. Cell-mediated responses, like antibody responses are controlled by feedback inhibition and by suppressor systems that can inhibit both T and B cell responses.

Some of the types of interference that were mentioned for antibodies are also relevant to cell mediated immunity. Low levels of virus antigen (item 3, Table I), covering up of viral antigen (item 6, Table I) or antibody-mediated loss of viral antigen (item 5, Table I) on the cell surface will obviously result in protection from cell-mediated lysis of the infected cell. Also the infection may be characterized by a weak (item 4, Table I) or slowly evolving (item 7, Table I) cell-mediated response to the infection. As with antibody responses there will be genetic determinants of the cell-mediated immune responses.

But infectious viruses are a great deal more than carriers of antigens. Because of their almost unique ability to invade tissues and infect cells without producing inflammation and necrosis, they are capable of subtle influences on immune responses. Macrophages, which are strategically placed to monitor the body surfaces, fluids and cavities, take up viruses as they do other micro-organisms. In most cases the phagocytosed virus is inactivated and antigenic components are prepared for delivery in small amounts to neighbouring lymphocytes. At this stage, macrophages exercise a controlling influence on the induction of the immune response. Strict controls on the movement and handling of antigens are probably vital in the lymphoid tissue zones where these responses are generated. Viruses however, sometimes disobey the rules and disturb this well-ordered process by invading lymphoid tissues and infecting the very macrophages and lymphocytes in which the immune response is unfolding. It has been suggested (Mims, 1978) that if as a result of this, the immune responses to the infecting virus can be weakened and made less effective, then it is likely that many viruses will have "learnt" how to do this. Perhaps it is no accident that all the successful persistent viruses invade or persist in lymphoreticular tissues (Table II).

Put simply, it could be that the most audacious way of *evading* immune defences is by *invading* the site and cells where these defences are generated and controlled. There are various ways in which this could be achieved, but generally studies of these matters are in their infancy. They will proceed hand in hand with advances in basic immunology. A clearer picture will emerge when we can identify and allocate function to all the lymphocyte subsets or understand the immunological activities of macrophages, and when we have unravelled the control mechanisms of immune responses. For the moment we

TABLE II.
Infection of lymphoreticular tissues by viruses exhibiting systemic infection or persistence.

Virus	Host
Adenoviruses (L)	Man
EB virus (L)	Man
Cytomegalovirus (L)	Man etc.
Leukaemia virus (ML)	Mouse etc.
Visna virus (LM)	Sheep
LCM virus (LM)	Mouse
Varicella-zoster virus (L)	Man
Thymic necrosis (L)	Mouse
Measles (L)	Man
Rubella (LM)	Man
Lactic dehydrogenase virus (LM)	Mouse
Aleutian disease virus (M)	Mink
Equine infectious anaemia (M)	Horse
African swine fever virus (M)	Pig

L, lymphocytes known to be infected; M, macrophages known to be infected.

can do little more than list the things that are theoretically possible.

The close interaction of systemic and persistent virus infections with lymphoreticular tissues is reflected in two interesting ways. First, a generalized immunosuppression to unrelated antigens is a common although usually temporary feature in these infections (for review see Notkins, 1970), and this suggests interference with immune function. Second, autoimmune phenomena are quite common, for instance in EB virus and cytomegalovirus infections. Whether this is due to polyclonal B cell activation or suppressor effects, it suggests a degree of immunological chaos.

The following mechanisms are available by which viruses infecting lymphoid tissue can influence immune responses to their own advantage (Table III).

(1) Local liberation of large amounts of virus antigen. This will happen whenever there is productive infection in lymphoreticular tissues, and it is likely to interfere with the normal induction of an immune response. It might theoretically expose lymphocytes to large amounts of virus antigen and induce suppression or tolerance. One set of observations is relevant to this argument (Greene and Bach, 1978; Greene and Weiner, 1980). When in the normal course of events antigens encounter immune cells adjacent to body surfaces the immune response begins by the stimulation of lymphoid cells in peripheral

TABLE III

How viruses in lymphoreticular tissues can interfere with immune responses.

Virus activity	Possible result
Replication and liberation of large amounts of viral antigen in lymphoreticular tissues	Tolerance? Switch from cell-mediated to antibody response
Replication in macrophages	Defects in antigen handling or presentation Immune response becomes less effective
Replication in lymphocytes	Alterations in lymphocyte behaviour Interference with protein synthesis (differentiation, antibody production) in lymphocytes
Replication in lymphocytes specifically responsive to viral surface antigens	Dysfunction or destruction of specifically antiviral lymphocytes leads to their clonal deletion
Viral interaction with suppressor cell systems	Effects on suppressor functions of T cells and macrophages Could be specific for viral antigens
Viral interaction with lymphocytes and macrophages	Switch from cell-mediated to antibody response or vice versa May favour infecting virus

sites such as lymph nodes. This results in mainly cell-mediated immune responses. In contrast, when antigens are experimentally presented by the intravenous route, the central lymphoid tissue (spleen etc.) is stimulated first, and this reversal of the normal sequence suppresses the cell-mediated response and leads to the production of large amounts of antibody. Evidently too much antigen in the wrong place can unbalance immune responses.

(2) Viruses may multiply in macrophages, which then fail to carry out the correct handling and processing of viral antigens. There are indications that this occurs in mice infected with LDH virus. Macrophages are infected and this is associated with a very poor antibody response and persistence of virus throughout the life of the infected animal (Isakov, pers. comm.).

(3) Viruses may multiply in immunocompetent lympocytes. The sensitivity

of various classes of lymphocytes to virus infections is now being charted. This might upset lymphocyte movement through tissues, or interfere with lymphocyte function in other ways. Viruses such as herpes simplex or rubella inhibit protein synthesis in the host cell and will obviously interfere with lymphocyte function. They may affect the differentiation of T cells, interfere with the helper function of T cells (Pelton *et al.*, 1980) or inhibit the synthesis of antibodies by B cells. It has been shown for instance, that when infectious herpes simplex virus is added to mouse lymphocytes the immune response to herpes simplex (as well as to unrelated) antigens is adversely affected without the virus undergoing a full replicative cycle in infected cells (Plaeger-Marshall, 1978).

(4) Viruses may multiply in lymphocytes that are specifically responsive to the antigens of the infecting virus. A few B and T lymphocytes would have surface components that reacted specifically with the antigens on the virus surface. These cells would be present in increasing numbers following clonal expansion as the immune response to the virus develops. The antigen-reactive surface components would act as virus receptors, favouring infection of these lymphocytes in particular. If the infection killed or otherwise interfered with their immune function it would amount to a clonal deletion of antigen-specific T or B cells. Clonal deletion has been suggested as a factor in the suppression of specific cytotoxic T cell responses in mice persistently infected with LCM virus (Dunlop and Blanden, 1977). In this instance the virus is known to infect T cells but is noncytopathic. Destruction of LCM-reactive cells that become infected could theoretically occur by "suicide" if the cell membrane was internalized. Alternatively such cells could either lyse each other, or be lysed by noninfected LCM-reactive T cells (a phenomenon that has been demonstrated *in vitro*).

Interestingly enough, several viruses have been shown to infect resting lymphocytes but replication in the infected cell is halted until it differentiates and divides. Measles virus, for instance, infects peripheral blood lymphocytes of man *in vitro*, and will remain in the infected cell for as long as 1–2 weeks without replicating. When phytohaemagglutinin (PHA) is added to induce DNA synthesis and mitosis the virus begins to replicate (Lucas *et al.*, 1978). Similar events have been shown to occur with vesicular stomatitis virus.

(5) Viruses might interact with suppressor T cells, infecting them and perhaps interfering with their function. Suppressor effects could be induced by the formation of suppressor macrophages or soluble suppressor factors in serum, although some of the latter effects may be attributable to immune complexes. So far, in most reports (e.g. Israel *et al.*, 1980) viruses have been shown to induce immunologically nonspecific repression, as tested for instance by the inhibition of concanavalin A (con A) or PHA-driven mitogenesis in mouse spleen cells. Reports of antigen-specific suppression are beginning to

appear and these are more likely to be relevant to my theme, because there is the possibility of suppression of responses to the antigens of the infecting virus (Liew and Russell, 1980).

Interactions between viruses and T cells are receiving much attention, and research workers are identifying T cell subsets that are susceptible to virus infection. Measles virus, for instance, has been shown to replicate in mitogenically stimulated T_G (suppressor) cells and T_M (helper) cells from human peripheral blood (Huddlestone *et al.*, 1980). Also some viruses have been shown to activate suppressor T cells (Tosato *et al.*, 1979; Rinaldo *et al.*, 1980). Such interactions would surely result in immunoregularly disturbances, some of which might benefit the infecting virus.

(6) Viruses acting on lymphoreticular cells in any of the above ways could not only cause ineffective antibody or cell-mediated immune responses to the infected virus, but also cause a change in the balance of this response. For some virus infections (e.g. poliomyelitis, certain arboviruses) antibodies are the most important defence mechanism whereas for most others (herpes-type viruses, poxviruses etc.) cell-mediated immune defences are more important. If an infecting virus induced a swing to a less important type of response, so that, for instance, EB virus, induced antibody formation rather than cell-mediated immunity, or poliomyelitis induced cytotoxic T cells rather than neutralizing antibodies, this would favour the virus infection. There would be an equally important result if the immune response were diverted to irrelevant rather than relevant (i.e. surface) virus antigens.

VIRUS INTERFERENCE WITH IMMUNE RESPONSES BY INFECTION OF PRIVILEGED SITES WHERE THESE RESPONSES ARE LESS EFFECTIVE

Many viruses infect body sites that give the virus protection at the topographical level from immune forces. This has been discussed elsewhere in relation to persistent viruses (Mims, 1978) and should be mentioned as a method of evasion of antiviral defences. Viruses that persist in glands and other body surfaces discharging to the outside world are able to spread to the exterior and infect other individuals. This is true of the skin with wart and papillomaviruses, feather follicles with Marek's disease virus, kidney tubules with cytomegalovirus (CMV) and polyomaviruses or salivary glands in vampire bats with rabies. At the same time the virus is protected from circulating antibodies which fail to reach the lumenal surface of infected cells where virus is being released. Viruses often show a striking polarity in epithelial cells, viral antigens and budding being confined to the lumenal surface of the cell (Boulan and Sabatini, 1978). The infected cell also escapes attack by sensitized lymphocytes which are unable to traverse the basement membrane and the epithelial cell sheet unless there is local inflammation or cell damage. In so far as this can be regarded as a virus "strategy", could it also apply to many "hit-and-run" virus infections of epithelial surfaces, especially those involving the respiratory and intestinal tracts? Perhaps the idea should not be pressed too far, because most viruses are obliged to infect epithelial surfaces simply because they must be discharged to the exterior if they are to infect other individuals.

The nervous system is another site that is to some extent protected from immune defences. Antiviral forces are less effective in the nervous system and in man this site is infected by SSPE, persistent papovavirus (progressive multifocal leucoencephalopathy) and varicella-zoster (dorsal root ganglia) infections.

REFERENCES

Adler, R., Glorioso, J. C., Cossman, J. and Levine, M. (1978). Possible role of Fc receptors on cells infected and transformed by herpes virus: escape from immune lysis. *Infection and Immunity* 21, 442–447.

Albrecht, P. (1978). Immune control in experimental subacute sclerosing panencephalitis. *American Journal of Clinical Pathology* (Suppl.) 70, 175–184.

Baucke, R. B. and Spear, P. G. (1979). Membrane proteins specified by herpes simplex virus. V. Identification of an Fc-binding glycoprotein. *Journal of Virology* 32, 779–789.

Boulan, E. R. and Sabatini, D. D. (1978). Asymmetric budding of viruses in epithelial monolayers. Model system for study of epithelial polarity. *Proceedings of the National Academy of Science, U.S.A.* 75, 5071–5075.

Dunlop, M. B. C. and Blanden, R. V. (1977). Mechanisms of suppression of cytotoxic T cell responses in murine lymphocytic choriomeningitis virus infection. *Journal of Experimental Medicine* 145, 1131–1143.

Furukawa, T., Hornberger, E., Sakuma, S. and Plotkin, S. A. (1975). Demonstration of immunoglobulin G receptors induced by human cytomegalovirus. *Journal of Clinical Microbiology* 2, 332–336.

Greene, M. I. and Bach, B. A. (1979). The physiological regulation of immunity: differential regulatory contributions of peripheral and central lymphon compartments. *Cell Immunology* 45, 446–451.

Greene, M. I. and Weiner, H. L. (1980). Delayed hypersensitivity in mice infected with reovirus. II. Induction of tolerance and suppressor T cells to viral-specific gene products. *Journal of Immunology* 125, 283–287.

Halstead, S. B. (1979). *In vivo* enhancement of dengue virus infection in Rhesus monkeys by passively transferred antibody. *Journal of Infectious Diseases* 140, 527–533.

Hooks, J. J., Burns, W., Hayashi, I., Gels, S. and Notkins, A. L. (1976). Viral spread in the presence of meutralizing antibody: mechanisms of persistence in foamy virus infections. *Infection and Immunity* **14**, 1172–1178.

Huddlestone, J. R., Lampert, P. W. and Oldstone, M. B. A. (1980). Virus-lymphocyte interactions: infection of T_G and T_M sub-sets by measles virus. *Clinical Immunology and Immunopathology* **15**, 502–509.

Israel, E., Beiss, B. and Wainberg, M. A. (1980). Viral abrogation of lymphocyte mitogenesis: induction of a soluble factor inhibitory to cellular proliferation. *Immunology* **40**, 77–85.

Katz, F. E. and Steward, M. W. (1975). The genetic control of antibody affinity in mice. *Immunology* **29**, 543–548.

Lampert, P. W., Joseph, B. S. and Oldstone, M. B. A. (1975). Antibody-induced capping of measles virus antigens on plasma membrane studied by electron microscopy. *Journal of Virology* **15**, 1248–1255.

Liew, F. Y. and Russell, S. M. (1980). Delayed-type hypersensitivity to influenza virus. *Journal of Experimental Medicine* **151**, 799–814.

Lucas, C. J., Ubeis-Postma, J. C., Rezee, A. and Galama, J. M. (1978). Activation of measles virus from silently infected human lymphocytes. *Journal of Experimental Medicine* **148**, 940–952.

Mims, C. A. (1978). General features of persistent virus infections. *Postgraduate Medical Journal* **54**, 581–586.

Notkins, A. L., Mage, M., Ashe, W. K. and Madar, S. (1968). Neutralization of sensitized laetic dehydrogenase virus by anti-γ-globulin. *Journal of Immunology* **100**, 314–320.

Notkins, A. L., Mergenhagen, S. and Howard, R. (1970). Effect of virus infections on the function of the immune system. *Annual Review of Microbiology* **24**, 525–538.

Ogata, M. and Shigeta, S. (1979). Appearance of Immunoglobulin G Fc receptor in cultured human cells infected with varicella-zoster virus. *Infection and Immunity* **26**, 770–774.

Peiris, J. S. M. and Porterfield, J. S. (1979). Antibody-mediated enhancement of Flavivirus replication in macrophage-like cell lines. *Nature* **282**, 509–511.

Pelton, B. K., Duncan, I. B. and Denman, A. M. (1980). Herpes simplex virus depresses antibody production by affecting T cell function. *Nature* **284**, 176–177.

Plaeger-Marshall, S. and Smith, J. W. (1978). Inhibition of mitogen and antigen-induced lymphocyte blastogenesis by herpes simplex virus. *Journal of Infectious Diseases* **138**, 506–511.

Rinaldo, C. R., Carney, W. P., Richter, B. S., Black, P. H. and Hirsch, M. S. (1980). Mechanisms of immunosuppression in cytomegaloviral mononucleosis. *Journal of Infectious Diseases* **141**, 488–495.

Ross, S. S. C., Parker, J. C., Rowe, W. P. and Robbins, M. L. (1979). Biology of mouse thymic virus, a herpes virus of mice, and the antigenic relationship to mouse cytomegalovirus. *Infection and Immunity* **28**, 1186–1195.

Tosato, G., Magrath, I., Koski, I., Dooley, N. and Blaese, M. (1979). Activation of suppressor T cells during Epstein–Barr virus induced infectious mononucleosis. *New England Journal of Medicine* **301**, 1133–1137.

Weiner, H. L. and Fields, B. N. (1977). Neutralization of reovirus: the gene responsible for the neutralization antigen. *Journal of Experimental Medicine* **146**, 1305–1310.

Westmoreland, D. and Watkins, J. F. (1974). The IgG receptors induced by herpes simplex virus: studies using radioiodinated IgG. *Journal of General Virology* 24, 167–178.

DISCUSSION

Mogensen I should like to start with your first mechanism by which viruses may evade host defences, namely that virus infections might induce non-neutralizing or poorly-neutralizing antibodies. To me it is interesting that the examples listed (the lactic dehydrogenase virus, the aleutian disease virus, the equine infectious anaemia virus and the lymphocytic choriomeningitis virus) are all viruses which are known to persistently infect macrophages. Do you see any relationship between these two phenomena?

Mims Only in the sense that macrophages have moved to the centre of immunology, both in the induction process and the effector process of immune responses. Obviously, viruses by infecting macrophages could influence antibody responses, but one can do no more than say that this is the sort of thing that could be happening.

Stuart-Harris It would be very churlish of me not to thank you, Professor Mims, for producing such a broad prospectus of your views on how viruses evade the action of defence mechanisms, and you have been very fundamental about this and comprehensive also. There are aspects, of course, of what you term "defence" about which one can quibble. For instance, the evidence that antibodies are defensive is derived almost entirely from those instances where re-infection is being sought by a new virus of the same type as before, and not by the actual virus which is inducing the primary infection. My first question to you then would be, how exactly do you visualize a virus as overwhelming the defence in the most ultimate way by killing the animal? Could you just tell us how viruses do, in fact, kill animals or men?

Mims To go first to the question of killing, I am glad to hear you ask that because it has always intrigued me. As you imply, very often a patient or an animal can die and you are not really quite sure how it worked out that way. There are some good examples where the mechanisms are clear and perhaps I will focus all my answer in terms of poliomyelitis. This virus replicates in anterior horn cells, inhibits macromolecular synthesis and ultimately kills them. If enough anterior horn cells are involved, there is enough interference with muscle activity to result in paralysis and, as we know from the old days of polio, this can lead to death in a fairly direct way if only by respiratory failure. So that is a fair example. There are one or two other examples such as the acute myocarditis caused by cardioviruses. However, I do agree, and you have made a good point, that most of the time we cannot identify the terminal events that cause death.

On the other question about antibodies and do they in fact protect, I have to accept that in many cases—and, as you will know, respiratory infections are one of them—the whole infection can be over before the antibodies have really got around to doing very much.

If I can come back to poliomyelitis again, it is quite clear that primary infection of the intestinal tract with the shedding of poliovirus in the faeces can occur in all unprotected people. But what matters for pathogenicity is that the virus leaves the intestine, travels free in the plasma to the central nervous system where it passes across cerebral and spinal cord capillaries and does its work in neurones. At that critical time while it is in the blood it is vulnerable to the action of antibodies, and antibodies in the blood have a critical action in protecting from disease. This is clearest from the experiments of nature where the agammaglobulinaemics show a striking susceptibility to paralytic poliomyelitis.

Stuart-Harris Thank you very much for those comments. I think you will agree that neutralizing antibodies are not necessarily a primary method of defence against all viruses. One is talking about viruses as though they are all going to behave the same way and, of course, the one thing which everybody knows is that they all behave entirely differently from each other. You have given SSPE as an example of antibody-mediated loss of virus from the infected cell surface. I wonder whether that is really fair in view of the new work which has come out, particularly that from the Rockefeller Institute by Dr Choppin. The fact that virus persists in the brain and evades antibody does not represent the true state of affairs, because the virus is locked in the brain by dint of the fact that it is defective, being without its M protein and therefore unable to escape from the cell. May I ask if you accept this particular interpretation of SSPE?

Mims I agree that the virus spreads directly by cell-to-cell transit, and this is one possible reason why the evolution of this particular infection takes such a long time. However, in SSPE the capping phenomenon could have some significance because it gives infected cells an insusceptibility to immune attack. On the other hand, it has been shown *in vitro* that SSPE-infected cells, even though you add no antibody to them, can be susceptible to complement destruction. So you have to ask about this possibility in the central nervous system. However, Dr Albrecht and his colleagues, have shown that in cerebrospinal fluid you do not have complement. They could not detect complement in cerebrospinal fluid, even when they induced inflammatory events inside a monkey's brain so that the concentrations of IgG were raised ten- to twenty-fold in cerebrospinal fluid.

Williams I was interested in the neutralizing antibody acting as an enhancing antibody. I was wondering about the kinetics of antibody production here. Does it explain why in dengue and some other virus infections the second attack is worse than the first or in other virus infections why there are two separate episodes of illness with the one infection?

Mims Yes, as you may know, dengue haemorrhagic fever is important in South East Asia where children in particular have a serious disease with major organ involvement, haemorrhage, circulatory failure and shock, kidney troubles and other effects. For a long time people thought this was purely a matter of antigen–antibody complexes, complement activation, disseminated intravascular coagulation and so on, but this story is not holding up too well. However, if one of the main susceptible cell types is a mononuclear cell and if antibodies help virus to get into this cell, you have a possible mechanism by which a second attack is worse than the first one. As Sir Charles has implied, there may not be very much antibody early in an infectious process, but if you have a preceding dengue infection then perhaps, because of shared antigens, an anamnestic response would occur, so that quite early in that second infection you have a lot of antibody. This could influence the amount of replication of dengue in susceptible mononuclear cells. This is the sort of interpretation Dr Halstead and his colleagues are giving.

Beale I would like to support one of the things you were talking about, which is the specific suppression of viral antigens and other antigens by suppressor T cells. Dr Liew in our laboratory has recently reported two examples of this, one of them concerns influenza virus which I might talk about a little bit later on, and the other concerns *Leishmania tropica* where delayed-type hypersensitivity is the important immune response, both for cure and for protection. Dr Howard and Dr Liew have shown, by passive transfer experiments, that strains of mice which die from *Leishmania tropica* develop specific T suppressor cells and if they transfer specific DTH cells the animals can be protected or cured as the case may be. That is a specific example of what you were talking about

Mims That is very interesting. My examples from virology concern LCM virus in mice, and the work of Howard Weiner and his group who have got some very nice information about suppressor cells in reovirus infections. Unfortunately, studies of virus replication in lymphocytes have always been rather artificial. When you take out peripheral blood lymphocytes and add the virus nothing very much happens, so you have to stimulate them with a mitogen like PHA and then they will support virus replication. One interesting thing—and this principle at least could be very important—is that you can take a peripheral blood lymphocyte (this is work from Dr Lucas and his colleagues in West Africa), and infect them *in vitro* with measles virus and nothing will happen because the cells are in a resting state as isolated from the peripheral blood. If you then keep them for a couple of weeks in culture and at the end of that time treat them with a mitogen like PHA measles antigen is now expressed on the surface of the lymphocyte as seen by fluorescence and measles virus nucleocapsids are seen by electron microscopy. This seems important because the virus can stay around for more than a week, doing nothing, until PHA is added when virus synthesis will occur and the other events which we have been talking about. This has been shown also for vesicular stomatitis virus.

Smith With regard to the fact that virulent viruses seem to grow better in animals than attenuated viruses, is there any evidence that when cells are infected with virulent viruses there are less antigens on the outside of that cell than when an attenuated strain infects similar cells?

Mims Do you mean less antigens per cell or less antigens in the whole infected animal?

Smith Less antigens per cell. There seem to be methods available for examining the antigenic content of cell membranes. Would it be possible to experiment with attenuated and virulent viruses to see if the virulent viruses produce less antigens on cell membranes and hence the cells may not be so prone to immunospecific defence mechanisms?

Mims One of the problems is that as soon as you take cells out of the body the tropisms and other phenomena may change. A classic example of that comes from poliovirus. If you inject a monkey peripherally with poliovirus there is no growth of the virus in its kidney. If you take a monkey and inject the virus directly into its kidney there is still no growth in the kidney. But take the kidney out, dissociate and spread the cells on glass, and you have the standard system for growing poliovirus and doing plaque assays. To return to your question, I know of no relevant evidence except the work done by Choppin and others on SV5 virus and perhaps this is not all that relevant! When the virus replicated successfully in a cell and matured by budding without cytopathic effect, the cell was OK, but in another cell type nucleocapsids accumulated under the cell membrane and something went wrong with the system. The virus was not released by budding and the cell died. But this is a long way from virulence and antigen density and does not answer the sort of question you ask.

Peters I suppose you might argue on first principles that in so far as pathology in virus infections is due to immunological mechanisms then the extent to which the virus is reflected on the surface of the cell must inevitably influence it. Without expression, there could be no immunopathological reaction.

Mims No, I am not sure that is entirely true, because even if the virus is never expressed on the surface of the cell you could get viral antigens shed if the cell disintegrated, with antigen–antibody complexes formed, and a lot of immunopathology.

Peters I was referring specifically to cytolytic events which are immunopathological in origin.

Mims I do agree there.

Anderson I would just like to make one comment concerning the expression of viral antigens at the cell surface. You have pointed out several very cunning mechanisms whereby the virus appears to be hiding from the immune response. I think it is worth bearing in mind that the virus is hiding quite effectively from us as well. We use our fluorescent antibody techniques to detect viral antigens on the surface of infected cells, but there are now several examples of the expression of viral antigens on the surface of cells which cannot be detected by serological techniques but which nevertheless are recognizable by immune cells, T cells in particular.

Mims I have to confess my total ignorance; you must tell us about it. Is it just that the antisera used in the immunofluorescence test is not of the right specificity or of high enough titre, or whatever?

Anderson One example that comes to mind is work being done in Bristol with Epstein–Barr virus. Various antigens are produced during infection. One of these, LYDMA, cannot be detected by serology, although it is recognized by lymphoid cells. In answer to your question it is, of course, possible that we have not yet produced the right antiserum to detect this antigen. There is a second example which involves coxsackie B virus. This is work published by the Woodruffs, where fibroblasts were infected with coxsackie virus. No surface antigen was demonstrable by fluorescent antibody techniques but nevertheless these infected cells were susceptible to cytolysis by coxsackie-sensitized killer T cells.

Mims There is always the problem as to whether those new antigens are necessarily virus-coded and it is not always easy to show that they are. Nevertheless, as you say, as long as the infected cell is recognized and there is cell destruction, that is good enough.

Williams Professor Mims, you implied when you were talking about cell mediated immunity that viruses always went for the lymphoreticular system. Was I mistaken in thinking you said that?

Mims No. What I said is that all the persistent viruses, the ones that stay around in the body and obviously evade host defences, seem to be characterized by their ability to invade, and often persist in, lymphoid tissues.

Williams But what about persistent neurotrophic viruses, for example? Does that apply to them?

Mims Yes. By persistent neurotrophic viruses we think of measles in SSPE, we think of JC virus, a human papovavirus, and we think of scrapie, if that is a virus.

Williams Where are they persisting?

Mims In lymphoid tissues. Let us take SSPE. Dr Valdimarsson is more of an expert on SSPE than I am, but this virus, although it causes a persistent central nervous system infection, has also been isolated from lymphoid tissues, at least on one occasion. It is not unreasonable to suppose that it stays around in lymphoid tissue and did so in the earlier stages when it was setting things up for persistence.

Williams But what about anterior horn cells and ganglion cells for herpes?

Mims Well, this virus persists there, too. Herpes simplex virus may persist in ganglion cells because it has done something about immune defences. Very few viruses go to one cell type only. There are exceptions, but they nearly always do more than one thing.

In my table on interference with antibody responses I have put a column giving the status of each item. Perhaps status is the wrong word. It means how important I think these particular mechanisms are. Some have no mark against them at all because it is no more than a suggestion, whereas others seem to be of some importance, and I have given them one or two pluses.

I like lists and, as I have said before, they are important when we look at infectious disease from this novel, inverted point of view, asking what the microbe is doing about host defences. When you categorize and make out a list you can identify things that can actually be put to the test. I think that is one good thing about lists, even if in a year or so many of the things on this list get crossed off and other things added to it.

Stuart-Harris Could I jump in at this stage and say, please interpret for us how the hepatisis B virus persists? Is it, in fact, one of those lymphoreticular cell infections?

Mims That is a very good point, because I do not know! I have always been interested in extrahepatic manifestations of hepatitis B infection. Unfortunately, nearly all these are immune complex mediated, the prodromal allergy, the vasculitis and so on, and not due to local viral replication. Hepatic cells are the only ones we know to be infected but certainly there are perturbations in immune responses and I would like to suggest that at some stage this virus is present in lymphoid tissues. Peripheral lymphatics drain nearly all tissues of the body and viruses replicating in the liver will be delivered to lymphoreticular tissues, for instance local lymph nodes, quite early on. Then the opportunities for interactions with immune defences occur.

One trouble with hepatitis B is that there is no simple way in which you can test for infectious virus. The only thing you can do, as has been done recently with saliva and semen from infected individuals, is inject it into an expensive primate such as a chimpanzee. Thirty years ago they estimated the amount of virus present in the blood of man by injecting dilutions of the blood into volunteers, checking out who got hepatitis, and thus obtaining an end point. The amount of heptatitis B virus in serum was about 10^6 infection doses per ml. There is no ways these days that you can do that, but I would like to see somebody do something about the relevance of lymphoid tissues in hepatitis B infection.

Wilton I should like to ask Professor Mims where he sees the release of the glycoprotein 70 from murine leukaemia viruses fitting into this story and whether there is now any similar human example of immunosuppressive protein being released in this way.

Mims I know the mouse system, but human leukaemia viruses are still, as far as I am concerned, a big question mark. You may find reverse transcriptases in bone marrows, you may even isolate viruses from human tissues, but so far there is no generally accepted human leukaemia virus. The ones isolated are either primate derived or of uncertain status. So, although this interesting substance you refer to may be important in a mouse, I know nothing—nor, I suppose, does anybody else—about such things in man.

Wilton You were talking about the immune perturbation in hepatitis. I think the immune perturbation in most immune complex diseases is due to the antibody in the complex, not necessarily to the antigen. That is the first point.

The second point is that you were talking about the admittedly highly theoretical possibility of virus antigens being expressed on intracellular membranes such as the phagosome and you said this might be one way in which the macrophage would be diverted from presenting the right sort of antigen to the lymphocyte. I am not entirely sure we know that much about antigen presentation by macrophages and whether it is actually a surface phenomenon. Is the right antigen the one that is on the surface of the macrophage and not the one that it has taken intracellularly? I am not sure you could go that far even speculatively at this moment.

Mims Perhaps I did not make myself clear enough. All I wanted to imply for those viruses that mature on intracellular vacuoles is that it could thereby give them some resistance to destruction by cytotoxic T cells, antibody plus complement and so on, as long as the antigens were not on the external plasma membrane surface. I did not want to imply that that in itself was going to affect handling and presentation of antigens. It might do, but as you have said we do not know enough to judge whether that matters.

Vaccines in Relation to Microbial Mechanisms that Interfere with Host Defences

A. J. BEALE

Wellcome Research Laboratories, Beckenham, Kent, UK.

In this volume a great deal of information has been summarized dealing with the subtle means that microbes have evolved to evade the defence mechanisms of the host.

For the most part these mechanisms are to enable the microbe to establish and reproduce itself so that it can be transmitted to a new host. Later immune mechanisms are established that prevent re-infection or a second attack. It is this natural immunity that gave the impetus to vaccination, first with living modified microbes and later with killed microbes, or antigens extracted from them. These antigenic components extracted from microorganisms are often the very components responsible for the perturbations in the host response. The key for the vaccine researcher is to identify and isolate the crucial protective components away from other deleterious components. In this way the immune response to a component of the microbe can be more effective than natural immunity. Although for many microbial infections a living vaccine made from microorganisms found empirically of lower virulence, for example, by passage in a foreign environment is most effective, it is an aspiration and a goal to believe that if we know enough about the immune response and the protective components of the microbe then a killed vaccine can be developed.

There are several steps involved in the logical development of a vaccine and some of them are enumerated below:

(1) Knowledge of the portal of entry of the microbe and pathogenesis of the disease;

(2) The components of the immune response crucial for clinical immunity;

(3) The identity of the immunogen: means of measurement and production.

Some of the problems and solutions in the development of vaccines are discussed. The classical, successful vaccines that represent the high technology in medicine are the toxoids, best exemplified by those for diphtheria and tetanus (Thomas, 1975). Circulating toxin is not the whole story of these diseases, but antitoxin is sufficient to confer clinical immunity. Indeed, with present knowledge the use of formalin to detoxify the vaccine is no longer necessary. Vaccine against diphtheria could be achieved using the isolated nontoxic receptor portions of the toxin molecule, and these native proteins might be even more effective as vaccines than existing toxoids (Collier, 1975).

A more recent example of a vaccine based on a toxoid is that used in the prevention of pig bel. The elucidation of the role of *Clostridium welchii* type C in the necrotizing enterocolitis in Papua, New Guinea and its prevention by toxoid is now well known (Lawrence *et al.*, 1979). The importance of this disease as an insight into bowel disease due to other *Clostridia*, for example, *Cl. difficile* is also now generally recognized. The results of trials of toxoid are shown in Table I.

TABLE I.
Protective effect of two doses of *Cl. welchii* type C vaccine against pig bel.

Vaccine	Deaths	Cases	
		No.	Per 10 000
Unvaccinated	5	30	23·4
Tetanus toxoid	1	21	22·6
Cl. welchii	0	3	3·2

Data by courtesy of Dr P. D. Walker.

The adhesins that are responsible for the attachment of *Escherichia coli*, for example, to the gut wall can be used to prevent neonatal diarrhoea in animals by immunizing the dam with vaccines containing purified K88 and K99 antigens (Nagy *et al.*, 1978). So far, the importance of these adhesins in the pathogenesis of diarrhoea in man is less clearly established. The alternative approach, which is oral immunization, is just beginning to be investigated and the principles established. Much of the basic work has been done with cholera and the use of subtoxic quantities of toxin as an oral vaccine seems at least possible. An emerging problem is the possible immunosuppressive effect of malnutrition and other infections in those populations who are most in need of immunity. Unfortunately, the indications from work in animals are discouraging (Barry and Pierce, 1979).

One vaccine that is very effective in the developed countries giving substantial gut immunity is oral polio vaccine. In developing countries the results are far inferior, but the reasons are not clear. The virus fails to colonize the gut and to produce a serological response. It also fails to prevent disease so that it does not establish itself sufficiently in the gut to produce local immunity; and this may be due to the immunosuppressive effect of infections and malnutrition. The most plausible explanation for this lies in the complex patterns of interference observed between vaccine viruses and other microbial infections of the gut in developing countries. These have been studied extensively in England by Hale *et al.* (1961).

The problem in tropical countries can be overcome by the use of killed polio vaccine; the products now available are of greater purity and are adjusted as to potency of all three types. Although these vaccines give a much inferior gut immunity they lead to very effective protection against the disease, and at least for countries like Holland and those in Scandinavia, they also provide a herd immunity. Initial studies with highly potent killed polio vaccine in tropical countries are promising (Salk *et al.*, 1978).

The identification of the immunogen is also of key importance for vaccine development and is not always straightforward. The importance of toxins is clear enough but the importance of aggressins and the elucidation of their role in immunity, and therefore for vaccine production took many years to achieve. For example, the now classical work of Harry Smith and his colleagues led to the production of an effective extract vaccine for anthrax using the concept of the "*in vivo*" growth to identify crucial components in virulent organisms required for satisfactory protection (Smith and Stoner, 1967).

In virus diseases the identification of the protective antigenic components for immunity has also proved important. Two examples will suffice. The first is vaccinia virus. Many years ago Boulter showed that very high titre antiserum could be prepared in animals using killed vaccinia. Titres of neutralizing antibody were far higher than those produced by living vaccinia but compared with convalescent serum this hyperimmune serum raised by killed vaccinia was less effective for the prevention or cure of rabbitpox in rabbits (Boulter, 1969). Similarly killed vaccinia as a vaccine was less effective. Later analysis by Appleyard *et al.* (1971) showed that the explanation lay in the presence of a new antigen acquired by the virus as it left the cytoplasm and became extracellular virus. Antibodies to this antigen on extracellular virus are essential for the prevention of spreading virus infections in a sheet of cells caused by fully infectious virus and for prevention of disease *in vivo*. It is certain that other components of the immune response, especially cell mediated immunity are vital for the control of infection. However, antibody of the correct sort is a sufficient bar to infection and confers immunity.

The prevention of measles by killed vaccine had seemed a very rational approach to the prevention of this disease because the vaccine could be given in early childhood in combination with other vaccines. In this way active immunity might be produced under cover of maternal immunity and possible reactions to living vaccine would be avoided. In the event, the killed vaccine was shown to produce clinical hypersensitivity rather than clinical immunity. The explanation for this problem was first elucidated by Norrby (1975), who showed that antibodies to haemolysin were produced by natural infection and by living vaccine but that they were absent after killed vaccine and even more striking, they were absent after a killed/living vaccine schedule of immunization. Later Merz *et al.*, (1980) showed that for the parainfluenza virus SV5 the fusion protein was the essential antigen required to raise antibodies which would prevent spreading infection in a sheet of cells caused by cell to cell spread. Extracellular virus is neutralized by antibodies to the haemagglutinin. As with vaccinia there is a crucial antigen that must be present in a killed vaccine, and again despite the importance of other components of the immune response, these antibodies alone are crucial for protective immunity.

The means for controlling influenza virus infection still evade us but there are some clues from experiments of nature as well as deliberate experiment. First, contrary to popular belief, the duration of immunity is long and solid as shown, for example, by the age distribution of influenza during the recent outbreak due to the re-emergence of H_1N_1 virus similar to the strains present in the 1950s. Thus, there were virtually no cases of influenza in individuals over 23 years who had been through the H_1N_1 outbreak. A second clue is the fact that an attack of influenza seemed to provide a better immunity within a drift series in the Christ's Hospital study, (Table II) whereas killed vaccine merely postponed the inevitable (Hoskins *et al.*, 1979). There is clearly a factor missing in influenza immunity when a killed vaccine is used, perhaps similar to the story of killed vaccinia or measles vaccines. The missing component may not be an antigen as in those examples, but a component of the host response, for example, delayed type hypersensitivity (DTH), cytotoxic T cell activity (Hackett *et al.*, 1980) or local immunity at the mucosal surface. Alternatively the response to the protective component may be diverted by antigenic deviation of immune response or by competition. Liew and Russell (1980) have shown that DTH does occur with influenza, but that it is normally suppressed by antigen-

TABLE II.

Protective effect of natural infection with influenza virus Christ's Hospital study.

Number (and per cent) of children with (+) and without (−) initial antibody who became infected on successive exposure

Natural HA antibody on entry	Case 42/72	Case PC	Case Vic	Total
−148	−103	−81	−66	
			+15 (18·5%)	83/148 (56%)
		+22 (21%)	−22	
	+45 (30%)	−45	−44	
			+1 (2%)	
+171	−162	−146	−113	
			+33 (23%)	58/171 (34%)
		+16 (10%)	−16	
	+9	−9	−9	

Data by courtesy of Dr Joan Davies.

specific T suppressor cells. The idea that LDTH might be accentuated so as to give a better and broader protection has not so far proved to be true for influenza although similar studies by Howard *et al.* (1980) referred to by Liew and Russell (1980) have shown the importance of delayed type hypersensitivity for cure and prevention of *Leishmania tropica*. Similarly, Russell and Liew (1979) have observed significant adjuvant effects of the matrix protein. So far influenza immunity remains a riddle and a challenge, which may be solved by new approaches, for example involving genetic manipulation to identify the components vital for immunity.

The scope for vaccine development coming from increased knowledge of the host response and in particular in the strategies microbes employ to evade host defences, which are the subject of this colloquium, gives great encouragement to the development of a new generation of vaccines. When this knowledge is coupled to the powerful new techniques for searching for protective antigens illustrated by monoclonal antibodies and genetic manipulation, the prospects become very exciting. For example, a strategy for the development of a malaria vaccine using a mouse model could be as follows. First, to raise monoclonal antibodies to merozoites and select those producing passive protection. The monoclonal antibodies are then used to identify, characterize, measure and purify the antigen, which is then used for active immunization. The final stage, when the earlier steps have been accomplished, is to produce antigen by the techniques of genetic manipulation. The future for vaccine development is bright.

REFERENCES

Appleyard, G., Hapel, A. J. and Boulter, E. A. (1971). An antigenic difference between intracellular and extracellular rabbitpox virus. *Journal of General Virology* **13**, 9–17.

Barry, W. S. and Pierce, N. F. (1979). Protein deprivation causes reversible impairment of mucosal immune response to cholera toxoid/toxin in rat gut. *Nature* **281**, 64–65.

Boulter, E. A. (1969). Protection against poxviruses. *Proceedings of the Royal Society of Medicine* **62**, 295–297.

Collier, R. J. (1975). Diphtheria toxin: mode of action and structure. *Bacteriological Reviews* **39**, 54–85

Hackett, C. J., Askonas, B. A., Webster, R. G. and van Wyke, K. (1980). Quantitation of influenza virus antigens on infected target cells and their recognition by cross-reactive cytotoxic T cells. *Journal of Experimental Medicine* **151**, 1014–1025.

Hale, J. H., Lee, L. H. and Gardner, P. S. (1961). Interference patterns encountered when using attenuated poliovirus vaccines. *British Medical Journal* **2**, 728–732.

Hoskins, T. W., Davies, J. R., Smith, A. J., Miller, C. L. and Allchin, A. (6 January

1979). Assessment of inactivated influenza-A vaccine after three outbreaks of influenza A at Christ's Hospital. *The Lancet* **i**, 33–35.

Howard, J. G., Hale, C. and Liew, F. Y. (1980). Immunological regulation of experimental cutaneous Leishmaniasis. III. Nature and significance of specific suppression of cell-mediated immunity in mice highly susceptible to *Leishmania tropica*. *Journal of Experimental Medicine* **152**, 594–607.

Lawrence, G., Shann, F., Freestone, D. S. and Walker, P. D. (3 February 1979). Prevention of necrotising enteritis in Papua, New Guinea by active immunization. *Lancet* **i**, 227–230.

Liew, F. Y. and Russell, S. M. (1980). Delayed-type hypersensitivity to influenza virus. *Journal of Experimental Medicine* **151**, 799–814.

Merz, D. C., Scheid, A. and Choppin, P. W. (1980). Importance of antibodies to the fusion glycoprotein of paramyxoviruses in the prevention of spread of infection. *Journal of Experimental Medicine* **151**, 275–288.

Nagy, L. K., Walker, P. D., Bhogal, B. S. and Mackenzie, T. (1978). Evaluation of *Escherichia coli* vaccines against experimental enteric colibacillosis. *Research in Veterinary Science* **24**, 39–45.

Norrby, E. (1975). Occurrence of antibodies against envelope components after immunization with formalin inactivated and live measles vaccine. *Journal of Biological Standardization* **3**, 375–380.

Russell, S. M. and Liew, F. Y. (1979). T cells primed by influenza virion internal components can co-operate in the antibody response to haemagglutinin. *Nature* **280**, 147–148.

Salk, J., Cohen, H., Fillastre, C., Stoeckel, P., Rey, J.-L., Schlumberger, M., Nicolas, A., van Steenis, G., van Wezel, A. L., Triau, R., Saliou, P., Barry, L. F., Morceau, J.-P. and Merieux, C. (1978). Killed poliovirus antigen titration in humans. XV International Congress for Biological Standardization. Vaccinations in the Developing Countries, pp. 119–132. S. Karger, Basel.

Smith, H. and Stoner, H. B. (1967). Anthrax toxic complex. *Federation Proceedings* **26**, 1554–1557.

Thomas, L. (1975). "The Lives of a Cell", pp. 35–42. Bantam Books.

DISCUSSION

Mims I would like to refer to a few points in Dr Beale's talk in terms of the title of this symposium. The message seems to be that with all these microbial perturbations of immune responses, the vaccine strategy is as follows. First you can take a live replicating virus or bacterium and use that as your vaccine. In this case it must not produce disease and presumably also it must be less capable of producing these immunological disturbances. Nevertheless it often turns out that this live vaccine strain will persist in the body. This is so for Marek's disease vaccine, where the vaccinated chicken is persistently infected for life with the live virus. But this somehow interferes with subsequent infection with the virulent virus.

Second, with the killed vaccines—and this is clearer from Dr Beale's talk—you have to extract the antigens which really are the protective antigens. It is fascinating to hear of the differences between haemagglutinins and fusion factors from the myxo- and paramyxoviruses. Once upon a time, we all thought that it was haemagglutinins that mattered and now we can identify a specific fusion-factor antigen, we purify it and raise specific antibodies which are protective. When the vaccine contains only antigens we presumably avoid the perturbations of immunity which might interfere with the actions of the vaccine because these are produced by the whole infectious entity. Of course, monoclonal antibodies turn out to be an important practical way of isolating with great purity the required antigen.

Smith I think the results of pig bel illustrate a point that came up when Professor Arbuthnott was speaking about the role of toxin in perturbation of host defences. The fact that you get protection against infection by immunizing against the lethal toxin probably means that the toxin is acting at the early stages of an infection to inhibit the host defences as well as killing the host at the end of infection. By producing antibodies against the toxin you stop the early attack of the disease. Another example occurs in anthrax. The toxin that is responsible for death in anthrax inhibits phagocytes at the start of infection. By using a component of the toxin as a vaccine, antibody is produced which neutralizes the toxin at the early stages of infection and effective protection is obtained.

The second point is that the effectiveness of the *Pseudomonas* vaccine is probably dependent upon the polysaccharide slime material on the outside of the bacteria which is a potent inhibitor of phagocytic ingestion. Other bacterial vaccines like the pneumococcus vaccine and the plague vaccine rely on raising antibodies to the capsular and slime materials whose function in infection is to inhibit ingestion by phagocytes. Probably the best example of these materials are the meningococcal polysaccharides.

Williams Can I ask what is the infecting dose of anthrax or pig bel and how much of this toxin the organisms are producing?

Smith I do not know about pig bel, but I do know about anthrax in animals. You can infect with 10 organisms of some strains.

Williams And how much toxin will that produce?

Smith I cannot give it to you in concrete terms but they produce a small amount of toxin because you get oedema at the site of injection. If you immunize by one of the toxin components antibody is produced which will neutralize that toxin. But let me say that if you put in a massive dose of anthrax organisms you can break through that immunity.

Williams I am talking about the animal with no antibodies at this point. It must be producing quite a lot of toxin if 10 organisms can inhibit phagocytosis.

Smith A lot of toxin is produced at the end of infection but only a small amount at the start. When the organism is growing in the blood-stream an enormous amount of toxin is produced and that leads to death. But in the initial lesion, only a small amount of toxin is produced and its primary function, in my view, is antiphagocytic, not toxic.

Mims Can I just make a comment about pig bel, because that was brought up and you may not know about it. This is a disease seen in Papua New Guinea where pigs are eaten. Unfortunately, in the method of cooking the pig is often judged to be cooked when it has stopped squeaking. I am exaggerating slightly I admit, but it may be undercooked and as a result of this you eat a large number of clostridia initially present in the intestines and the dose could be enormous.

Williams In those circumstances one can imagine a toxin being able to act as an antiphagocytic factor, but where there are just 10 organisms one wonders whether there might not be something else interfering with phagocytosis.

Smith Undoubtedly there is. It is the capsular polyglutamic acid on anthrax bacilli but that is not antigenic so you cannot use it to make the vaccine.

Wilton I think the point that Professor Smith is making is that these small numbers of bacteria are producing a sublethal dose of toxin. However, almost by definition—which is what Professor Arbuthnott said yesterday—there are log orders of magnitude of difference between toxicity and interference with an event which determines whether the infection is going to take off, such as chemotaxis or phagocytosis. I am reminded of Ashley Miles, who pointed out that it was the first two or three hours which basically determined whether an infection was going to go on or whether it was going to be aborted.

Smith Ashley Miles said that 30 years ago and it is still as true now as it was then. He always stressed that because he dealt primarily with skin infections and he could determine what would happen within two or three hours.

Easmon I should like to ask Dr Beale how he thinks we are going to overcome the problem, when you go for purified components, when the virulence factor may be a very poor immunogen.

Beale I do not know how we are going to overcome it. I think we are going to wait and see. The example that Professor Smith has already raised about anthrax, where a nonantigenic factor is very important in the disease, illustrates the problem which you can face, but in that example the successful vaccine can be made using antigenic components. Certainly, one of the potential problems for a malaria antigen made by genetic manipulation is very low immunogenicity. It is for that reason that we are devoting such a lot of attention to adjuvants and the means of presentation of the antigenic material to attempt to forestall the problem.

Easmon How do you think that product liability laws, where they exist, are going to influence future development of vaccines?

Beale You mean in relationship to acceptable adjuvants?

Easmon Both adjuvants and purified antigens.

Beale As Sir Charles knows only too well, the problem of not only litigation but public acceptance of vaccines is a very serious threat that hangs over the whole programme of immunization. On the whole, I believe that purified antigens may well prove to be more immunogenic than less immunogenic. There are several examples of that. Earlier, Dr Wilton was talking about the antigens of murine leukaemia where there are components of the virus that are immunosuppressive, and the extracted material is in fact more antigenic. So far we have been rather impressed by the very small amounts of pure antigen that are immunogenic. However, you are quite right: there may be serious problems waiting round the corner.

Potter The only adjuvant studied extensively in man to date is aluminium hydroxide, which has been shown to enhance the immune response of animals to influenza vaccines; however, in two separate studies aluminium hydroxide failed to enhance antibody titres in man. I await with interest the results of volunteer studies of your adjuvant.

A second point from your paper relates to the work of Dr Hoskins and his colleagues at Christ's Hospital. Studies by Dr Beare at Salisbury have suggested that live influenza vaccines give a more solid immunity than killed virus vaccines and this is indicated by the Christ's Hospital experiences. It would be a tragedy if further studies with live influenza vaccines were dropped for legalistic reasons before the relative value of live vaccines was known.

Arbuthnott Dr Beale mentioned *E. coli* diarrhoea and cholera. In the first case he showed clearly that you could protect piglets with a vaccine containing the adhesin K88. Would he like to comment on enterotoxin as a protective antigen in *E. coli* and on the present position regarding cholera vaccine, either in relation to the surface antigens or to the enterotoxin?

Beale Can I go back to the influenza problems first? I agree with you that mice are not necessarily the best possible model for doing experiments with influenza virus, but they do have the merit that one is able to analyse the immune response more thoroughly. For example, the work on delayed hypersensitivity that Liew and Russell did would be almost impossible to do in other models. We are hoping to move progressively in the development of our influenza vaccine, first to ferrets and then to horses. Finally, if all goes well we shall think about using it in man.

I have been very keen to persuade the group at Christ's Hospital to use living influenza vaccines, but as you know the problems there are very great because virulence is multifactorial and it is not possible to predict that you have got an acceptable living virus strain without experiments in man. So I think there are major problems about getting live influenza vaccines accepted. I have had the simple faith, going back to a point that Professor Mims made, that if you know enough you ought to be able to do with a killed antigen what you can do with a living vaccine. It is just a question of knowing enough. At the moment we do not know enough about influenza by a long way.

Going on to Professor Arbuthnott's questions about cholera and *E. coli*, I have not got very much to say. We have been trying to do studies out in Bangladesh against cholera using both toxin and improved whole antigen vaccines, but there are great problems in organizing such trials and I am afraid we have not got very far. As for enterotoxins for *E. coli*, part of the problem there is the poor antigenicity of these factors.

Mims Perhaps we should refer to the nonspecific resistance that was dealt with in the course of earlier papers. I mention it because of the respiratory virus infections, where the antigenc diversity is so tremendous that apart from influenza and one or two others I do not think there is any possibility of producing specific vaccines. The old Bernard Shaw statement was that we should "stimulate the phagocytes", a good example of the induction of nonspecific resistance to infections. Few of us die of these respiratory infections, but, as was said earlier, economically they are very important in western society.

Smith I have been asked to sum up, but it is silly to try to summarize such a wide-ranging discussion. I will confine myself to five points.

Firstly, I do not think there is much doubt that both viruses and bacteria perturb the host defences and with regard to overall pathogenicity this capacity is just as much important as ability to grow within the host.

Secondly, with regard to bacteria, we do know quite a lot about the determinants of this perturbation in biochemical terms. This applies particularly to toxins and the capsular materials that inhibit ingestion by phagocytes and we are beginning to know something about the determinants of intracellular survival and growth within phagocytes.

Thirdly, with regard to viruses, we know that perturbation occurs but the biochemical basis for it is unknown at the moment.

The fourth point is that I believe—and I admit it is a bias—that we could learn in virology a lot more about the chemical basis of this perturbation if we adopted one of the classical approaches to the problems of pathogenicity that has been successful in bacteriology. This is to make comparisons between virulent and attenuated strains of the same virus in relation to perturbation of defences.

Last of all, it is pretty obvious, as shown by Dr Beale, that you can protect against infectious disease by having immunological methods that neutralize these perturbers of host defence. I see no reason why you could not also accomplish this chemically with drugs.

Index